Type 1 Diabetes

Editor

OSAGIE EBEKOZIEN

ENDOCRINOLOGY AND METABOLISM CLINICS OF NORTH AMERICA

www.endo.theclinics.com

Consulting Editor
ROBERT RAPAPORT

March 2024 • Volume 53 • Number 1

ELSEVIER

1600 John F. Kennedy Boulevard • Suite 1800 • Philadelphia, Pennsylvania, 19103-2899

http://www.theclinics.com

ENDOCRINOLOGY AND METABOLISM CLINICS OF NORTH AMERICA Volume 53, Number 1
March 2024 ISSN 0889-8529, ISBN 13: 978-0-443-12899-8

Editor: Taylor Hayes
Developmental Editor: Saswoti Nath

Endocrinology and Metabolism Clinics of North America (ISSN 0889-8529) is published quarterly by Elsevier Inc., 360 Park Avenue South, New York, NY 10010-1710. Months of issue are March, June, September, and December. Periodicals postage paid at New York, NY and additional mailing offices. Subscription prices are USD 419.00 per year for US individuals, USD 100.00 per year for US students and residents, USD 486.00 per year for Canadian individuals, USD 532.00 per year for international individuals, USD 100.00 per year for Canadian students/residents, and USD 245.00 per year for international students/residents. For institutional access pricing please contact Customer Service via the contact information below. To receive student/resident rate, orders must be accompanied by name of affiliated institution, date of term, and the signature of program/residency coordinator on institution letterhead. Orders will be billed at individual rate until proof of status is received. Foreign air speed delivery is included in all *Clinics* subscription prices. All prices are subject to change without notice. **POSTMASTER:** Send address changes to *Endocrinology and Metabolism Clinics of North America*, Elsevier Health Sciences Division, Subscription Customer Service, 3251 Riverport Lane, Maryland Heights, MO 63043. **Customer Service: Telephone: 1-800-654-2452** (U.S. and Canada); **1-314-447-8871** (outside U.S. and Canada). **Fax: 1-314-447-8029. E-mail: journalscustomerservice-usa@elsevier.com (for print support); journalsonlinesupport-usa@elsevier.com (for online support).**

Reprints. For copies of 100 or more, of articles in this publication, please contact the Commercial Rights Department, Elsevier Inc., 360 Park Avenue South, New York, NY 10010-1710; phone: +1-212-633-3874; fax: +1-212-633-3820; E-mail: reprints@elsevier.com.

Endocrinology and Metabolism Clinics of North America is covered in *MEDLINE/PubMed (Index Medicus), EMBASE/Excerpta Medica, Current Contents/Clinical Medicine, Current Contents/Life Sciences, Science Citation Index, ISI/BIOMED, BIOSIS,* and *Chemical Abstracts.*

Contributors

CONSULTING EDITOR

ROBERT RAPAPORT, MD
Professor of Pediatrics, Emma Elizabeth Sullivan Professor of Pediatric Endocrinology and Diabetes, Icahn School of Medicine at Mount Sinai, Director Emeritus, Division of Pediatric Endocrinology and Diabetes, Mount Sinai Kravis Children's Hospital, New York, New York

EDITOR

OSAGIE EBEKOZIEN, MD, MPH, CPHQ
Chief Medical Officer, T1D Exchange, QI and Population Health Department, Boston, Massachusetts

AUTHORS

SHIVANI AGARWAL, MD, MPH
Associate Professor, Fleischer Institute for Diabetes and Metabolism, Montefiore Medical Center, NY Regional Center for Diabetes Translation Research, Albert Einstein College of Medicine, Bronx, New York

HALIS KAAN AKTURK, MD
Associate Professor of Medicine and Pediatrics, Barbara Davis Center for Diabetes, University of Colorado, Aurora, Colorado

EMILY BREIDBART, MD
Assistant Professor, Department of Pediatrics, Division of Pediatric Endocrinology, NYU Grossman School of Medicine, Hassenfeld Children's Hospital at NYU Langone Health, New York, New York

SAMANTHA A. CARREON, PhD
Fellow, Baylor College of Medicine, Texas Children's Hospital, Houston, Texas

LAURYN CHOLEVA, MD, MSc
Assistant Professor of Pediatrics, Division of Pediatric Endocrinology and Diabetes, Department of Pediatrics, Icahn School of Medicine at Mount Sinai, New York, New York

INDIA COLE, MHA
James M. Anderson Center for Health Systems Excellence, Cincinnati Children's Hospital Medical Center, Cincinnati, Ohio

SARAH D. CORATHERS, MD
Clinical Director, Division of Endocrinology, Director, Quality Scholars Program, James M. Anderson Center for Health Systems, Excellence Associate Professor, UC Department of Pediatrics, University of Cincinnati College of Medicine, Cincinnati, Ohio

OSAGIE EBEKOZIEN, MD, MPH, CPHQ
Chief Medical Officer, T1D Exchange, QI and Population Health Department, Boston, Massachusetts

JULIA ELLIS, BS
Pritzker Department of Psychiatry and Behavioral Health, Ann and Robert H. Lurie Children's Hospital of Chicago, Chicago, Illinois

KATHRYN L. FANTASIA, MD, MSc
Assistant Professor of Medicine, Section of Endocrinology, Diabetes and Nutrition, Department of Medicine, Boston University Chobanian & Avedisian School of Medicine, Boston Medical Center, Department of Medicine, Evans Center for Implementation and Improvement Sciences (CIIS), Boston, Massachusetts

MARISSA A. FELDMAN, PhD
Assistant Professor of Psychiatry and Behavioral Sciences, Johns Hopkins University, Saint Petersburg, Florida

MARY PAT GALLAGHER, MD
Associate Professor, Department of Pediatrics at NYU Grossman School of Medicine Director, Pediatric Diabetes Center, Department of Pediatrics, Division of Pediatric Endocrinology, NYU Grossman School of Medicine, Hassenfeld Children's Hospital at NYU Langone Health, New York, New York

KIMBERLY P. GARZA, PhD, MPH
Assistant Professor of Sociology and Public Health, Roanoke College, Salem, Virginia

PATRICIA GOMEZ, MD
Assistant Professor, Department of Pediatrics, Division of Pediatric Endocrinology, University of Miami Miller School of Medicine, Miami, Florida, USA

JODY B. GRUNDMAN, MD, MPH
Assistant Professor of Pediatrics, Children's National Hospital, Washington, DC

HOLLY HARDISON, BS
Quality Improvement Coordinator, T1D Exchange, Boston, Massachusetts

MICHAEL A. HARRIS, PhD
Professor of Pediatrics, Oregon Health & Science University, Harold Schnitzer Diabetes Health Center, Portland, Oregon

KELSEY J. HART, DNP, RN
James M. Anderson Center for Health Systems Excellence, Cincinnati Children's Hospital Medical Center, Cincinnati, Ohio

MARISA E. HILLIARD, PhD
Professor, Baylor College of Medicine, Texas Children's Hospital, Houston, Texas

KELSEY HOWARD, PhD
Assistant Professor of Psychiatry and Behavioral Sciences, Pritzker Department of Psychiatry and Behavioral Health, Ann and Robert H. Lurie Children's Hospital of Chicago, Department of Psychiatry and Behavioral Sciences, Northwestern University Feinberg School of Medicine, Chicago, Illinois

JENIECE ILKOWITZ, RN, MA, CDCES
Pediatric Diabetes Center, NYU Langone Health, New York, New York

MANMOHAN K. KAMBOJ, MD
Professor of Pediatrics, The Ohio State University College of Medicine, Division Chief, Section of Endocrinology, Director of Quality Improvement for Endocrinology, Nationwide Children's Hospital, Columbus, Ohio

RACHEL LONGENDYKE, MD
Fellow Physician, Children's National Hospital, Washington, DC

SHIDEH MAJIDI, MD, MSCS
Associate Professor of Pediatrics, Children's National Hospital, Washington, DC

FAISAL S. MALIK, MD, MSHS
Department of Pediatrics, University of Washington School of Medicine, Seattle Children's Research Institute, Center for Child Health, Behavior, and Development, Seattle, Washington

MONA MANSOUR, MD, MS
Professor of Pediatrics, University of Cincinnati College of Medicine, Department of Pediatrics, Associate Director, Population Health, CCHMC, Division of General and Community Pediatrics, Medical Director Community Engagement - HealthVine, Medical Director CCHMC Coordinated School Strategy, Cincinnati Children's Hospital Medical Center, University of Cincinnati, Cincinnati, Ohio

CHRISTINE MARCH, MD, MS
Assistant Professor, Division of Pediatric Endocrinology and Diabetes, University of Pittsburgh, UPMC Children's Hospital of Pittsburgh, Pittsburgh, Pennsylvania

PRIYANKA MATHIAS, MD
Assistant Professor, Fleischer Institute for Diabetes and Metabolism, Albert Einstein College of Medicine, Montefiore Medical Center, Bronx, New York

ALEXIS M. McKEE, MD
Assistant Professor, Division of Endocrinology, Metabolism and Lipid Research, Washington University in St. Louis School of Medicine, St Louis, Missouri

CYNTHIA E. MUÑOZ, PhD, MPH
Associate Professor, Department of Pediatrics, Keck School of Medicine of USC, University of Southern California, Los Angeles, California

ANN MUNGMODE, MPH
Quality Improvement Program Manager, T1D Exchange, Boston, Massachusetts

ORI ODUGBESAN, MD, MPH
T1D Exchange, QI and Population Health Department, Boston, Massachusetts

AMY OHMER
International Children's Advisory Network, Atlanta, Georgia

JACLYN L. PAPADAKIS, PhD
Northwestern University Feinberg School of Medicine, Pritzker Department of Psychiatry and Behavioral Health, Ann and Robert H. Lurie Children's Hospital of Chicago, Chicago, Illinois

MARIA PESANTEZ, MD
Fellow, Jackson Memorial Hospital, Miami, Florida

ELIZABETH A. PYATAK, PhD, OTR/L, CDCES
Director of the Lifestyle Redesign® Knowledge Mobilization Initiative, and Associate Professor, Chan Division of Occupational Science and Occupational Therapy, Ostrow School of Dentistry, University of Southern California, Los Angeles, California

ROBERT RAPAPORT, MD
Professor of Pediatrics, Emma Elizabeth Sullivan Professor of Pediatric Endocrinology and Diabetes, Icahn School of Medicine at Mount Sinai, Director Emeritus, Division of Pediatric Endocrinology and Diabetes, Mount Sinai Kravis Children's Hospital, New York, New York

JENNIFER K. RAYMOND, MD, MCR
Chief, Division of Endocrinology, Diabetes and Metabolism, Associate Professor of Pediatrics, Keck School of Medicine of USC Division of Pediatric Endocrinology, Children's Hospital Los Angeles, Los Angeles, California

NICOLE RIOLES, MA
Senior Director of Clinical Partnerships, T1D Exchange, Boston, Massachusetts

JANINE SANCHEZ, MD
Professor of Pediatrics, Director, Pediatric Diabetes, Pediatric Endocrinology, University of Miami Miller School of Medicine, Miami, Florida

JENNA B. SHAPIRO, PhD
Assistant Professor of Psychiatry and Behavioral Sciences, Pritzker Department of Psychiatry & Behavioral Health, Ann and Robert Lurie Children's Hospital of Chicago, Department of Psychiatry & Behavioral Sciences, Northwestern University Feinberg School of Medicine, Chicago, Illinois, USA

MADELEINE SUHS, BS
Pritzker Department of Psychiatry and Behavioral Health, Ann and Robert H. Lurie Children's Hospital of Chicago, Chicago, Illinois

DEVIN W. STEENKAMP, MD
Director of Clinical Diabetes, Assistant Professor of Medicine, Section of Endocrinology, Diabetes and Nutrition, Department of Medicine, Boston University Chobanian & Avedisian School of Medicine, Boston Medical Center, Boston, Massachusetts

AMANDA TERRY, PhD
Assistant Professor of Psychiatry and Behavioral Sciences, Pritzker Department of Psychiatry and Behavioral Health, Ann and Robert H. Lurie Children's Hospital of Chicago, Department of Psychiatry and Behavioral Sciences, Northwestern University Feinberg School of Medicine, Chicago, Illinois

FRANCESCO VENDRAME, MD, PhD
Department of Medicine, Division of Endocrinology, Diabetes and Metabolism, University of Miami Miller School of Medicine, Miami, Florida

KATHRYN W. WEAVER, MD
Department of Medicine, University of Washington School of Medicine, Seattle, Washington

JILL WEISSBERG-BENCHELL, PhD, CDCES
Professor of Psychiatry and Behavioral Sciences, Pritzker Department of Psychiatry and Behavioral Health, Ann and Robert H. Lurie Children's Hospital of Chicago, Department of Psychiatry and Behavioral Sciences, Northwestern University Feinberg School of Medicine, Chicago, Illinois

PATIENCE H. WHITE, MD, MA
Professor, Department of Medicine and Pediatrics, George Washington University School of Medicine

MEREDITH WILKES, MD
Assistant Professor of Pediatrics, Division of Pediatric Endocrinology and Diabetes, Department of Pediatrics, Icahn School of Medicine at Mount Sinai, New York, New York

RISA M. WOLF, MD
Associate Professor, Department of Pediatrics, Division of Endocrinology, Johns Hopkins School of Medicine, Baltimore, Maryland

HOWARD A. WOLPERT, MD
Director of Diabetes Care Delivery and Innovation, Clinical Professor of Medicine, Section of Endocrinology, Diabetes and Nutrition, Department of Medicine, Boston University Chobanian & Avedisian School of Medicine, Boston Medical Center, Boston, Massachusetts

VICKIE WU, MD
Fellow, Division of Pediatric Endocrinology and Diabetes, Department of Pediatrics, Icahn School of Medicine at Mount Sinai, New York, New York

NANA-HAWA YAYAH JONES, MD
Assistant Professor, Division of Pediatric Endocrinology, Cincinnati Children's Hospital Medical Center, University of Cincinnati, Cincinnati, Ohio, USA

Contents

Type 1 diabetes (T1D) management has evolved over the last decade. Innovations and groundbreaking research have paved the way for improved outcomes for people with T1D. One of the major T1D focused research network that has supported real-world research studies in the United States is the T1D Exchange Quality Improvement Collaborative (T1DX-QI) Network.T1DX-QI is a large multicenter network of 55 T1D clinics that uses quality improvement, health equity framework, and population health principles to improve outcomes for people with T1D. This article summarizes insights from T1DX-QI clinical and population health improvement studies.

Those with concerning signs or symptoms should be evaluated for type 1 diabetes (T1D). Those with first-degree relatives with T1D or based on the presence of high-risk genes are at increased risk and benefit from screening. Universal screening should be considered in light of new potential therapies to delay disease progression. Although oral glucose tolerance test is the gold standard for T1D staging, there are multiple tools available when oral glucose tolerance test is not feasible. Risk score calculations increase the ability to predict disease progression. Testing should be repeated when symptoms of overt diabetes mellitus are not present.

Changes in physical growth, neurocognitive development, and pubertal maturation are some of the challenges to achieving blood glucose targets in children with type 1 diabetes mellitus. To optimize glycemic outcomes, a comprehensive approach is crucial to address psychosocial needs, expand the use of diabetes technology, and diminish health inequities.

> Young adults experience multiple developmental transitions across social, educational, vocational, residential, and financial life domains. These transitions are potential competing priorities to managing a chronic condition such as type 1 diabetes and can contribute to poor psychosocial and medical outcomes. In this narrative review, we describe population outcomes of young adult populations and the unique considerations associated with managing type 1 diabetes in young adulthood. We provide an overview of the current evidence-based strategies to improve care for young adults with type 1 diabetes and recommendations for future directions in the field.

> A growing body of literature finds persistent problems in the provision of recommended health care transition services, as well as adverse outcomes associated with the lack of these services in emerging adults with type 1 diabetes. The Six Core Elements of Health Care Transition offers a structured approach to the phases of health care transition support for both pediatric and adult diabetes practices. This article reviews strategies to incorporate the Six Core Elements into ambulatory diabetes care to support successful health care transition for emerging adults with type 1 diabetes.

> Individuals living with type 1 diabetes (T1D) from medically underserved communities have poorer health outcomes. Efforts to improve outcomes include a focus on team-based care, activation of behavior change, and enhancing self-management skills and practices. Advanced diabetes technologies are part of the standard of care for adults with T1D. However, health care providers often carry implicit biases and may be uncomfortable with recommending technologies to patients who have traditionally been excluded from efficacy trials or have limited real-world exposure to devices. We review the literature on this topic and provide an approach to address these issues in clinical practice.

> Recent years witnessed advancements in diabetes technologies and therapeutics. People with type 1 diabetes have more options to control their blood glucose, prevent hypoglycemia, and spend more time with their loved ones. Newer diabetes technologies and therapeutics improve the quality of life and boost the confidence of people with type 1 diabetes. In parallel to changes in the diabetes technology field, stem cell research

has been evolving. Gene editing and production of β cells from stem cells are ongoing. The current focus of cure studies is how to increase the survival of cells produced with stem cells. New adjunctive therapies are under development.

Nana-Hawa Yayah Jones, India Cole, Kelsey J. Hart, Sarah Corathers, Shivani Agarwal, Ori Odugbesan, Osagie Ebekozien, Manmohan K. Kamboj, Michael A. Harris, Kathryn L. Fantasia, and Mona Mansour

Type 1 diabetes management is intricately influenced by social determinants of health. Economic status impacts access to vital resources like insulin and diabetes technology. Racism, social injustice, and implicit biases affect equitable delivery of care. Education levels affect understanding of self-care, leading to disparities in glycemic outcomes. Geographic location can limit access to health care facilities. Stressors from discrimination or financial strain can disrupt disease management. Addressing these social factors is crucial for equitable diabetes care, emphasizing the need for comprehensive strategies that go beyond medical interventions to ensure optimal health outcomes for all individuals with type 1 diabetes.

Jenna B. Shapiro, Kimberly P. Garza, Marissa A. Feldman, Madeleine C. Suhs, Julia Ellis, Amanda Terry, Kelsey R. Howard, and Jill Weissberg-Benchell

The intensive demands of diabetes care can be difficult for youth with type 1 diabetes and their families to integrate into daily life. Standards of care in pediatric diabetes highlight the importance of evidence-based psychosocial interventions to optimize self-management behaviors and psychological well-being. The current review summarizes select systematic reviews and meta-analyses on evidence-based behavioral health interventions in pediatric diabetes. Interventions include strategies to strengthen youth psychosocial skills, improve family dynamics and caregiver mental health, enhance health and mental health equity, and address psychosocial factors related to diabetes technology use.

Rachel Longendyke, Jody B. Grundman, and Shideh Majidi

Type 1 diabetes is associated with both acute and chronic complications. Acute complications include diabetic ketoacidosis and severe hypoglycemia. Chronic complications can be microvascular or macrovascular. Microvascular complications include retinopathy, nephropathy, and neuropathy. The pathophysiology of microvascular complications is complex. Hyperglycemia is a common underlying risk factor, underscoring the importance of optimizing glycemic management. Patients with type 1 diabetes are also at increased risk of macrovascular complications including coronary artery disease and vascular disease. The American Diabetes Association provides screening guidelines for chronic complications of diabetes. Adherence to these guidelines is an important aspect of diabetes care.

The coronavirus disease 2019 (COVID-19) pandemic disrupted health care, creating challenges for people with diabetes and health care systems. Diabetes was recognized as a risk factor for severe disease early in the pandemic. Subsequently, risk factors specific for people with type 1 diabetes were identified, including age, hemoglobin A1c level, and lack of continuous glucose monitoring . Telemedicine, especially when accompanied by diabetes data, allowed effective remote care delivery. However, pre-existing racial disparities in access to diabetes technology persisted and were associated with worse outcomes. Events of the COVID-19 pandemic underscore the importance of continuing to develop flexible and more equitable health care delivery systems.

Type 1 diabetes (T1D) is associated with an increased risk of cardiovascular disease (CVD). CVD occurs much earlier in people with T1D than in the general population, and several risk factors have been identified some of which are modifiable. Risk prediction models and imaging tests to detect early signs of CVD have not been extensively validated. Strategies to promote cardiovascular health (CVH) in T1D include identifying risk factors, early treatment to achieve CVH targets, and improving the education of health care providers and people with T1D.

The integration of stakeholder engagement (SE) in research, quality improvement (QI), and clinical care has gained significant traction. Type 1 diabetes is a chronic disease that requires complex daily management and care from a multidisciplinary team across the lifespan. Inclusion of key stakeholder voices, including patients, caregivers, health care providers and community advocates, in the research process and implementation of clinical care is critical to ensure representation of perspectives that match the values and goals of the patient population. This review describes the current framework for SE and its application to research, QI, and clinical care across the lifespan.

ENDOCRINOLOGY AND METABOLISM CLINICS OF NORTH AMERICA

SERIES OF RELATED INTEREST

Medical Clinics
https://www.medical.theclinics.com
Primary Care: Clinics in Office Practice
https://www.primarycare.theclinics.com/

VISIT THE CLINICS ONLINE!
Access your subscription at:
www.theclinics.com

Foreword

Type 1 Diabetes

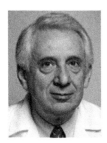

Robert Rapaport, MD
Consulting Editor

Diabetes affects an ever-increasing number of people both in the United States and worldwide. In children and young adults, Type 2 diabetes has shown a remarkable increase over the last two decades. Still, most children and youth affected by diabetes have Type 1 diabetes (T1DM). The incidence and prevalence of T1DM have increased and continue to increase both nationally and internationally. Hence it is appropriate that an issue of *Endocrinology and Metabolism Clinics of North America* be dedicated to T1DM. I could not have had a better partner in the design of this issue than Dr Osagie Ebekozien, who leads the relatively recently formed T1DM Exchange Quality Improvement Collaborative, which now includes a network of 55 endocrinology clinics in the United States. Since its inception in 2016, the collaborative yielded exceptional quality data that inform the current state of T1DM management in the United States. Members of the collaborative have published numerous high-quality papers in peer-reviewed publications that continue to provide information and tools that aid health care providers in T1DM. The 13 articles contained in this issue aptly summarize a range of topics, such as screening and diagnosing T1DM to improvements in management procedures using the latest in diabetes technology to optimize glycemic outcomes in children and youth while considering social determinants of health and psychological aspects necessary to comprehensively care for this population. Articles also deal with acute and chronic complications, school issues, as well as unique management challenges during difficult periods, such as the COVID-19 pandemic. I want to congratulate Dr Ebekozien and the contributing members of the issue for providing a

Endocrinol Metab Clin N Am 53 (2024) xv–xvi
https://doi.org/10.1016/j.ecl.2023.11.002
0889-8529/24/© 2023 Published by Elsevier Inc.

comprehensive compendium that will serve to educate and enlighten health care pro-viders caring for patients with T1DM.

Robert Rapaport, MD
Icahn School of Medicine at Mount Sinai
Division of Pediatric Endocrinology and Diabetes
Kravis Children's Hospital at Mount Sinai
New York, NY 10029, USA

E-mail address:
robert.rapaport@mountsinai.org

Preface

The Evolving Landscape of Type 1 Diabetes Management

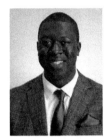

Osagie Ebekozien, MD, MPH, CPHQ
Editor

Type 1 diabetes (T1D) care in the United States has evolved in the last decade.[1] The global incidence of T1D is estimated to be 15 per 100,000 people, while prevalence is 5.9 per 10,000.[2] By 2040, T1D is projected to impact 13.5 to 17.4 million people.[3]

I am privileged to serve as the guest editor for this March 2024 issue of *Endocrinology and Metabolism Clinics of North America* with a timely focus on *Type 1 Diabetes*. We explore the evolving landscape of T1D care in the United States and share practical insights for clinicians.

I thank T1D Exchange Quality Improvement Collaborative (T1DX-QI) faculty contributors for authoring the articles and T1DX-QI peer-reviewers and the publication committee for providing critical feedback.

T1DX-QI is a T1D population health research and quality improvement network of 55 US endocrinology clinics. T1DX-QI includes over 200 active faculty endocrinologists and care team members serving more than 85,000 people with T1D (PwT1D).[4–6] In the first article of this series, I discuss clinical and population health improvement insights from the T1DX-QI network.

The screening and diagnosis of T1D have evolved especially with the approval of a new medication that can successfully delay T1D onset (Teplizumab). Gomez and Sanchez share the new state of science as it relates to screening, monitoring, and diagnosis of T1D.

Successful management of T1D across the lifespan has unique challenges, needs, and opportunities. Wu and colleagues discuss strategies to optimize outcomes in children; Mathias and colleagues explore the benefit of care customization for young adults with T1D, and Malik and colleagues review how an evidence-based framework can support the best practices in pediatric to adult care transition among PwT1D. Steenkamp and colleagues provide insights on successful approaches to support T1D care improvement among marginalized adults with T1D.

Endocrinol Metab Clin N Am 53 (2024) xvii–xix
https://doi.org/10.1016/j.ecl.2023.09.005
0889-8529/24/© 2023 Published by Elsevier Inc.

Diabetes technologies are revolutionizing T1D care outcomes.[7,8] Akturk and McKee review diabetes therapies and technologies that can support the management of T1D. Diabetes technologies don't relieve all the burdens of T1D care; one major area of need that requires attention is the psychosocial care. In this issue, Shapiro and colleagues explore insights from the literature on T1D and psychosocial management.

Despite major innovations in T1D care, unfortunately PwT1D still experience major complications as deliberated by Longendyke and colleagues and Pesantez and colleagues in a comprehensive review of cardiovascular health for PwT1D.

T1D care, like other chronic diseases, was significantly impacted by the COVID-19 pandemic.[9,10] Breidbart and Gallagher provide a synopsis on relevant clinical insights for managing PwT1D in the age of COVID-19.

COVID-19 amplified inequities in care outcomes[11-13] and expanded the significance of addressing social determinants of health as addressed in the review by Jones and colleagues.

Finally, we can't improve outcomes for PwT1D without actively engaging them in care transformation. Rioles and colleagues review practical strategies on how best to engage PwT1D in research and quality improvement and to change processes in endocrinology clinics.

I hope you find these articles insightful and actionable. I am grateful to everyone that contributed to the success of the series, including the authors, editorial staff, and consulting editor, Dr Robert Rapaport.

DISCLOSURE STATEMENT

Osagie Ebekozien is a member of the Medtronic and Sanofi Advisory Board and receives consultation and speaker fees from Medtronic Diabetes, Sanofi and Vertex Pharmaceuticals. He is P.I on research supported by Medtronic Diabetes, MannKind Pharmaceuticals, Dexcom, Abbott, Vertex Pharmaceuticals, Janssen Pharmaceuticals. All financial support from industry has been through his employer (T1D Exchange).

Osagie Ebekozien, MD, MPH, CPHQ
T1D Exchange
101 Federal Street
Boston, MA 02110, USA

John D Bower School of Population Health
University of Mississippi
Jackson, MS 39216, USA

E-mail address:
oebekozien@t1dexchange.org

REFERENCES

1. Mungmode A, Hardison H, Rioles N, et al. Diabetes Population Health Innovations in the Age of COVID-19: Insights From the T1D Exchange Quality Improvement Collaborative. J Clin Outcomes Manag 2022;29(5):185–92.

2. Mobasseri M, Shirmohammadi M, Amiri T, et al. Prevalence and incidence of type 1 diabetes in the world: a systematic review and meta-analysis. Health Promot Perspect 2020;10(2):98–115.

3. Gregory GA, Robinson TIG, Linklater SE, et al. Global incidence, prevalence, and mortality of type 1 diabetes in 2021 with projection to 2040: a modelling study. Lancet Diabetes Endocrinol 2022;10(10):741–60.
4. Alonso GT, Corathers S, Shah A, et al. Establishment of the T1D Exchange Quality Improvement Collaborative (T1DX-QI). Clin Diabetes 2020;38(2):141–51.
5. Majidi S, Rioles N, Agarwal S, et al, Collaborative TDEQI. Evolution of the T1D Exchange Quality Improvement Collaborative (T1DX-QI): using real-world data and quality improvement to advance diabetes outcomes. Clin Diabetes 2022;41(1): 32–4.
6. Weinstock RS, Prahalad P, Rioles N, et al. T1D Exchange Quality Improvement Collaborative: a learning health system to improve outcomes for all people with type 1 diabetes. Clin Diabetes 2021;39(3):251–5.
7. Noor N, Kamboj MK, Triolo T, et al. Hybrid closed-loop systems and glycemic outcomes in children and adults with type 1 diabetes: real-world evidence from a U.S.-based multicenter collaborative. Diabetes Care 2022;45(8):e118–9.
8. Noor N, Norman G, Sonabend R, et al. An Observational Crossover Study of People Using Real-Time Continuous Glucose Monitors Versus Self-Monitoring of Blood Glucose: Real-World Evidence Using EMR Data From More Than 12,000 People With Type 1 Diabetes. J Diabetes Sci Technol 2023. https://doi.org/10.1177/19322968231178017. 19322968231178017.
9. Wolf RM, Noor N, Izquierdo R, et al. Increase in newly diagnosed type 1 diabetes in youth during the COVID-19 pandemic in the United States: a multi-center analysis. Pediatr Diabetes 2022;23(4):433–8.
10. Beliard K, Ebekozien O, Demeterco-Berggren C, et al. Increased DKA at presentation among newly diagnosed type 1 diabetes patients with or without COVID-19: data from a multi-site surveillance registry. J Diabetes 2021;13(3):270–2.
11. Ebekozien O, Agarwal S, Noor N, et al. Inequities in diabetic ketoacidosis among patients with type 1 diabetes and COVID-19: data from 52 US clinical centers. J Clin Endocrinol Metab 2021;106(4):e1755–62.
12. Lavik AR, Ebekozien O, Noor N, et al. Trends in type 1 diabetic ketoacidosis during COVID-19 surges at 7 US centers: highest burden on non-Hispanic black patients. J Clin Endocrinol Metab 2022;107(7):1948–55.
13. Noor N, Ebekozien O, Levin L, et al. Diabetes technology use for management of type 1 diabetes is associated with fewer adverse COVID-19 outcomes: findings from the T1D Exchange COVID-19 Surveillance Registry. Diabetes Care 2021; 44(8):e160–2.

Improving Outcomes for People with Type 1 Diabetes Through Collaboration
Summary of Type 1 Diabetes Exchange Quality Improvement Collaborative Studies

Osagie Ebekozien, MD, MPH, CPHQ[a,b,*], Ann Mungmode, MPH[a],
Holly Hardison, BS[a], Robert Rapaport, MD[c]

KEYWORDS

- Type 1 diabetes • Population health • Quality improvement • Health equity

KEY POINTS

- Type 1 Diabetes Exchange Quality Improvement Collaborative (T1DX-QI) is a network of 55 type 1 diabetes and 10 type 2 diabetes clinical centers in the United States.
- T1DX-QI uses real-world data, benchmarking, and quality improvement to drive collaborative change.
- Insights from major learning networks like T1DX-QI can contribute to diabetes population health improvement.

INTRODUCTION

People with type 1 diabetes (PwT1D) make a myriad of decisions daily that are impacted by several psychological and physiologic states.[1] Acute and chronic complications in the sea of life transitions make managing T1Ds (T1D) burdensome and challenging.[2,3]

In the United States, the estimated economic cost of diabetes management is more than $300 billion annually.[4] Studies show that the most of the people with diabetes including PwT1D do not meet the American Diabetes Association standards for glycemic outcomes.[5,6] Coordinated efforts to understand health outcomes, identify process inefficiencies, and effectively implement solutions can reduce the burden of disease for PwT1D.

There are several organizations and large population-based networks working to expand our understanding and drive improvement in T1D outcomes globally.[7] One

[a] T1D Exchange, Boston, MA, USA; [b] University of Mississippi School of Population Health, Jackson, MS, USA; [c] Department of Pediatrics at Icahn School of Medicine; Mount Sinai Kravis Children's Hospital, New York, NY, USA
* Corresponding author. 100 Federal Street, Boston 02110.
E-mail address: oebekozien@t1dexchange.org

Endocrinol Metab Clin N Am 53 (2024) 1–16
https://doi.org/10.1016/j.ecl.2023.10.001
0889-8529/24/© 2023 Elsevier Inc. All rights reserved.
endo.theclinics.com

of the US-focused T1D research organizations is the T1D Exchange (www.t1dexchange.org). T1D Exchange is a Boston-based nonprofit with a mission to improve outcomes for the PwT1D through analyzing real-world evidence and driving collaborative change.

In 2010, T1D Exchange established the T1D Exchange clinic registry (T1DX-Research) that was coordinated by the JAEB Center.[8] T1DX-Research clinics participated in epidemiologic studies, clinical trials, and real-world outcome studies.

A landmark study from the T1DX-Research found worse mean glycated hemoglobin (HbA1c) outcomes in 2016 to 2018 as compared with 2010 to 2012. This finding was alarming considering the advancement in diabetes technology and standards of care in that period.[9] Furthermore, other international registries that incorporated quality assurance, benchmarking, and quality improvement (QI) reported improved outcomes.[10]

In 2016, through funding support from the Loena M and Harry B Helmsley Charitable Trust, T1D Exchange established the T1D Exchange Quality Improvement Collaborative (T1DX-QI). T1DX-QI started as a pilot with 10 centers focused on population health by advancing health equity, real-world studies, and QI. T1DX-QI has grown to a network of 55 T1D and 10 type 2 diabetes (T2D) centers as at the time of writing this article.[11–13] **Fig. 1** illustrates the geographic distribution of the T1DX-QI centers.

POPULATION HEALTH RESEARCH INSIGHTS FROM TYPE 1 DIABETES EXCHANGE QUALITY IMPROVEMENT COLLABORATIVE

Since 2020, the T1DX-QI has contributed a wide, multidimensional impact on collaborative centers and the larger diabetes community. Overall population health insights from T1DX-QI studies have been categorized into four key domains as summarized below.

Electronic Medical Record Data are an Effective Source for Real-World Studies on Type 1 Diabetes Outcomes

T1DX-QI centers share de-identified electronic medical records (EMRs) data of more than 120 variables with the coordinating office at least monthly.[14–17] T1DX-QI centers work with the coordinating office to map EMR data fields to corresponding variables in the T1DX-QI data specification, which are validated monthly for data quality assurance.

This real-world data support center-to-center benchmarking, population health insights, and QI studies. T1DX-QI has supported diabetes device coverage advocacy and national quality measures using insights from its' real-world studies. Findings from relevant T1DX-QI EMR data from real-world studies are summarized in **Table 1**. Major insights include.

1. Diabetes technologies can improve glycemic outcomes and are associated with reduced complications for PwT1D.[18–20]
2. There are several modifiable (eg, the use of diabetes technology, depression, body mass index) and non-modifiable factors (eg, race, ethnicity) that directly impact glycemic outcomes for PwT1D.[21–24]
3. There are various opportunities for population health improvement and learning from benchmarking with other international T1D registries.[7,18]

A Comprehensive Data Sharing Infrastructure Can Support Surveillance and Emerging Needs

Coordinated data sharing efforts are a key component of effective population health improvement. Standardized data collection supports real-time decision-making for

T1D Exchange Quality Improvement Collaborative

Type 1 Diabetes Clinics

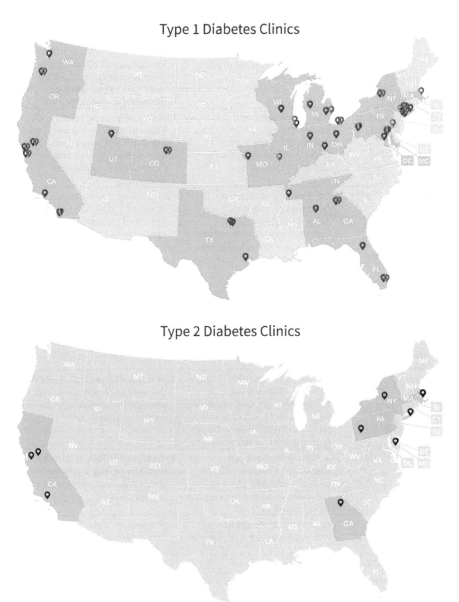

Type 2 Diabetes Clinics

Fig. 1. T1D and T2D participating centers. (*Courtesy of* T1D Exchange Quality Improvement Collaborative.)

the deployment of resources, targeted interventions, and future activities in public health emergencies.[25]

When COVID-19 emerged in March 2020, the T1DX-QI swiftly initiated a data sharing program dedicated to quantifying the impact of the pandemic on PwT1D.

Table 1
Type 1 diabetes exchange quality improvement collaborative real-world data relevant studies

Author Date	Title	Key Findings
Akturk et al,[21] 2022	Factors Associated with Improved Hemoglobin A1c among Adults with Type 1 Diabetes in the United States	Obesity, positive screen for depressive symptoms, public insurance, and minority race were associated with reduced odds for optimal glycemic outcomes for adult PwT1D.
Demeterco-Berggren et al,[22] 2022	Factors Associated with Achieving Target HbA1c in Children and Adolescents with Type 1 Diabetes: Findings from the T1DX-QI Collaborative	Children and young adults with T1D and HbA1c <7% were more likely to be privately insured, non-Hispanic White, and effectively using diabetes technology.
DeSalvo et al,[60] 2021	Patient demographics and clinical outcomes among type 1 diabetes patients using continuous glucose monitors: Data from T1D Exchange real-world observational study	PwT1D using continuous glucose monitors (CGM) had less severe outcomes including diabetes ketoacidosis (DKA) and severe hypoglycemia (SHE) and had better glycemic outcomes compared with those not using CGM.
DeSalvo et al,[18] 2022	Transatlantic Comparison of Pediatric Continuous Glucose Monitoring use in the DPV Initiative and T1D Exchange Quality Improvement Collaborative	CGM users have lower HbA1c values compared with non-CGM users both in the United States and Germany.
Ebekozien et al,[59] 2023	Seven Years Trends (2016–2022) in Glycemic Outcomes and Technology Use for Over 48,000 People with Type 1 Diabetes from the T1D Exchange Quality Improvement Collaborative	HbA1c trends have significantly decreased in a positive direction, whereas diabetes device use has increased in use.
Garey et al,[23] 2022	The association between depression symptom endorsement and glycemic outcomes in adolescents with type 1 diabetes	Approximately 30% of adolescents had mild or major depressive symptoms, with an increased risk for DKA.
Lanzinger et al,[7] 2022	A collaborative comparison of international pediatric diabetes registries	Collaboration, data, and active benchmarking are all key components to successful registry development in diabetes care.
Lee et al,[24] 2021	Feasibility of Electronic Health Record Assessment of Six Pediatric Type 1 Diabetes Self-Management 2 Habits and Their Association with Glycemic Outcomes	Six habits related to the effective use of diabetes technologies are associated with improved glycemic outcomes in PwT1D.

(continued on next page)

Table 1
(continued)

Author Date	Title	Key Findings
Mungmode et al,[17] 2022	Making Diabetes Electronic Medical Record Data Actionable: Promoting Benchmarking and Population Health Improvement Using the T1D Exchange Quality Improvement Portal Collaborative	The T1DX-QI benchmarking Portal allows data sharing between clinical centers and is a centralized platform for resource sharing to improve outcomes for PwT1D.
Noor et al,[19] 2023	An Observational Crossover Study of people using Real-Time Continuous Glucose Monitors (CGMs) vs Self-Monitoring of Blood Glucose (SMBG): Real-World Evidence using EMR Data from over 12,000 people with Type 1 Diabetes	PwT1D who switched from self-monitoring of blood glucose to CGM had elevated HbA1c value.
Noor et al,[20] 2022	Hybrid Closed Loop Systems and Glycemic Outcomes in Children and Adults with Type 1 Diabetes: Real World Evidence from U.S. Based Multi-Center Collaborative	Hybrid closed-loop system use is associated with increased time in range and lower HbA1c for PwT1D.

T1DX-QI centers shared data on symptoms, complications, and outcomes for PwT1D and COVID-19 as part of a multicenter surveillance study.[26]

Results from the multiyear COVID-19 study are summarized in **Table 2** and major highlights briefly outlined below.

1. PwT1D had an increased risk for thromboembolism and hospitalizations as compared with people without diabetes.[27,28]
2. T1DX-QI identified contributors to adverse outcomes for PwT1D with COVID-19. Contributors include the presence of other comorbidities, age, baseline HbA1c, and so forth.[29–34]
3. Clinical findings and outcomes on newly diagnosed PwT1D during the COVID-19 pandemic[35,36] were identified and shared broadly to support clinical care management.

Type 1 Diabetes Outcomes Can Be Improved by Reducing Variations and Optimizing Workflows

QI is a systematic approach to examine processes to improve patient outcomes, care, and clinic workflow.[37] T1DX-QI centers use QI methods and tools to understand local center practices, identify contributing factors, and test potential solutions. Participation in an learning health system (LHS) like the T1DX-QI allows centers to rapidly learn from dozens of relevant and simultaneous initiatives, and swiftly incorporate best practices and lessons learned for prompt translation of best practices into real-world processes.

The T1DX-QI has published multiple manuscripts on QI frameworks and initiatives, as summarized in **Table 3**. Using process improvement frameworks, T1DX-QI centers have.

Table 2
Type 1 diabetes exchange quality improvement collaborative COVID-19 surveillance relevant studies

Author Date	Title	Key Findings
Alonso et al,[33] 2021	Diabetic ketoacidosis drives COVID-19-related hospitalizations in children with type 1 diabetes	Elevated baseline HbA1c is the major association for COVID-19 hospitalization and diabetes ketoacidosis (DKA) among children with T1D.
Beliard et al,[36] 2021	Increased DKA at presentation among newly diagnosed type 1 diabetes patients with or without COVID-19: Data from a multi-site surveillance registry	Over 60% of new-onset T1D diagnosis with or without COVID-19 presented with DKA.
Demeterco-Berggren et al,[32] 2022	Age and Hospitalization Risk in People with Type 1 Diabetes and COVID-19: Data from the T1D Exchange Surveillance Study	PwT1D age 40 years and older with COVID-19 had greater risk for hospitalizations.
Ebekozien et. al, [26] 2020	Type 1 Diabetes and COVID-19: Preliminary Findings From a Multicenter Surveillance Study in the US	Over half of patients with COVID-19 presented with hyperglycemia and roughly 30% had DKA.
Gallagher et al,[31] 2022	Differences in COVID-19 outcomes among patients with type 1 diabetes: first vs late surges	PwT1D with COVID-19 had increased adverse events in the first surge compared with those during the later surge.
Lee et al,[61] 2021	Adoption of Telemedicine for Type 1 Diabetes Care During the COVID-19 Pandemic	The COVID-19 pandemic led to an increased adoption in telemedicine visits during the pandemic.
Mann et al,[29] 2022	Comorbidities increase COVID-19 hospitalization in young people with type 1 diabetes	The presence of additional comorbidities along with T1D led to an increased risk of hospitalization in adults and pediatrics PwT1D and COVID-19.
Miyazaki et al,[62] 2023	Association between health insurance type and adverse outcomes for children and young adults with Type 1 Diabetes and SARS-CoV-2	Publicly insured PwT1D with COVID-19 had an increased risk of hospitalization.
Noor et al,[34] 2021	Diabetes Technology Use for management of type 1 diabetes (T1D) is associated with fewer adverse COVID-19 outcomes: Findings from the T1D Exchange COVID-19 Surveillance Registry	PwT1D with evidence of diabetes device use had lower rates of DKA and hospitalizations with COVID-19 compared with without documented use of diabetes devices.
O'Malley et al,[63] 2021	COVID-19 Hospitalization in Adults with Type 1 Diabetes: Results from the T1D Exchange Multi-Center Surveillance Study	Continuation of care and glucose baseline should be prioritized to optimize care for PwD.

(continued on next page)

Table 2 (continued)		
Author Date	**Title**	**Key Findings**
Tallon et al,[28] 2023	Diabetes status and other factors as correlates of risk for thrombotic and thromboembolic events during SARS-CoV-2 infection: A nationwide retrospective case-control study using *Cerner Real-World Data*	PwT1D had an increased risk for thromboembolic events during COVID-19 illness than those without diabetes.
Tallon et al,[27] 2022	Impact of diabetes status and related factors on COVID-19-associated hospitalization: A nationwide retrospective cohort study of 116,370 adults with SARS-CoV-2 infection	The increased risk in hospitalization for T1D compared with T2D needs further research and inquiry.
Wolf et al,[35] 2022	Increase in newly diagnosed type 1 diabetes in youth during the COVID-19 pandemic in the US: A multi-center analysis	There was an increase of T1D diagnosis and DKA presentation during the COVID-19 pandemic than in the previous year (2019).

1. Illuminated variations in clinical processes and structures, such as QI capacity,[37] clinic staffing,[38] and barriers to telemedicine implementation[39] and smart insulin pen prescription.[40]
2. Improved the rates of continuous glucose monitors (CGM) and insulin pumps prescription, depression screening, and so forth.[41–43]
3. The mean HbA1c for PwT1D in the T1DX-QI network in 2022 to 2023 (n = 81,455) was favorable improved at 8.1% compared with the mean HbA1c in 2016 to 2017 of 8.8% (0.7% improvement; $P < .01$) (**Fig. 2**).

Type 1 Diabetes Outcomes Can be Improved by Advancing Health Equity and Supporting Advocacy

Health inequities persist in many disease states, including diabetes, despite recent improvements in glycemic outcomes and improved diabetes technology prescriptions.[44] Even in well-intentioned efforts, improvements may not be equitably experienced by race, ethnicity, sexual orientation, immigration status, and other determinants of health.[45,46]

To advance diabetes health equity, the T1DX-QI organizes a multipronged approach[47] to identify and effectively address inequities, as summarized in **Table 4**.

1. It is critical to illuminate inequities in diabetes' health outcomes[48–51] and technology use. For example, T1DX-QI studies have demonstrated that non-Hispanic Black (NHB) PwT1D were more likely to experience diabetes ketoacidosis (DKA) as compared with non-Hispanic White PwT1D.[48,49] In addition, studies from the T1DX-QI show that NHB children with T1D experience higher HbA1c, higher rates of DKA, and severe hypoglycemia.[50]
2. Diabetes centers can adapt traditional approaches and tools to advance health equity in QI and research spaces.[52,53]
3. Inequities in T1D outcomes should be addressed with multiple approaches including addressing provider bias[54] and inequity in clinical, insurance, and pharmacy or durable medical equipment prescription processes.[55]

Table 3
Type 1 diabetes exchange quality improvement collaborative clinic practice variations and quality improvement relevant studies

Author Date	Title	Key Findings
Alonso et al,[14] 2020	Establishment of the T1D Exchange Quality Improvement Collaborative (T1DX-QI)	The T1DX-QI promoted collaboration and shared learning using QI methodologies to improve outcomes for PwD.
Corathers et al,[43] 2023	Implementation of Psychosocial Screening into Diabetes Clinics: Experience from the Type 1 Diabetes Exchange Quality Improvement Network	Diabetes outcomes are not solely measured by HbA1c and total person health including psychosocial aspects should be incorporated into care.
Gallagher et al,[38] 2023	Variations in Clinic Staffing for Adult and Pediatric Diabetes Centers in the US: Data from T1D Exchange	Staffing ratios trend more favorably in the pediatric T1D centers as compared with adult centers indicating a high level of disparities.
Gandhi et. al, [64] 2023	Insulin Pump Utilization 2017–2021 for over 22,000 Children and Adult with Type 1 Diabetes: Multi-Center Observational Study	Insulin pump utilization has increased 7% over the past 5 years.
Ginnard et al,[65] 2021	Quality Improvement in Diabetes Care: A Review of Initiatives and Outcomes in the T1D Exchange QI Collaborative	T1DX-QI quality improvement studies have resulted in improved care processes.
Grimaldi et al,[66] 2023	Connecting from Afar: Implementation of remote data sharing for patients with Type 1 diabetes on insulin pump therapy	Encouraging patients to sign up for the portal during clinic visits led to an uptake of patients sharing pump data.
Lee et al,[39] 2023	Institutional Barriers to the Successful Implementation of Telemedicine for Type 1 Diabetes Care	Telemedicine rates remained 20% higher than rates pre-pandemic despite a decrease in rates during the start of the pandemic.
Lyons et al,[42] 2021	Increasing Insulin Pump Use among 12–26 Year Olds with Type 1 Diabetes: Results from the T1D Exchange Quality Improvement Collaborative	Insulin pump uptake increased by 13% over a 22-month intervention testing period.
Marks et al,[37] 2022	Baseline Quality Improvement Capacity of 33 Endocrinology Centers Participating in the T1D Exchange QI Collaborative	It is essential to invest in QI capacity specifically in centers that are smaller in size, serve adult patients, or serve minoritized groups.
Ospelt et al,[40] 2022	Facilitators and Barriers to Smart Insulin Pen Use: A mixed-method study of multidisciplinary stakeholders from diabetes teams in the United States	Most providers agreed that the potential benefits of smart insulin pen use outweigh the barriers.

(continued on next page)

Table 3
(continued)

Author Date	Title	Key Findings
Peter et al,[67] 2023	Prevalence of fear of hypoglycemia in adults with type 1 diabetes using a newly developed screener and clinician's perspective on its implementation	Fear of hypoglycemia is prevalent in PwD and is a leading factor in how diabetes is managed.
Prahalad et al,[41] 2021	Multi-Clinic Quality Improvement Initiative Increases Continuous Glucose Monitoring Use Among Adolescents and Young Adults with Type 1 Diabetes	CGM uptake increased by 21% over a 22-month intervention testing period.

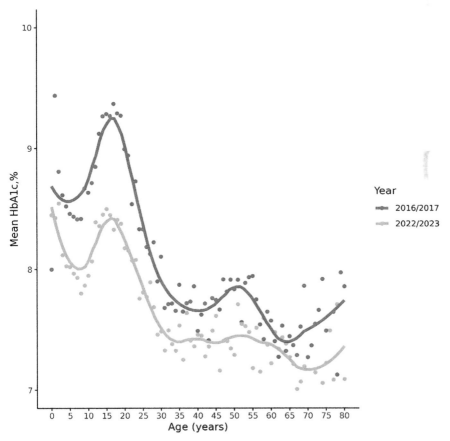

Fig. 2. Improvement in mean HbA1c (*n* = 81,455) from the T1DX-QI 2016/2017 as compared with 2022/2023. (*Courtesy of* T1D Exchange Quality Improvement Collaborative.)

Table 4
Type 1 Diabetes Exchange Quality Improvement Collaborative health equity and population health improvement advocacy relevant studies

Author Date	Title	Key Findings
Ebekozien,[55] 2023	Roadmap to Achieving Continuous Glucose Monitoring Equity: Insights from the T1D Exchange	CGM equity is determined by the removal of barriers and intentionally undoing injustices in the current system.
Ebekozien et al,[53] 2022	Achieving Equity in Diabetes Research: Borrowing from the Field of Quality Improvement Using A Practical Framework and Improvement Tools	A 10-step framework coupled with the lived experience perspective is an effective way to create equitable care and management.
Ebekozien et al,[52] 2020	Equitable Post-COVID-19 Care: A Practical Framework to Integrate Health Equity in Diabetes Management	Health equity can be addressed using the 10-step framework to identify barriers and create solutions to expand care in an equitable way.
Ebekozien et al,[48] 2021	Inequities in Diabetic Ketoacidosis among Patients with Type 1 Diabetes and COVID-19: Data from 52 US Clinical Centers	In PwD with a COVID-19 diagnosis, non-Hispanic Black (NHB) patients had a greater presentation of DKA compared with non-Hispanic White (NHW) patients.
Ebekozien et. al, [47] 2022	Addressing Type 1 Diabetes Health Inequities in the United States: Approaches from the T1D Exchange QI Collaborative	T1DX-QI is actively addressing health inequities and intentionally collaborating with stakeholders to close the disparity gap using a comprehensive multistep framework.
Khan et al,[68] 2023	Advancing Diabetes Quality Measurement in the Era of Continuous Glucose Monitoring	As diabetes technology evolves, the direction of care to be comprehensive and equitable should adapt as well.
Lavik et.al, [49] 2022	Trends in type 1 diabetic ketoacidosis during COVID-19 surges at seven US centers: highest burden on non-Hispanic Blacks	NHB experienced diabetes ketoacidosis (DKA) at a higher proportion compared with NHW in both 2019 and 202 during the COVID-19 pandemic.
Majidi et al,[50] 2021	Inequities in Health Outcomes in Children and Adults with Type 1 Diabetes: Data from the T1D Exchange Collaborative	Significant differences were seen in NHW and NHB patients including DKA presentation, limited technology, and severe hypoglycemia episodes in the latter group.

(continued on next page)

Table 4
(continued)

Author Date	Title	Key Findings
Odugbesan et al,[54] 2022	Implicit Racial-Ethnic and Insurance Mediated Bias to Recommending Diabetes Technology: Insights from T1D Exchange Multi-Center Pediatric and Adult Diabetes Provider Cohort	Diabetes technology prescription is influenced by provider implicit bias based on insurance and race/ethnicity.
Odugbesan et al, [58] 2023	Increasing Continuous Glucose Monitor (CGM) Use for Non-Hispanic Black and Hispanic Patients with Type 1 Diabetes (T1D): Results from the T1D Exchange Quality Improvement Collaborative Equity Study	The disparities between NHW and NHB CGM users were reduced by 5% and NHW and Hispanic patients was reduced by 6%.
Ospelt et al,[51] 2023	The Impact of Climate Change on People Living with Diabetes: A Scoping Review	Negative outcomes enhanced by climate change can lead to severe complications or even death for PwD.
Walker et al,[69] 2023	Addressing Global Inequity in Diabetes: International Progress	Interventions to address health equity in minority groups require multilevel practices along with a shift of framework and clinic practice.

DISCUSSION

Although presented in separate categories here, each of the above-described domains contributes to improving care for PwT1D. The infrastructure of a multicenter improvement collaboration, including expertise in data integration, analysis, visualization, QI, health equity, and broader network coordination, serves to support population health improvement.

Through an extensive and validated data sharing process, the T1DX-QI has examined real-world trends, benchmarked outcomes across centers, and identified specific opportunities for improvement. T1DX-QI resources support centers to test and implement local success stories and spread best practices throughout the network. Intentional adaptations of frameworks and approaches support health equity. The existing capabilities support this work in the face of unprecedented public health emergencies like the COVID-19 pandemic to implement expeditious surveillance.

There is urgency in multicenter T1D collaboration that is driven by the increase incidence of diabetes,[56] COVID-19 exacerbated inequities, and persistence of avoidable barriers to care.[57]

The T1DX-QI model of sharing, networking, and collaboration has demonstrated improvement in T1D population health outcomes and equity.[58,59] There is strength in collaboration to improve the outcomes and reduce inefficiencies in T1D management.

CLINICS CARE POINTS

- Real-world data can provide valuable clinical insights to type 1 diabetes care management.
- Diabetes technologies are associated with improved outcomes for people with type 1 diabetes.
- Clinic efficiency and effectiveness can be improved with quality improvement methodology.
- Inequities in type 1 diabetes can be reduced with collaboration and care process changes.

DISCLOSURE

Osagie Ebekozien is a member of the Medtronic and Sanofi Advisory Board and receives consultation and speaker fees from Medtronic Diabetes, Sanofi, and Vertex Pharmaceuticals. He is PI on research supported by Medtronic Diabetes, MannKind Pharmaceuticals, Dexcom, United States, Abbott, Vertex Pharmaceuticals, Janssen Pharmaceuticals, United States. All financial support from industry has been through his employer (T1D Exchange).

FUNDING STATEMENT

T1DX-QI is supported through grants from the Leona M and Harry B Helmsley Charitable Trust, United States and JDRF, United States.

ACKNOWLEDGMENTS

The authors acknowledge T1DX-QI Principal Investigators and Team members.

REFERENCES

1. Atkinson MA, Eisenbarth GS, Michels AW. Type 1 diabetes. Lancet 2014; 383(9911):69–82.
2. Longendyke R, Grundman J, Majidid S. Acute and chronic outcomes of type 1 diabetes. Endocrinol Metab Clin North Am 2023; https://doi.org/10.1016/j.ecl. 2023.09.004.
3. Pesantez M, Ebekozien O, Vendrame F. Type 1 diabetes and cardiovascular health. Endocrinol Metab Clin North Am 2023; https://doi.org/10.1016/j.ecl.2023.07.003.
4. Prevention CfDCa. Diabetes Fast Facts 2023 Available at: https://www.cdc.gov/diabetes/basics/quick-facts.html#:~:text=More%20than%2037%20million%20people,(and%20may%20be%20underreported).
5. Wang L, Li X, Wang Z, et al. Trends in Prevalence of Diabetes and Control of Risk Factors in Diabetes Among US Adults, 1999-2018. JAMA 2021;326(8):704–16.
6. Miller KM, Foster NC, Beck RW, et al, T1D Exchange Clinic Network. Current state of type 1 diabetes treatment in the U.S.: updated data from the T1D Exchange clinic registry. Diabetes Care 2015;38(6):971–8.
7. Lanzinger S, Zimmermann A, Ranjan AG, et al, Australasian Diabetes Data Network ADDN, Danish Registry of Childhood and Adolescent Diabetes DanDiabKids, Diabetes prospective follow-up registry DPV, Norwegian Childhood Diabetes Registry NCDR, National Paediatric Diabetes Audit NPDA, Swedish Childhood Diabetes Registry Swediabkids, T1D Exchange Quality Improvement Collaborative T1DX-QI, and SWEET initiative. A collaborative comparison of international pediatric diabetes registries. Pediatr Diabetes 2022;23(6):627–40.

8. Beck RW, Tamborlane WV, Bergenstal RM, et al, T1D Exchange Clinic Network. The T1D Exchange Clinic Registry. J Clin Endocrinol Metabol 2012;97(12):4383–9.
9. Foster NC, Beck RW, Miller KM, et al. State of Type 1 Diabetes Management and Outcomes from the T1D Exchange in 2016-2018. Diabetes Technol Therapeut 2019;21(2):66–72.
10. Albanese-O'Neill A, Grimsmann JM, Svensson AM, et al. Changes in HbA1c Between 2011 and 2017 in Germany/Austria, Sweden, and the United States: A Lifespan Perspective. Diabetes Technol Therapeut 2022;24(1):32–41.
11. Mungmode A, Hardison H, Rioles N, et al. Diabetes Population Health Innovations in the Age of COVID-19: Insights From the T1D Exchange Quality Improvement Collaborative. J Clin Outcome Manag 2022;29(5).
12. Majidi S, Rioles N, Agarwal S, et al. Evolution of the T1D Exchange Quality Improvement Collaborative (T1DX-QI): Using Real-World Data and Quality Improvement to Advance Diabetes Outcomes. Clin Diabetes 2022;41(1):32–4.
13. Agarwal S, Rioles N, Majidi S, et al. Commentary on the T1D exchange quality improvement collaborative learning session November 2022 abstracts. J Diabetes 2022;14(11):780–2.
14. Alonso GT, Corathers S, Shah A, et al. Establishment of the T1D Exchange Quality Improvement Collaborative (T1DX-QI). Clin Diabetes 2020;38(2):141–51.
15. Weinstock RS, Prahalad P, Rioles N, et al. T1D Exchange Quality Improvement Collaborative: A Learning Health System to Improve Outcomes for All People With Type 1 Diabetes. Clin Diabetes 2021;39(3):251–5.
16. Prahalad P, Rioles N, Noor N, et al, T1DX-QI Collaborative. T1D exchange quality improvement collaborative: Accelerating change through benchmarking and improvement science for people with type 1 diabetes. J Diabetes 2022; 14(1):83–7.
17. Mungmode A, Noor N, Weinstock RS, et al. Making Diabetes Electronic Medical Record Data Actionable: Promoting Benchmarking and Population Health Improvement Using the T1D Exchange Quality Improvement Portal. Clin Diabetes 2022;41(1):45–55.
18. DeSalvo DJ, Lanzinger S, Noor N, et al. Transatlantic Comparison of Pediatric Continuous Glucose Monitoring Use in the Diabetes-Patienten-Verlaufsdokumentation Initiative and Type 1 Diabetes Exchange Quality Improvement Collaborative. Diabetes Technol Therapeut 2022;24(12):920–4.
19. Noor N, Norman G, Sonabend R, et al. An Observational Crossover Study of People Using Real-Time Continuous Glucose Monitors Versus Self-Monitoring of Blood Glucose: Real-World Evidence Using EMR Data From More Than 12,000 People With Type 1 Diabetes. J Diabetes Sci Technol 2023. 19322968231178017.
20. Noor N, Kamboj MK, Triolo T, et al. Hybrid Closed-Loop Systems and Glycemic Outcomes in Children and Adults With Type 1 Diabetes: Real-World Evidence From a U.S.-Based Multicenter Collaborative. Diabetes Care 2022;45(8):e118–9.
21. Akturk HK, Rompicherla S, Rioles N, et al. Factors Associated With Improved A1C Among Adults With Type 1 Diabetes in the United States. Clin Diabetes 2022; 41(1):76–80.
22. Demeterco-Berggren C, Ebekozien O, Noor N, et al. Factors Associated With Achieving Target A1C in Children and Adolescents With Type 1 Diabetes: Findings From the T1D Exchange Quality Improvement Collaborative. Clin Diabetes 2022;41(1):68–75.
23. Garey CJ, Clements MA, McAuliffe-Fogarty AH, et al. The association between depression symptom endorsement and glycemic outcomes in adolescents with type 1 diabetes. Pediatr Diabetes 2022;23(2):248–57.

24. Lee JM, Rusnak A, Garrity A, et al. Feasibility of Electronic Health Record Assessment of 6 Pediatric Type 1 Diabetes Self-management Habits and Their Association With Glycemic Outcomes. JAMA Netw Open 2021;4(10):e2131278.

25. Kringos D, Carinci F, Barbazza E, et al, HealthPros Network. Managing COVID-19 within and across health systems: why we need performance intelligence to coordinate a global response. Health Res Pol Syst 2020;18(1):80.

26. Ebekozien OA, Noor N, Gallagher MP, et al. Type 1 Diabetes and COVID-19: Preliminary Findings From a Multicenter Surveillance Study in the U.S. Diabetes Care 2020;43(8):e83–5.

27. Tallon EM, Ebekozien O, Sanchez J, et al. Impact of diabetes status and related factors on COVID-19-associated hospitalization: A nationwide retrospective cohort study of 116,370 adults with SARS-CoV-2 infection. Diabetes Res Clin Pract 2022;194:110156.

28. Tallon EM, Gallagher MP, Staggs VS, et al. Diabetes status and other factors as correlates of risk for thrombotic and thromboembolic events during SARS-CoV-2 infection: A nationwide retrospective case-control study using Cerner Real-World Data. BMJ Open 2023;13(7):e071475.

29. Mann EA, Rompicherla S, Gallagher MP, et al. Comorbidities increase COVID-19 hospitalization in young people with type 1 diabetes. Pediatr Diabetes 2022; 23(7):968–75.

30. Maahs David M, Todd Alonso G, Gallagher Mary Pat, et al. Comment on Gregory et al. COVID-19 Severity Is Tripled in the Diabetes Community: A Prospective Analysis of the Pandemic's Impact in Type 1 and Type 2 Diabetes. Diabetes Care 2021. https://doi.org/10.2337/dc20-3119.

31. Gallagher MP, Rompicherla S, Ebekozien O, et al. Differences in COVID-19 outcomes among patients with type 1 diabetes: first vs later surges. J Clin Outcomes Manag 2022;29(1):27–31.

32. Demeterco-Berggren C, Ebekozien O, Rompicherla S, et al. Age and Hospitalization Risk in People With Type 1 Diabetes and COVID-19: Data From the T1D Exchange Surveillance Study. J Clin Endocrinol Metab 2022;107(2):410–8.

33. Alonso GT, Ebekozien O, Gallagher MP, et al. Diabetic ketoacidosis drives COVID-19 related hospitalizations in children with type 1 diabetes. J Diabetes 2021;13(8):681–7.

34. Noor N, Ebekozien O, Levin L, et al. Diabetes Technology Use for Management of Type 1 Diabetes Is Associated With Fewer Adverse COVID-19 Outcomes: Findings From the T1D Exchange COVID-19 Surveillance Registry. Diabetes Care 2021;44(8):e160–2.

35. Wolf RM, Noor N, Izquierdo R, et al. Increase in newly diagnosed type 1 diabetes in youth during the COVID-19 pandemic in the United States: A multi-center analysis. Pediatr Diabetes 2022;23(4):433–8.

36. Beliard K, Ebekozien O, Demeterco-Berggren C, et al. Increased DKA at presentation among newly diagnosed type 1 diabetes patients with or without COVID-19: Data from a multi-site surveillance registry. J Diabetes 2021;13(3):270–2.

37. Marks BE, Mungmode A, Neyman A, et al. Baseline Quality Improvement Capacity of 33 Endocrinology Centers Participating in the T1D Exchange Quality Improvement Collaborative. Clin Diabetes 2022;41(1):35–44.

38. Gallagher MP, Noor N, Ebekozien O. Variations in Clinic Staffing for Adult and Pediatric Diabetes Centers in the United States: Data From T1D Exchange. Endocr Pract 2023;29(8):678–9.

39. Lee JM, Ospelt E, Noor N, et al. Institutional Barriers to the Successful Implementation of Telemedicine for Type 1 Diabetes Care. Clin Diabetes 2023. https://doi.org/10.2337/cd23-0056. Online ahead of print.
40. Ospelt E, Noor N, Sanchez J, et al. Facilitators and Barriers to Smart Insulin Pen Use: A Mixed-Method Study of Multidisciplinary Stakeholders From Diabetes Teams in the United States. Clin Diabetes 2022;41(1):56–67.
41. Prahalad P, Ebekozien O, Alonso GT, et al, T1D Exchange Quality Improvement Collaborative Study Group. Multi-Clinic Quality Improvement Initiative Increases Continuous Glucose Monitoring Use Among Adolescents and Young Adults With Type 1 Diabetes. Clin Diabetes 2021;39(3):264–71.
42. Lyons SK, Ebekozien O, Garrity A, et al, T1D Exchange Quality Improvement Collaborative Study Group. Increasing Insulin Pump Use Among 12- to 26-Year-Olds With Type 1 Diabetes: Results From the T1D Exchange Quality Improvement Collaborative. Clin Diabetes 2021;39(3):272–7.
43. Corathers S, Williford DN, Kichler J, et al. Implementation of Psychosocial Screening into Diabetes Clinics: Experience from the Type 1 Diabetes Exchange Quality Improvement Network. Curr Diabetes Rep 2023;23(2):19–28.
44. EBEKOZIEN O, NOOR N, KAMBOJ MK, et al. 167-OR: Inequities in Glycemic Outcomes for Patients with Type 1 Diabetes: Six-Year (2016–2021) Longitudinal Follow-Up by Race and Ethnicity of 36,390 Patients in the T1Dx-QI Collaborative. Diabetes 2022;71 (Supplement_1).
45. Quality Improvement Efforts Under Health Reform, Hasnain-Wynia R. How To Ensure That They Help Reduce Disparities—Not Increase Them. Health Aff 2011;30(10):1837–43.
46. Lion KC, Faro EZ, Coker TR. All Quality Improvement Is Health Equity Work: Designing Improvement to Reduce Disparities. Pediatrics 2022;149(Supplement 3).
47. Ebekozien O, Mungmode A, Odugbesan O, et al, T1DX-QI Collaborative. Addressing type 1 diabetes health inequities in the United States: Approaches from the T1D Exchange QI Collaborative. J Diabetes 2022;14(1):79–82.
48. Ebekozien O, Agarwal S, Noor N, et al. Inequities in Diabetic Ketoacidosis Among Patients With Type 1 Diabetes and COVID-19: Data From 52 US Clinical Centers. J Clin Endocrinol Metab 2021;106(4):e1755–62.
49. Lavik AR, Ebekozien O, Noor N, et al. Trends in Type 1 Diabetic Ketoacidosis During COVID-19 Surges at 7 US Centers: Highest Burden on non-Hispanic Black Patients. J Clin Endocrinol Metab 2022;107(7):1948–55.
50. Majidi S, Ebekozien O, Noor N, et al, T1D Exchange Quality Improvement Collaborative Study Group. Inequities in Health Outcomes in Children and Adults With Type 1 Diabetes: Data From the T1D Exchange Quality Improvement Collaborative. Clin Diabetes 2021;39(3):278–83.
51. Ospelt E, Hardison H, Mungmode A, et al. The Impact of Climate Change on People Living with Diabetes: A Scoping Review. Clin Diabetol 2023;12(3):186–200.
52. Ebekozien O, Odugbesan O, Rioles N, et al. Equitable post-COVID-19 care: a practical framework to integrate health equity in diabetes management. J Clin Outcome Manag 2020;27(6):256–9.
53. Ebekozien O, Mungmode A, Buckingham D, et al. Achieving Equity in Diabetes Research: Borrowing From the Field of Quality Improvement Using a Practical Framework and Improvement Tools. Diabetes Spectr 2022;35(3):304–12.
54. Odugbesan O, Addala A, Nelson G, et al. Implicit Racial-Ethnic and Insurance-Mediated Bias to Recommending Diabetes Technology: Insights from T1D Exchange Multicenter Pediatric and Adult Diabetes Provider Cohort. Diabetes Technol Therapeut 2022;24(9):619–27.

55. Ebekozien O. Roadmap to Achieving Continuous Glucose Monitoring Equity: Insights from the T1D Exchange. Diabetes Spectrum 2023;36:320–6.
56. Prevention CfDCa. National Diabetes Statistics Report, 2022, Available at: https://www.cdc.gov/diabetes/data/statistics-report/index.html., Accessed September 27, 2023.
57. Sherry Glied and Benjamin Zhu. Not So Sweet: Insulin Affordability over Time Commonwealth Fund, 2020, Available at: https://www.commonwealthfund.org/publications/issue-briefs/2020/sep/not-so-sweet-insulin-affordability-over-time, Accessed September 27, 2023.
58. Odugbesan O, Mungmode A, Rioles N, et al. Increasing Continuous Glucose Monitor (CGM) Use for Non-Hispanic Black and Hispanic Patients with Type 1 Diabetes (T1D): Results from the T1D Exchange Quality Improvement Collaborative Equity Study. Clin Diabetes 2023; https://doi.org/10.2337/cd23-0050.
59. Ebekozien O, Mungmode A, Sanchez J, et al. Seven Years Trends (2016-2022) in Glycemic Outcomes and Technology Use for Over 48,000 People with Type 1 Diabetes from the T1D Exchange Quality Improvement Collaborative. Diabetes Technol Therapeut 2023. https://doi.org/10.1089/dia.2023.0320. Online ahead of print.
60. DeSalvo DJ, Noor N, Xie C, et al. Patient Demographics and Clinical Outcomes Among Type 1 Diabetes Patients Using Continuous Glucose Monitors: Data From T1D Exchange Real-World Observational Study. J Diabetes Sci Technol 2023;17(2):322–8.
61. Lee JM, Carlson E, Albanese-O'Neill A, et al. Adoption of Telemedicine for Type 1 Diabetes Care During the COVID-19 Pandemic. Diabetes Technol Therapeut 2021;23(9):642–51.
62. Miyazaki B, Ebekozien O, Rompicherla S, et al. Association between health insurance type and adverse outcomes for children and young adults with Type 1 Diabetes and SARS-CoV-2. Diabetes Spectr 2023;230002. https://doi.org/10.2337/ds23-0002. Online ahead of print.
63. O'Malley G, Ebekozien O, Desimone M, et al. COVID-19 Hospitalization in Adults with Type 1 Diabetes: Results from the T1D Exchange Multicenter Surveillance Study. J Clin Endocrinol Metab 2021;106(2):e936–42.
64. Gandhi K, Ebekozien O, Noor N, et al. Insulin Pump Utilization 2017-2021 for over 22,000 Children and Adult with Type 1 Diabetes: Multi-Center Observational Study. Clin Diabetes 2023; https://doi.org/10.2337/cd23-0055.
65. Ginnard OZB, Alonso GT, Corathers SD, et al, T1D Exchange Quality Improvement Collaborative Study Group. Quality Improvement in Diabetes Care: A Review of Initiatives and Outcomes in the T1D Exchange Quality Improvement Collaborative. Clin Diabetes 2021;39(3):256–63.
66. Grimaldi M, Cardenas L, Saenz AM, et al. Connecting From Afar: Implementation of Remote Data-Sharing for Patients With Type 1 Diabetes on Insulin Pump Therapy. Clin Diabetes 2023;41(3):442–5.
67. Peter ME, Rioles N, Liu J, et al. Prevalence of fear of hypoglycemia in adults with type 1 diabetes using a newly developed screener and clinician's perspective on its implementation. BMJ Open Diabetes Res Care 2023;11(4).
68. Khan M, Wahid N, Musser T, et al. Advancing Diabetes Quality Measurement in the Era of Continuous Glucose Monitoring. Sci Diabetes Self Manag Care 2023; 49(2):112–25.
69. Walker AF, Graham S, Maple-Brown L, et al. Interventions to address global inequity in diabetes: international progress. Lancet 2023;402(10397):250–64.

Type 1 Diabetes Screening and Diagnosis

Patricia Gomez, MD[a],*, Janine Sanchez, MD[b]

KEYWORDS

- T1D screening • T1D screening programs • T1D staging and risk of progression
- T1D diagnosis

KEY POINTS

- Deciding who and how to screen for T1D has broad clinical and research implications.
- Several screening programs exist with goals of early detection of T1D and possible entry into prevention and/or new-onset trials.
- In pediatric patients at increased risk of T1D, OGTT is the gold standard for disease staging and assisting in predicting risk of progression, especially when incorporated in a T1D risk score.
- Unless overt symptoms of DM are present at diagnosis, testing should be repeated to confirm the diagnosis.

WHO TO EVALUATE FOR TYPE 1 DIABETES

Those with Concerning Signs and/or Symptoms

Type 1 diabetes (T1D) is one of the most common chronic diseases of childhood and adolescence, with an estimated worldwide prevalence of approximately 1.52 million people younger than age 20 living with the condition as of 2022. In 2022, the T1D Index estimated that 35,000 of T1D-related deaths were in undiagnosed people younger than 25 years old.[1] It is critical that health care providers be aware and attentive to the symptoms of T1D to ensure a timely diagnosis. In general, patients with polyuria, polydipsia, nocturia, and/or unexplained weight loss should be screened for T1D. Additional findings may include abdominal pain, nausea, emesis, blurred vision, lethargy, decreased appetite, and irregular breathing. Detection of symptoms is challenging in young patients so close attention should be given to anthropometric data during well and sick visits.

At Risk Based on Family History

The risk of T1D is approximately 0.4% in the overall population. Risk increases if one has a relative with T1D.[2] This information is useful to guide screening patterns and

[a] Department of Pediatrics, Division of Pediatric Endocrinology, University of Miami Miller School of Medicine, 1601 NW 12th Avenue, Suite 3044A, Miami, FL 33136, USA; [b] Pediatric Diabetes, Pediatric Endocrinology, University of Miami Miller School of Medicine, 1601 NW 12th Avenue, Suite 3044A, Miami, FL 33136, USA
* Corresponding author.
E-mail address: pgomez5@med.miami.edu

Endocrinol Metab Clin N Am 53 (2024) 17–26
https://doi.org/10.1016/j.ecl.2023.09.008
0889-8529/24/© 2023 Elsevier Inc. All rights reserved.

counseling of families. The estimated lifetime risk depends on which relative has T1D, as further described next.

- Sibling of person with T1D: 6.7% according to data from the nationwide Childhood Diabetes in Finland (DiMe) study.[3]
- Child of mother with T1D: 3.4%, according to data from the Familial Autoimmune and Diabetes (FAD) Study based out of Pittsburgh, Pennsylvania.[4]
- Child of father with T1D: 4.9%, according to data from the FAD.[4]
- Twins with person with T1D:
  - Monozygotic twin: 65% in long-term follow-up studies, according to data obtained from patients identified at the Joslin Diabetes Center, the Barbara Davis Center for Childhood Diabetes, and through the Diabetes Prevention Trial–Type 1 Diabetes.[5]
  - Dizygotic twin: Risk is similar to nontwin siblings, according to patient data from the Joslin Diabetes Center, the Barbara Davis Center for Childhood Diabetes, and the Diabetes Autoimmunity Study in the Young (DAISY).[6]

Potential Universal Screening, Considering New Therapies

The recent Food and Drug Administration (FDA) approval of teplizumab-mzwv (TZIELD) indicated for stage 2 T1D brings into question the consideration of universal screening for T1D. The age and method of screening would likely generate great debate and true universal screening would be challenging. **Fig. 1** provides a pictorial summary of who to screen for T1D.

SCREENING PROGRAMS

The Environmental Determinants of Diabetes in the Young (TEDDY) Study is a consortium responsible for creating and implementing studies to investigate the potential triggers and/or protective factors of T1D in children with higher risk genes. The clinical centers recruit subjects as neonates from the general population and newborn first-degree relatives of someone with T1D. Neonates are enrolled if they have a predetermined risk of T1D of 3% (general population) or 10% (those with first-degree relatives with T1D), based on genetic testing (HLA genotype). Subjects are followed for 15 years or until they develop islet autoimmunity and/or T1D. Participants have blood samples collected every 3 months for 4 years followed by every 6 months until 15 years old. Other samples collected include drinking water, nasal swabs, stools samples, toenail clippings, and urine. Historical data are collected, and diet, illnesses, allergies, vaccinations, psychosocial stressors, gestational events, and toxins. As of 2022, 8667 children have participated to date worldwide of which 435 have been diagnosed with T1D. Notable findings have included the role of non-HLA genetic factors in the development of T1D[7] and the importance of the order of appearance of autoantibodies in predicting the risk of developing T1D.[8]

TrialNet is an international multidisciplinary network of scientists whose overarching goal is to cure diabetes. There are more than 100 participating locations worldwide. Relatives of people with T1D or those who have tested positive for at least one T1D-related autoantibody can receive free risk screening through TrialNet in the Pathway to Prevention risk screening study. The testing is performed either with an in-home test kit or in a laboratory and tests for five autoantibodies. Those with one diabetes-related autoantibody are advised to repeat antibody testing in 1 year. Those with two or more autoantibodies are advised to have an oral glucose tolerance test (OGTT) performed to determine if dysglycemia is present and whether they qualify for available prevention studies. Prevention studies through TrialNet are aimed at

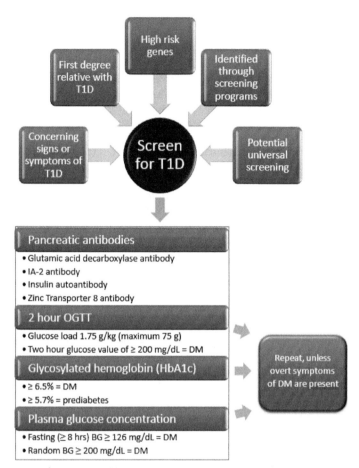

Fig. 1. Screening for T1D. BG, blood glucose; DM, diabetes mellitus.

slowing or preventing diabetes in people who are in early stage T1D, defined as having two or more T1D-related autoantibodies. Studies are also ongoing for those with newly diagnosed T1D, with the goal of maximally preserving the person's insulin production. Participants who develop T1D during a TrialNet prevention study can join the Long-Term Investigative Follow-up in TrialNet (LIFT) study for ongoing monitoring. Participants who completed a new-onset study are also eligible to join the LIFT study. Those participating in LIFT have a visit at a TrialNet location yearly to complete a health status questionnaire and laboratory evaluations. TrialNet is unique in that it is following participants with T1D in all phases: before, during, and after being diagnosed with T1D.

T1Detect is a population awareness and education program created by the Juvenile Diabetes Research Foundation. T1Detect's goals are to make the public aware of the importance of T1D screening, how to obtain screening, and what to do with the results of the screening.

Autoimmunity Screening for Kids (ASK) is a research program located at the Barbara Davis Center for Diabetes at the University of Colorado. This program offers free screening for T1D and celiac disease to all children in the United States, ages 1 to 17 years old. Goals of ASK include early detection of T1D, monitoring and education of children at increased risk of T1D, trialing therapies to prevent diabetes, and maximizing treatment and monitoring of children with undiagnosed celiac disease. Participants who live more than 15 miles from a screening site can perform at-home screening.

The Fr1da Study was created in 2015 at the Helmholtz Diabetes Center Institute of Diabetes Research. It is the world's largest population-based screening for T1D in children. All children ages 2 to 10 years old who live in Bavaria, Germany are eligible for islet autoantibody testing. Children with a first- or second-degree relative with T1D can receive autoantibody testing between 1 and 21 years old. Children can participate twice in the study if they are within the included age ranges. The main goal of the Fr1da study is to diagnose T1D in children while they are in a presymptomatic stage to prevent diabetic ketoacidosis, improve early onset education, assist with creating standards for early diagnosis of T1D, and detect children who may benefit from immune-based therapies. Two other relevant studies currently being conducted at the Helmholtz Diabetes Center Institute of Diabetes Research are Freder1k and SINT1A. Freder1K is a free and optional newborn screening program completed within the first week after birth to determine the infant's genetic predisposition of T1D. SINT1A is a prevention study for infants with increased risk of T1D, investigating the efficacy of a probiotic *Bifidobacterium infantis*. Freder1k and SINT1A are part of the Global Platform for the Prevention of Autoimmune Diabetes (GPPAD), which is a European platform aimed at identifying infants with increased genetic risk of T1D and performing prevention trials. GPPAD research sites are in Belgium, Germany, Poland, Sweden, and the United Kingdom, with the coordination center being located at Helmholtz Munich.

Fig. 2 provides a summary of some of the T1D screening programs available.

WAYS TO SCREEN ASYMPTOMATIC PARTICIPANTS

- The HLA complex is involved in the immune process of antigen presentation and is therefore critical in the pathogenesis of T1D. The combination of specific alleles of HLA class II genes confers about 50% of the genetic risk of T1D. The highest risk of T1D is linked to DR4-DQ8 and DR3-DQ2 haplotypes, whereas DR2 is protective of T1D. Less than 10% of people with high-risk HLA haplotypes develop T1D.[9] Other genes that confer increased risk of T1D include insulin, PTPN22, and CTLA4.[10]
- Islet cell autoantibodies have an important role as principal markers of pancreatic autoimmunity in T1D. These autoantibodies recognize antigens involved in the secretory machinery of pancreatic β cells.[11]
  - Glutamic acid decarboxylase antibody (GADA): Glutamic acid decarboxylase, particularly GAD65, is found in the cytoplasm of synaptic-like microvesicles. GAD65 is a critical enzyme involved in the synthesis of γ-aminobutyric acid (GABA). GABA is a main inhibitory neurotransmitter in the central nervous system. Despite multiple tissues using GABAergic systems, expression of GAD65 in humans has only been confirmed in pancreatic islet cells and in the central nervous system. The regulation of the GABAergic systems in the brain and pancreas differs. In the human pancreas, GAD65 is found mostly in β cells and in a minority of cells. GADA is the classic antibody detected in patients with latent autoimmune diabetes of the adult.[11]
  - IA-2 antibody (IA-2A): IA-2 is a receptor-type tyrosine phosphatase-like protein that is found on the membrane of secretory granules. Its biologic role is not completely understood, but it seems to ultimately influence insulin secretion,

Screening Programs

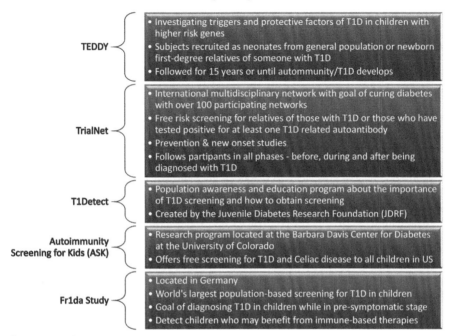

TEDDY
- Investigating triggers and protective factors of T1D in children with higher risk genes
- Subjects recruited as neonates from general population or newborn first-degree relatives of someone with T1D
- Followed for 15 years or until autommunity/T1D develops

TrialNet
- International multidisciplinary network with goal of curing diabetes with over 100 participating networks
- Free risk screening for relatives of those with T1D or those who have tested positive for at least one T1D related autoantibody
- Prevention & new onset studies
- Follows partipants in all phases - before, during and after being diagnosed with T1D

T1Detect
- Population awareness and education program about the importance of T1D screening and how to obtain screening
- Created by the Juvenile Diabetes Research Foundation (JDRF)

Autoimmunity Screening for Kids (ASK)
- Research program located at the Barbara Davis Center for Diabetes at the University of Colorado
- Offers free screening for T1D and Celiac disease to all children in US

Fr1da Study
- Located in Germany
- World's largest population-based screening for T1D in children
- Goal of diagnosing T1D in children while in pre-symptomatic stage
- Detect children who may benefit from immune-based therapies

Fig. 2. Screening Programs.

secretory granule synthesis/homeostasis, and beta-cell expansion. IA-2 expression is found at the mRNA and protein levels in several neuroendocrine cells, splenocytes, and the thymus. In the pancreas, IA-2 is only found in pancreatic islets (β, α, and δ cells) and is not seen in pancreatic exocrine tissue.[11]

o Insulin autoantibody (IAA): Insulin is contained within secretory granules and in humans is almost only expressed in the pancreatic β cells. At the mRNA and protein levels, insulin expression is also seen in thymic medullary epithelial cells. There are associations between specific polymorphic variants in the insulin gene and increased risk of T1D.[11]

o Zinc Transporter 8 antibody (ZnT8A): ZnT8 is found on the membrane of secretory granules. It seems to be essential for the accumulation of zinc into secretory granules and the appropriate maintenance of stored insulin. Polymorphisms of ZnT8 have been associated with increased risk of T2D, impaired glucose homeostasis, and altered rate of conversion of proinsulin to its mature hormone. ZnT8 expression in humans is mainly in the pancreas, at the mRNA and protein level. Within pancreatic islet cells, it is mainly found in beta cells.[11]

DISEASE STAGING AND RISK OF PROGRESSION

Almost all children with multiple islet cell autoantibodies eventually develop stage 3 T1D. Disease staging and ongoing monitoring is critical in this population.[12]

The 2-hour OGTT is the gold standard for T1D disease staging once multiple islet cell autoantibodies are present. Stage 1 is the presence of at least two autoantibodies with normal blood glucose levels and no symptoms. Stage 2 is the presence of at least two autoantibodies with abnormal glucose tolerance and typically no symptoms. Stage 3 is the presence of two autoantibodies, abnormal blood glucose values diagnostic of diabetes mellitus (DM), and typically symptoms of diabetes. Stage 4 is established T1D. The OGTT also aids in determining the risk of disease progression, either on its own or when used in risk score calculations. Most prevention trials require an OGTT for disease staging before being considered for inclusion. Alternatives to OGTT for disease staging and determining risk of progression include glycosylated hemoglobin (HbA$_{1c}$), continuous glucose monitoring (CGM), random venous plasma glucose, and self-monitoring of blood glucose, especially outside of a research setting.[12]

HbA$_{1c}$ has limitations when it comes to making an early diagnosis of T1D in the pediatric population. T1D can progress rapidly in this population. There is also the possibility of an underlying condition that may affect red blood cell turnover (eg, hemoglobinopathy), which may falsely lower the HbA$_{1c}$ in this group.[12] In the high-risk pediatric population, an HbA$_{1c}$ greater than or equal to 5.7% has a low sensitivity (<50%) and variable specificity to diagnose impaired glucose tolerance. In this same population, HbA$_{1c}$ greater than or equal to 6.5% has a very low sensitivity (24%–34%) and high specificity (98%–99%) to make a diagnosis of T1D. This was obtained from data from the DPT-1, TEDDY, TRIGR, and TrialNet Natural History studies. Across these studies, the positive predictive value of an HbA$_{1c}$ greater than or equal to 6.5% to predict development of T1D in this group ranged from 50% to 94%. Adjusting the current thresholds of HbA$_{1c}$, particularly in the high-risk pediatric population, may improve its utility in making an early diagnosis of diabetes.[13] An HbA$_{1c}$ in the normal range but that is increasing has shown some utility in making an early diagnosis of T1D.[14]

CGM has utility in monitoring patients at increased risk of developing T1D.[12] However, CGM usage is limited by cost and the lack of widespread accessibility. Average sensor glucose levels and increased glycemic variability are CGM metrics that are used to predict progression to clinical diabetes in high-risk patients. TA140 is the time spent with glucose levels greater than 140 mg/dL with a CGM. In data obtained from the Autoimmunity Screening for Kids (ASK) Study, autoantibody-positive children with TA140 greater than 10% had an 80% risk of progression to clinical diabetes in 1 year. In that same cohort, children who progressed to clinical diabetes within a median time range of 6 months were found to have significantly higher average CGM glucose levels, increased glycemic variability (including standard deviation, coefficient of variation, mean of daily differences, and mean amplitude of glycemic excursions), and increased time spent greater than 160 mg/dL.[15]

Random venous plasma glucose is an easy and low-cost tool that is used in monitoring high-risk patients.[12] In the Type 1 Diabetes Prediction and Prevention Project (DIPP), for those children with stage 1 T1D, the median time to diagnosis after a random plasma glucose greater than or equal to 140 mg/dL was 1 year (vs 0.7 years in those with impaired glucose tolerance during a 2-hour OGTT and 5.2 years in those with impaired fasting glucose).[16]

Self-monitoring of blood glucose is limited by the inability to confirm abnormal glucose values in real time. Pediatric data are insufficient regarding its functionality in predicting progression to clinical diabetes in high-risk patients.[12]

RISK CALCULATIONS AND TYPE 1 DIABETES RISK SCORES

- Islet autoantibodies and risk of progression: In genetically at-risk pediatric patients, progression to stage 3 T1D within 10 years in those with multiple autoantibodies is 69.7%, one autoantibody is 14.5%, and no autoantibodies is 0.4%. Progression to clinical disease is quicker in those who develop islet autoantibodies younger than 3 years of age.[17]

- HbA$_{1c}$ and risk of progression: In genetically at-risk pediatric patients with multiple islet autoantibodies, increase in HbA$_{1c}$ over time can aid in predicting progression to stage 3 T1D. Over a 3- to 12-month period, a 10% increase in HbA$_{1c}$ in this population increases the risk of progression to clinical disease by 5.7 times.[18]
- Diabetes Prevention Trial-Type 1 Risk Score (DPTRS): This score was created from data obtained from Diabetes Prevention Trial-Type 1 (DPT-1) and validated in the TrialNet Natural History Study (TNNHS), both of which included autoantibody-positive participants who were relatives of patients with T1D. Metrics included in the DPTRS calculation are C-peptide, values from 2-hour OGTT, age, and body mass index. A threshold of nine on the DPTRS score is highly predictive of those who will progress to stage 3 T1D within 2 years. The 2-year risk of progression was found to be 88% in this population. Because this threshold is typically reached well before diagnosis (on average >9 months before when diagnosis typically made), stimulated C-peptide levels are also higher in this population.[19]
- DPTRS60: This score was modified from the DPTRS and includes data obtained from a 1-hour OGTT versus the standard 2-hour OGTT. The DPTRS60 had a similar prediction rate of T1D at 5-year follow-up compared with DPTRS and was superior to a 2-hour glucose.[20]
- T1D Diagnostic Index60 (Index60): This is a pure metabolic index derived from 2-hour OGTT data from participants in DPT-1 and TNNHS. An Index60 value greater than or equal to 2.0 has potential utility in detecting the earlier stages of T1D.[21]
- M$_{120}$: This is a T1D disease prediction model based on a single blood sampling at 120 minutes during an OGTT. M$_{120}$ includes sex, age, body mass index, HbA$_{1c}$, IA-2A status, and OGTT metrics. M$_{120}$ was found to be at least as accurate as DPTRS, DPTRS60 or Index60 in the TrialNet population, while being more practical to obtain.[22]

CURRENT DIAGNOSTIC TOOLS USED IN MAKING THE DIAGNOSIS OF STAGE 3 TYPE 1 DIABETES

- Plasma glucose concentration:
  - Fasting (for at least 8 hours) value greater than or equal to 126 mg/dL in the presence of symptoms concerning for DM or confirmed on repeat testing.
  - Random value greater than or equal to 200 mg/dL in the presence of symptoms concerning for DM or confirmed on repeat testing.
- HbA$_{1c}$ greater than or equal to 6.5%, confirmed on repeat testing. HbA$_{1c}$ greater than or equal to 5.7% is consistent with prediabetes.
- 2-hour OGTT, using a glucose load of 1.75 g/kg (75 g maximum). Two-hour glucose value of greater than or equal to 200 mg/dL, confirmed on repeat testing.
- Fasting insulin level and C-peptide level may help distinguish between T1D and T2D at diagnosis.
- Blood or urine ketone levels to detect developing diabetic ketoacidosis.
- Islet cell autoantibodies:
  - GADA
  - IA-2 antibody (IA-2A)
  - IAA
  - ZnT8A
- Genetic testing for monogenic diabetes when the evaluation suggests that another form of diabetes is likely, such as when:

- ○ Islet autoantibodies are not present.
- ○ There is an autosomal-dominant family history of DM.
- ○ Diagnosis of DM is made within the first 6 to 12 months of life.
- ○ History of hyperinsulinism and associated hypoglycemia in infancy.
- ○ Low insulin requirements or prolonged honeymoon period.
- ○ Evaluation suggestive of T2D but patient is not obese and lacks signs of insulin resistance.
- ○ Other extrapancreatic features are present.

CLINICAL IMPLICATIONS AND RECOMMENDATIONS

- • Who should be evaluated for T1D (summarized in **Fig. 1**)?
  - ○ Everyone with concerning signs or symptoms, especially polyuria, polydipsia, nocturia, and/or unexplained weight loss, in whom a delay in diagnosis can have serious adverse effects.
  - ○ Those at increased risk based on family history, particularly first-degree relatives of someone with T1D.
  - ○ Participants identified through screening programs, such as TEDDY, TrialNet, ASK, and Fr1da.
  - ○ Those at high risk based on genetic profile, such as HLA haplotype and other genes that confer increased risk of T1D (insulin, PTPN22, and CTLA4).
  - ○ Those at high risk based on the presence of multiple islet autoantibodies (GADA, IA-2A, IAA, ZnT8A).
  - ○ Consideration for universal screening with the recent FDA approval of teplizumab-mzwv for stage 2 T1D. More broad screening efforts would also allow for earlier entry into ongoing prevention and new-onset T1D studies.
  - ○ The FDA-approved immunotherapy drug teplizumab-mzwv for the delay of T1D in at-risk individuals. TrialNet's Teplizumab Prevention Study was the first to show a clinical T1D diagnosis can be delayed an average of 2+ years in people at high risk.[23] Teplizumab-mzwv is a CD3-directed antibody indicated to delay the onset of stage 3 T1D in adults and pediatric patients aged 8 years and older with stage 2 T1D. Other studies to try to prevent or cure T1D that had some modest effect include using verapamil, abatacept, rituximab, alefacept, antithymocyte globulin, golimumab, imatinib, plasmid vector, and Vertex (Vx-880).
- • Goals of early evaluation and screening programs for T1D:
  - ○ Prevent diabetic ketoacidosis and associated severe complications.
  - ○ Smoother transition to initiation of insulin for the patient and the entire family.
  - ○ Possibility of inclusion in prevention and new-onset T1D trials.
  - ○ Potential treatment with teplizumab-mzwv for the treatment of stage 2 T1D.
- • Disease staging and risk of progression to stage 3 T1D:
  - ○ OGTT is the gold standard and typically required for entry into a prevention study.
  - ○ Caution should be taken in relying on the HbA_{1c} alone to diagnose early onset T1D, especially in high-risk patients. Change over time in HbA_{1c} is more informative in the early stages of T1D.
  - ○ CGM metrics, particularly TA140, is useful in predicting disease progression.
  - ○ A random plasma glucose is a low cost and more easily accessible option with informative value.
  - ○ T1D risk scores, which usually incorporate OGTT, can increase the ability to predict T1D progression. Examples of risk scores include DPTRS, DPTRS60, Index60, and M_{120}.

- Making the diagnosis of stage 3 T1D:
  - Most tests should be repeated to confirm the diagnosis, unless overt clinical symptoms are present.
  - Fasting plasma glucose greater than or equal to 126 mg/dL, random plasma glucose greater than or equal to 200 mg/dL, HbA_{1c} greater than or equal to 6.5%, and 2-hour glucose value of greater than or equal to 200 mg/dL on OGTT are typically used to make the diagnosis of DM.
  - Ancillary testing to assist in making a precise diagnosis: fasting insulin and C-peptide levels, blood or urine ketones, islet cell autoantibodies, and genetic testing.

CLINICS CARE POINTS

- If a patient has polyuria, polydipsia, nocturia, and/or unexplained weight loss, recommend evaluating for T1D.
- For new-onset T1D or if unsure of type of diabetes, recommend screening with islet cell antibodies (GADA, IA-2A, IAA, ZnT8A) and C-peptide.
- Those with first-degree relatives with T1D and/or high-risk genes should be screened for T1D.
- Those with stage 2 T1D may be candidates for therapy with teplizumab-mzwv.
- When making a diagnosis of T1D, most tests need to be repeated unless there are overt symptoms present.

DISCLOSURE

The authors have no financial relationships with any of the individuals, organizations, or products mentioned in this article.

REFERENCES

1. Ogle, G. D., Wang, F., Gregory, G. A., & Maniam, J. (2022). (rep.). Type 1 diabetes estimates in children and adults. Available at: https://diabetesatlas.org/idfawp/resource-files/2022/12/IDF-T1D-Index-Report.pdf.
2. Libman I, Haynes A, Lyons S, et al. ISPAD Clinical Practice Consensus Guidelines 2022: definition, epidemiology, and classification of diabetes in children and adolescents. Pediatr Diabetes 2022;23(8):1160–74.
3. Mrena S, Virtanen SM, Laippala P, et al. Models for predicting type 1 diabetes in siblings of affected children. Diabetes Care 2006;29(3):662–7.
4. Dorman JS, Steenkiste AR, O'Leary LA, et al. Type 1 diabetes in offspring of parents with type 1 diabetes: the tip of an autoimmune iceberg? Pediatr Diabetes 2000;1(1):17–22.
5. Redondo MJ, Jeffrey J, Fain PR, et al. Concordance for islet autoimmunity among monozygotic twins. N Engl J Med 2008;359(26):2849–50.
6. Redondo MJ, Rewers M, Yu L, et al. Genetic determination of islet cell autoimmunity in monozygotic twin, dizygotic twin, and non-twin siblings of patients with type 1 diabetes: prospective twin study. BMJ 1999;318(7185):698–702.
7. Törn C, Hadley D, Lee HS, et al. Role of type 1 diabetes-associated SNPs on risk of autoantibody positivity in the TEDDY Study. Diabetes 2015;64(5):1818–29.

8. Vehik K, Bonifacio E, Lernmark Å, et al. Hierarchical order of distinct autoantibody spreading and progression to type 1 diabetes in the TEDDY Study. Diabetes Care 2020;43(9):2066–73.

9. Primavera M, Giannini C, Chiarelli F. Prediction and prevention of type 1 diabetes. Front Endocrinol (Lausanne) 2020;11:248.

10. Aly TA, Ide A, Jahromi MM, et al. Extreme genetic risk for type 1A diabetes. Proc Natl Acad Sci U S A 2006;103(38):14074–9.

11. Lampasona V, Liberati D. Islet autoantibodies. Curr Diab Rep 2016;16(6):53.

12. Besser REJ, Bell KJ, Couper JJ, et al. ISPAD Clinical Practice Consensus Guidelines 2022: stages of type 1 diabetes in children and adolescents. Pediatr Diabetes 2022;23(8):1175–87.

13. Vehik K, Cuthbertson D, Boulware D, et al. Performance of HbA1c as an early diagnostic indicator of type 1 diabetes in children and youth. Diabetes Care 2012;35(9):1821–5.

14. Stene LC, Barriga K, Hoffman M, et al. Normal but increasing hemoglobin A1c levels predict progression from islet autoimmunity to overt type 1 diabetes: Diabetes Autoimmunity Study in the Young (DAISY). Pediatr Diabetes 2006;7(5):247–53.

15. Steck AK, Dong F, Geno Rasmussen C, et al. CGM metrics predict imminent progression to type 1 diabetes: Autoimmunity Screening for Kids (ASK) Study. Diabetes Care 2022;45(2):365–71.

16. Helminen O, Aspholm S, Pokka T, et al. OGTT and random plasma glucose in the prediction of type 1 diabetes and time to diagnosis. Diabetologia 2015;58(8):1787–96.

17. Ziegler AG, Rewers M, Simell O, et al. Seroconversion to multiple islet autoantibodies and risk of progression to diabetes in children. JAMA 2013;309(23):2473–9.

18. Helminen O, Aspholm S, Pokka T, et al. HbA1c predicts time to diagnosis of type 1 diabetes in children at risk. Diabetes 2015;64(5):1719–27.

19. Sosenko JM, Skyler JS, Mahon J, et al. The application of the diabetes prevention trial-type 1 risk score for identifying a preclinical state of type 1 diabetes. Diabetes Care 2012;35(7):1552–5.

20. Simmons KM, Sosenko JM, Warnock M, et al. One-hour oral glucose tolerance tests for the prediction and diagnostic surveillance of type 1 diabetes. J Clin Endocrinol Metab 2020;105(11):e4094–101.

21. Sosenko JM, Skyler JS, DiMeglio LA, et al. A new approach for diagnosing type 1 diabetes in autoantibody-positive individuals based on prediction and natural history. Diabetes Care 2015;38(2):271–6.

22. Bediaga NG, Li-Wai-Suen CSN, Haller MJ, et al. Simplifying prediction of disease progression in pre-symptomatic type 1 diabetes using a single blood sample. Diabetologia 2021;64(11):2432–44.

23. Herold K, Bundy B, Long A, et al, Type 1 Diabetes TrialNet Study Group. An anti-CD3 antibody, teplizumab, in relatives at risk for type 1 diabetes. N Engl J Med 2019;381:603–13.

Optimizing Glycemic Outcomes for Children with Type 1 Diabetes

Vickie Wu, MD, Lauryn Choleva, MD, MSc, Meredith Wilkes, MD*

KEYWORDS

- Type 1 diabetes mellitus • Technology • Psychosocial • Education

KEY POINTS

- Children with type 1 diabetes mellitus require psychosocial support and access to technologies to achieve glycemic targets.
- Multidisciplinary care is crucial for the prevention of acute complications as well as long-term macrovascular and microvascular complications.
- Continued quality improvement initiatives are needed to enhance diabetes technology uptake, improve education, and address psychosocial needs.

INTRODUCTION

Type 1 diabetes mellitus (T1D) is an autoimmune disease characterized by the progressive irreversible loss of pancreatic β-cell function resulting in insulin deficiency. The estimated number of new T1D cases in individuals aged 0 to 19 years increased from 128,900 to 149,500 globally from 2019 to 2021.[1] Because of near-total insulin deficiency, affected children are dependent on lifelong exogenous insulin. Changes in physical growth, neurocognitive development, and pubertal maturation are only some of the challenges to achieving adequate glycemic stability during childhood and adolescence. To optimize glycemic outcomes in children with T1D, a comprehensive approach is crucial (**Fig. 1**).

DEFINING GLYCEMIC OUTCOMES

There are multiple metrics to evaluate glycemic outcomes, including hemoglobin A1c (HbA1c), percentage of time in range (TIR) of blood glucoses, and frequency of acute and chronic diabetes-related complications. The American Diabetes Association (ADA) recommends assessing glycemic status at least biannually in patients who

Division of Pediatric Endocrinology and Diabetes, Department of Pediatrics, The Icahn School of Medicine at Mount Sinai, 1468 Madison Avenue, Box #1616, Annenberg Building, 4th Floor, New York, NY 10029, USA
* Corresponding author.
E-mail address: Meredith.wilkes@mountsinai.org

Endocrinol Metab Clin N Am 53 (2024) 27–38
https://doi.org/10.1016/j.ecl.2023.09.002   **endo.theclinics.com**

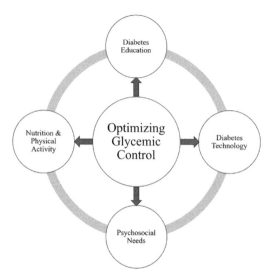

Fig. 1. Approaches to optimizing glycemic control.

meet glycemic goals, and at least quarterly in patients who do not meet treatment goals or whose treatment regimen was recently changed.[2]

Hemoglobin A1c

HbA1c is a measure of hemoglobin glycation and approximates mean glucose levels during the past 3 months. HbA1c can be used as a marker for glycemic goal; however, there are limitations to its use. Conditions influencing red blood cell turnover (such as thalassemia) may result in a discrepancy between a patient's HbA1c result and actual mean glucose levels.[3] Additionally, HbA1c does not provide data on acute hypoglycemic or hyperglycemic events or measure glycemic variability. Therefore, using HbA1c in conjunction with blood glucose monitoring can enhance glycemic management.

The most recent ADA guidelines recommend HbA1c goals to be individualized but a glycemic target of HbA1c less than 7% is considered appropriate for most children and adolescents with T1D.[4] The issue remains that only a minority of children achieve this goal. The T1D Exchange Quality Improvement Collaborative (T1DX-QI) is a multicenter learning health system in the United States that aims to improve T1D care through shared learning.[5] Among the diabetes clinics participating in the T1DX-QI, only 23% of adults and 18% of children with T1D had a HbA1c less than 7% from 2017 to 2022.[6,7] A higher HbA1c target may be more appropriate in those with hypoglycemia unawareness, history of severe hypoglycemia, inability to routinely check blood glucoses, or limited access to diabetes technology.[8]

Glucose Monitoring

Glucose monitoring is key to achieving target glucose range, whether through finger stick blood samples or continuous glucose monitoring (CGM). Children with T1D should monitor glucose levels 6 to 10 times daily including before consuming meals and carbohydrate-containing snacks, at bedtime, and as needed for safety.[4] CGM provides data on TIR, defined as the percentage of time a patient's blood glucoses are between 70 and 180 mg/dL. TIR aids providers in fine-tuning insulin dose adjustments and correlates well with HbA1c.[8] It is recommended for greater than 70% of daily readings to be in TIR, less than 4% of readings to be less than 70 mg/dL (defined as time below range), and less than 25% of readings to be greater than 180 mg/dL (defined as time above range).[9]

Acute Diabetes Complications

Acute diabetes complications include hypoglycemia and diabetes ketoacidosis (DKA). Hypoglycemia, defined as blood glucose less than 70 mg/dL, is the limiting variable with fine tuning doses for maintaining TIR. Symptoms include confusion, hunger, irritability, and tremor. Patients with T1D may have a blunted counterregulatory response or reduced autonomic response to hypoglycemia and experience hypoglycemia unawareness, placing them at risk for loss of consciousness, seizure, or death. Young children or those with conditions affecting neurocognitive ability are particularly at a higher risk because they may not be able to recognize or communicate these symptoms.

Chronic Diabetes Complications

Tight glycemic management in T1D delays the onset and progression of macrovascular and microvascular complications. The Diabetes Control and Complications Trial (DCCT), a prospective randomized controlled trial, compared intensive versus conventional diabetes treatment at the time of the study. Intensive treatment included insulin delivery with a pump or 3 or more insulin injections daily with self-monitoring of blood glucose at least 4 times per day, whereas conventional treatment consisted of 1 or 2 injections of insulin per day with daily self-monitoring of urine or blood glucose. The DCCT demonstrated that intensive glycemic control was associated with 39% to 76% reduction in onset and progression of microvascular complications and requirement for future ocular surgeries.[10,11] The DCCT also demonstrated a 41% reduction in all major cardiovascular and peripheral vascular events with intensive control, although not statistically significant.[10] Compared with patients in the conventional arm, those in the intensive arm had a 57% reduction in the risk of nonfatal myocardial infarctions, strokes, or cardiovascular death in a 9-year post-DCCT follow-up study.[12] As diabetes predisposes to accelerated arteriosclerosis, optimizing diabetes control as early in childhood can minimize these future events.[4]

APPROACH TO OPTIMIZING GLYCEMIC OUTCOMES: DIABETES EDUCATION

Quality structured diabetes education is crucial to the success of diabetes management. The education should optimize the patient and family's understanding of the condition and its treatment, assist with adjustment to living with the new diagnosis, and gradually empower the patient and family in promoting self-management.[13] It should be adapted to each patient's age and development as well as the family's learning style, existing knowledge, and goals. For people living in remote areas with minimal access to professional education locally, telemedicine is an alternative medium to provide education. Web-based educational resources can be a useful supplementation, especially those designed by manufacturing companies for device-specific patient education.

At the time of diagnosis, emotional stress can affect the patient and families' ability to learn and retain new skills. Therefore, emphasis should be placed on acquiring basic skills required to safely manage diabetes at home. Families should be provided with educational materials (ie, books, booklets, and smart phone applications) in the appropriate language and literacy level. At the follow-up visits, education should be reinforced and expanded.

A multidisciplinary team of health-care professionals including a pediatric endocrinologist, certified diabetes care and education specialist, nutritionist, psychologist, and social worker should deliver ongoing education. The team should have access to the latest advances in insulin therapy, diabetes technologies, and educational methods. Specialized diabetes centers should support professional education, which in-turn will improve the quality of diabetes education and standard of care delivered to patients.[14]

As many children spend the majority of their time in daycare programs or schools, child care and school personnel should be equipped with appropriate training and supplies to care for children with T1D, including the ability to support children using diabetes technology.[4,15] Increased sensitivity and inclusion surrounding special occasions, such as celebrations or field trips, are necessary so that these children can participate in school activities in an equitable manner.[15]

APPROACH TO OPTIMIZING GLYCEMIC OUTCOMES: NUTRITION AND PHYSICAL ACTIVITY

Nutrition therapy is an integral component to managing T1D.[4] Education should be initiated at diagnosis and reinforced at frequent intervals; it should include reading nutrition facts labels, carbohydrate counting, and balancing fat, protein, and carbohydrate consumption. Frequent assessments of nutrition and caloric intake by an experienced nutritionist are crucial to balance cardiovascular disease risk factors, weight status, and increased needs with growth and development. Nutrition counseling should be individualized and account for a multitude of factors including the child's food preference, the family's religious or cultural influences, and the family's finances and level of food security.

The American Academic of Pediatrics recommends for all youth at least 60 minutes daily of age-appropriate moderate-to-vigorous intensity physical activity.[16] Children with T1D require glucose monitoring before, during, and after physical activity and strategies should be developed to prevent hypoglycemia and hyperglycemia. Such strategies may include reducing basal insulin doses or using "exercise/activity mode" on an insulin pump as well as consuming complex carbohydrates before and/or after exercise.[4] Children with marked hyperglycemia (glucose level ≥350 mg/dL), moderate-to-large urine ketones, and/or β-hydroxybutyrate greater than 1.5 mmol/L should postpone intense activity because exercise can worsen these conditions.

APPROACH TO OPTIMIZING GLYCEMIC OUTCOMES: DIABETES TECHNOLOGY

Initial management of T1D includes self-monitoring of blood glucose several times daily along with exogenous insulin delivery. Insulin preparations include analogs that are short acting (human regular insulin), rapid acting (insulin lispro, insulin aspart, and insulin glulisine), ultrarapid acting (faster insulin aspart, insulin lispro-aabc, and inhaled human insulin), intermediate acting (neutral protamine hagedorn insulin [NPH] insulin), and long acting (insulin glargine, insulin detemir, and insulin degludec).[17] Advances in diabetes technology in the past few decades include CGM and devices that automate some insulin delivery. They should be offered to all children with T1D who are able to use the devices safely by themselves or with the support and/or supervision of a caregiver. The decision of which device to use should be made according to the child and family's individual circumstances and preferences, in addition to the clinicians' assessment.[4]

Continuous Glucose Monitoring

Although glucose meters measure glucose concentration from capillary blood, CGM devices are inserted into the subcutaneous fat and interstitial fluid is read via a small disposable glucose oxidase-coated electrode. The glucose in the interstitial fluid reacts with the glucose oxidase to generate hydrogen peroxide, resulting in an electrical current that is sent to a transmitter and translated to an estimate of blood glucose concentration.[18] The transmitter then relays the values to a receiver, other mobile device, and/or an insulin pump.[19] CGM provides near-immediate feedback on glycemic excursions and patterns, which affects insulin management and lifestyle modifications.

CGM use has shown significant benefits to achieving glycemic control. Lower mean HbA1c has been observed in youth and young adult CGM users compared with nonusers, regardless of insulin administration method.[20,21] A clinical trial randomizing adolescents and young adults with T1D to CGM or standard blood glucose meter use for 26 weeks showed a statistically significant improvement in HbA1c in CGM users.[22] Rates of severe hypoglycemia and DKA are also lower in CGM users compared with nonusers.[23]

Toddlers and preschool children tend to have unpredictable eating patterns and variable physical activity levels, making T1D care in this age group particularly challenging.[24] Additionally, they have wide glucose fluctuations and limited ability to identify symptoms of hypoglycemia or hyperglycemia.[25] CGM use in these children identifies glycemic patterns, decreases parental worry, increases parental confidence about child safety, and promotes other caregivers' involvement by allowing remote monitoring functionality.[26] Parents can also use CGM data retrospectively to improve their understanding of variables that may influence glucose levels, including time of day and types of food or physical activity.[26] Consistent CGM use in a 6-month randomized controlled trial of children aged less than 8 years with T1D did not show improvements in TIR compared with blood glucose meter use; however, the number of hypoglycemic events and amount of glucose variability were reduced in CGM users.[27]

Smart Insulin Pens

Smart insulin pens (SIPs) have a memory function that records the date, time, and amount of insulin administered. This record can be combined with CGM data and viewed by providers to enhance diabetes care.[19] SIP can calculate insulin doses if provided with blood glucose value and grams of carbohydrates being consumed, thereby having the potential to improve medication adherence. SIP can benefit young children by keeping track of when the last insulin dose was administered, which is helpful if there are multiple caregivers and potential gaps in communication. They can also benefit adolescents by increasing engagement and help track dose administration. In a one-arm prospective observational study of children with T1D using CGM in conjunction with SIPs for at least 12 months, the number of hypoglycemic events was reduced from baseline to follow-up.[28] Barriers to successful SIP use include lack of provider awareness and training and lack of patient education on SIP use.[29] Therefore, initiatives are needed to address these barriers while emphasizing the benefits of SIP use.

Insulin Pumps

Insulin delivery has changed dramatically during the past several decades, from syringes, pens, and open-loop pumps to now hybrid closed-loop pump systems (HCLS).[19,30,31] Continuous subcutaneous insulin infusion pumps infuse a rapid-acting insulin analog through a catheter at basal rates and additional bolus doses for hyperglycemia correction and carbohydrate coverage with preprogrammed correction factors and carbohydrate ratios.[19] The pump can be programmed to deliver variable basal amounts throughout the day, and multiple profiles can be established for different circumstances, including illness, menstruation, and physical activity. In comparison to a multiple daily injection regimen, insulin pump therapy in children has been associated with improved HbA1c and lower risks of severe hypoglycemia and DKA, with greater improvements in those with concomitant CGM use than in nonusers.[32,33]

Closed-loop insulin delivery links CGM data with an insulin pump to automate insulin delivery. Initial models of this technology suspend insulin delivery when sensor glucose level reaches or is predicted to reach a preset low threshold, called sensor-augmented pump therapy with predictive low-glucose suspend function.[19] Newer HCLS models allow for real-time adjustments in basal infusion rates in response to declining or increasing glucose levels.[18] HCLS has been associated with lower HbA1c and higher TIR, and the degree of HbA1c improvement is greater than that seen with sensor-augmented pump therapy, CGM, and insulin pump use without a closed-loop algorithm, or multiple daily injection regimen.[21,34,35]

In 2 randomized trials of young children with T1D who received HCLS compared with sensor-augmented pump therapy, HCLS resulted in higher TIR and lower HbA1c.[36,37] For example, in the HCLS group, the mean TIR increased from 56.7% at baseline to 69.3% during the 13-week follow-up period, compared with the standard care group, which included a CGM with either an insulin pump or multiple daily injections, of 54.9% at baseline to 55.9% at follow-up; the mean adjusted difference was 12.4% points, equivalent to approximately 3 hours daily.[37] HCLS may be especially beneficial for young children whose families may permit hyperglycemia for fear of hypoglycemia.[38] By reducing hyperglycemia permissive behaviors, young children can readily achieve target glycemic goals.

Although insulin pump therapy, and more recently HCLS, improves glycemic outcomes in children with T1D, it is important to consider the feasibility of using them and their psychosocial influence on patients and their families. Significant resources are required for educating families on ways to optimize the usage of pump therapy. Unsuspected pump failure may result in DKA, making it imperative that patients and their families learn how to prevent, recognize, and manage pump failures. Current studies report generally positive feedback on HCLS, including improved quality of life, sleep, confidence, and reduced anxiety about hypoglycemia and hyperglycemia.[35,39] Nevertheless, it is important to recognize the challenges of HCLS use in children, including alarm fatigue from frequent alarms, calibration difficulties, and wearing devices that are challenging to conceal from peers if they do not want to disclose their diagnosis.[40]

APPROACH TO OPTIMIZING GLYCEMIC OUTCOMES: PSYCHOSOCIAL NEEDS

A multidisciplinary team should provide support at the time of diagnosis of T1D and regular intervals thereafter in a developmentally appropriate and culturally sensitive manner.[4] The support should address social determinants of health (SDOH) and emotional, behavioral, or psychosocial factors that may pose a barrier to implementing treatment plans.[41] Screening for families' SDOH at routine diabetes appointments can identify unemployment and food or housing insecurity that may take precedence over intensive diabetes management, and these families should receive additional care from community health workers.

Family involvement is crucial in optimizing glycemic control throughout childhood and adolescence. Families may experience distress related to the burden of managing diabetes, including worry about hypoglycemia, future complications, and interrupted sleep.[42] Parental psychosocial functioning and adjustment may indirectly affect children's T1D outcomes.[43] Incorporating social support and building parental diabetes self-efficacy throughout all visits may build parental resilience and serve as a protective factor against diabetes-related distress.[27,44]

As the child develops and desires independence in their diabetes care, the multidisciplinary team must ensure appropriate transfer of self-management responsibilities and reinforce that the youth will still need supervision. Premature transfer of responsibilities or lack of adult supervision can result in suboptimal management, diabetes burnout, and worsening of glycemic outcomes.[4] The need for increasing autonomy in diabetes self-management along with the psychosocial changes that happen in adolescence can pose challenges to achieving optimal glycemic management.[15] Shared decision-making with adolescents, preventing diabetes-related family conflict, and providing adolescents time alone with providers may increase engagement and adoption of the management plan.

Depressive symptoms often coexist with T1D and are associated with an increased risk for elevated HbA1c and DKA.[45] Children and adolescents with T1D have a 2 to 3-fold greater prevalence of diabetes compared with peers without diabetes.[46] Furthermore, compared with children with HbA1c less than 7%, those with HbA1c greater than 7% were more likely to screen positive for depression or anxiety.[7] The perpetual cycle between mental health issues influencing diabetes management and vice-versa is important to recognize. It is imperative to routinely assess psychosocial health with tools such as the PHQ-2, generally starting at 7 to 8 years of age, and to refer to a mental health professional as soon as indicated.[4] If signs of disordered or disrupted eating are noted, the motivation behind these behaviors should be further explored to assess for mental distress or an underlying eating disorder.[47]

Racial, Ethnic, and Socioeconomic Disparities

Multiple studies have demonstrated racial/ethnic disparities in the health outcomes of children with T1D, with patients from groups that have been marginalized having a higher HbA1c and more acute complications.[48,49] Among children in the T1DX-QI with HbA1c less than 7%, 9% were non-Hispanic Black and 9% were Hispanic compared with 66% non-Hispanic White.[7] Compared with other racial/ethnic groups, non-Hispanic Black individuals had the highest rates of DKA before and during the coronavirus disease 2019 (COVID-19) pandemic; additionally, they were almost 4 times more likely to present in DKA during the COVID-19 pandemic compared with non-Hispanic Whites even after adjusting for sex, age, insurance status, and HbA1c.[50,51]

CGM and insulin pumps should be accessible to all patients with T1D as part of routine diabetes care.[21,23,34] In the T1DX-QI Collaborative, CGM use was highest in non-Hispanic White patients (50%), compared with Hispanic patients (38%) and non-Hispanic Black patients (18%), and these disparities existed even when stratifying by insurance type.[23] The same disparities were seen in HCLS use.[34] In a single-center cohort of children with T1D, non-Hispanic White patients were more likely to use both a CGM and insulin pump compared with no technology use; in contrast, Hispanic and non-Hispanic Black patients were more likely to not use technology.[21] Language differences may pose a barrier to managing T1D through technology use. Spanish-speaking patients in one study were found to have lower rates of CGM and insulin pump use than English-speaking patients, despite the center having a culturally sensitive Spanish language clinic.[21]

Disparities in diabetes technology utilization also exist across socioeconomic status (SES). Patients with private insurance are more likely to use CGM and insulin pumps than those with public insurance.[21,23] Using parental education level, insurance type, and annual income to create a composite SES score, patients with the lowest SES quintile had the lowest rates of CGM and pump use and highest HbA1c when compared with the other quintiles.[52] Even after adjusting for SES, insulin pump use was higher in non-Hispanic White children than in Hispanic and non-Hispanic Black children.[53]

The inequity in technology use by race/ethnicity may be contributing to the racial/ethnic disparities seen in glycemic outcomes. Additionally, the providers' perception of family's competence and implicit biases need to be studied so that these do not pose as additional barriers in equitable technology use.[54]

SUMMARY

Despite technological advances that have enhanced the capability to optimize glycemic management, many children with T1D are unable to meet the recommendations because of a multitude of barriers in SDOH, education, technology access, and psychosocial support. This has led to quality improvement initiatives such as the T1DX-QI, which focuses on areas such as care delivery, self-management, and psychosocial support.[55,56] One initiative increased CGM use in 12 to 26-year-old patients with T1D from 34% to 55% during 19 to 22 months using interventions such as coaching patients, training clinical teams, and provider engagement in advocacy efforts to promote CGM coverage by their state's Medicaid program.[57] Another initiative increased insulin pump adoption in 12 to 26-year-old patients with T1D by 13% by increasing in-person and telehealth technology education and improving clinic staff knowledge.[58] Although continued efforts are needed to develop processes that improve T1D care for all patients, emphasis needs to be placed on initiatives that eliminate racial, ethnic, and socioeconomic disparities.[59,60] Strategies are also needed to ensure equitable availability of insulin and technologies.

Achieving target blood glucose levels in children with T1D requires addressing the medical and psychosocial aspects of T1D. Additional quality improvement study is needed to reduce gaps in care delivery, psychosocial support, and health equity, such that diabetes care and quality of life can be improved for all children with T1D.

CLINICS CARE POINTS

- A multidisciplinary approach is necessary to achieve glycemic target in children with T1D.
- Hemoglobin A1c and TIR at goal reduce the risk of acute and chronic complications of diabetes.
- Technologies that have aided the management of T1D in children include continuous glucose monitors, SIPs, and insulin pumps.
- Use of diabetes technology in children with T1D has resulted in lower HbA1c and improved quality of life.
- Ongoing diabetes education, family support, and identification of SDOH are important to ensure adherence to diabetes treatment plans and reduction of barriers to glycemic targets.

DISCLOSURE

The authors have no commercial or financial conflicts of interest.

REFERENCES

1. Ogle GD, James S, Dabelea D, et al. Global estimates of incidence of type 1 diabetes in children and adolescents: results from the International Diabetes Federation Atlas, 10th edition. Diabetes Res Clin Pract. 2022;183:109083.

2. ElSayed NA, Aleppo G, Aroda VR, et al. Glycemic targets: standards of care in diabetes-2023. Diabetes Care 2023;46(Suppl 1):S97–110.
3. Kidney Disease: Improving Global Outcomes (KDIGO) Diabetes Work Group. KDIGO 2020 clinical practice guideline for diabetes management in chronic kidney disease. Kidney Int 2020;98(4s):S1–115.
4. ElSayed NA, Aleppo G, Aroda VR, et al. Children and adolescents: standards of care in diabetes-2023. Diabetes Care 2023;46(Suppl 1):S230–53.
5. Mungmode A, Noor N, Weinstock RS, et al. Making diabetes electronic medical record data actionable: promoting benchmarking and population health improvement using the T1D exchange quality improvement portal. Clin Diabetes 2022; 41(1):45–55.
6. Akturk HK, Rompicherla S, Rioles N, et al. Factors associated with improved A1C among adults with type 1 diabetes in the United States. Clin Diabetes 2022;41(1): 76–80.
7. Demeterco-Berggren C, Ebekozien O, Noor N, et al. Factors associated with achieving target A1C in children and adolescents with type 1 diabetes: findings from the T1D exchange quality improvement collaborative. Clin Diabetes 2022; 41(1):68–75.
8. Vigersky RA, McMahon C. The relationship of hemoglobin A1C to time-in-range in patients with diabetes. Diabetes Technol Therapeut 2019;21(2):81–5.
9. Battelino T, Danne T, Bergenstal RM, et al. Clinical targets for continuous glucose monitoring data interpretation: recommendations from the international consensus on time in range. Diabetes Care 2019;42(8):1593–603.
10. Nathan DM, Genuth S, Lachin J, et al. The effect of intensive treatment of diabetes on the development and progression of long-term complications in insulin-dependent diabetes mellitus. N Engl J Med 1993;329(14):977–86.
11. Aiello LP, Sun W, Das A, et al. Intensive diabetes therapy and ocular surgery in type 1 diabetes. N Engl J Med 2015;372(18):1722–33.
12. Nathan DM, Cleary PA, Backlund JY, et al. Intensive diabetes treatment and cardiovascular disease in patients with type 1 diabetes. N Engl J Med 2005;353(25): 2643–53.
13. Phelan H, Lange K, Cengiz E, et al. ISPAD clinical practice consensus guidelines 2018: diabetes education in children and adolescents. Pediatr Diabetes 2018;19: 75–83.
14. Chan JC, Lim L-L, Wareham NJ, et al. The lancet Commission on diabetes: using data to transform diabetes care and patient lives. Lancet 2020;396(10267): 2019–82.
15. Siminerio LM, Albanese-O'Neill A, Chiang JL, et al. Care of young children with diabetes in the child care setting: a position statement of the American Diabetes Association. Diabetes Care 2014;37(10):2834–42.
16. Lobelo F, Muth ND, Hanson S, et al. Council on sports medicine and fitness; section on obesity. physical activity assessment and counseling in pediatric clinical settings. Pediatrics 2020;145(3). e20193992.
17. Hirsch IB, Juneja R, Beals JM, et al. The evolution of insulin and how it informs therapy and treatment choices. Endocr Rev 2020;41(5):733–55.
18. Perkins BA, Sherr JL, Mathieu C. Type 1 diabetes glycemic management: Insulin therapy, glucose monitoring, and automation. Science 2021;373(6554):522–7.
19. Dovc K, Battelino T. Evolution of diabetes technology. Endocrinol Metab Clin N Am 2020;49(1):1–18.
20. DeSalvo DJ, Lanzinger S, Noor N, et al. Transatlantic comparison of pediatric continuous glucose monitoring use in the diabetes-patienten-verlaufsdokumentation

initiative and type 1 diabetes exchange quality improvement collaborative. Diabetes Technol Therapeut 2022;24(12):920–4.

21. Sawyer A, Sobczak M, Forlenza GP, et al. Glycemic Control in Relation to Technology Use in a Single-Center Cohort of Children with Type 1 Diabetes. Diabetes Technol Therapeut 2022;24(6):409–15.

22. Laffel LM, Kanapka LG, Beck RW, et al. Effect of continuous glucose monitoring on glycemic control in adolescents and young adults with type 1 diabetes: a randomized clinical trial. JAMA 2020;323(23):2388–96.

23. DeSalvo DJ, Noor N, Xie C, et al. Patient demographics and clinical outcomes among type 1 diabetes patients using continuous glucose monitors: data from T1D exchange real-world observational study. J Diabetes Sci Technol 2023;17(2):322–8.

24. Monaghan M, Bryant BL, Inverso H, et al. Young children with type 1 diabetes: recent advances in behavioral research. Curr Diabetes Rep 2022;22(6):247–56.

25. Streisand R, Monaghan M. Young children with type 1 diabetes: challenges, research, and future directions. Curr Diabetes Rep 2014;14(9):520. https://doi.org/10.1007/s11892-014-0520-2.

26. Hilliard ME, Levy W, Anderson BJ, et al. Benefits and barriers of continuous glucose monitoring in young children with type 1 diabetes. Diabetes Technol Therapeut 2019;21(9):493–8.

27. Strategies to Enhance New CGM Use in Early Childhood (SENCE) Study Group. A randomized clinical trial assessing continuous glucose monitoring (CGM) use with standardized education with or without a family behavioral intervention compared with fingerstick blood glucose monitoring in very young children with type 1 diabetes. Diabetes Care 2021;44(2):464–72.

28. Adolfsson P, Björnsson V, Hartvig NV, et al. Improved glycemic control observed in children with type 1 diabetes following the introduction of smart insulin pens: a real-world study. Diabetes Ther 2022;1–14.

29. Ospelt E, Noor N, Sanchez J, et al. Facilitators and barriers to smart insulin pen use: a mixed-method study of multidisciplinary stakeholders from diabetes teams in the United States. Clin Diabetes 2022;41(1):56–67.

30. Danne T, Phillip M, Buckingham BA, et al. ISPAD clinical practice consensus guidelines 2018: Insulin treatment in children and adolescents with diabetes. Pediatr Diabetes 2018;19:115–35.

31. Boughton CK, Hovorka R. New closed-loop insulin systems. Diabetologia 2021;64:1007–15.

32. Karges B, Schwandt A, Heidtmann B, et al. Association of insulin pump therapy vs insulin injection therapy with severe hypoglycemia, ketoacidosis, and glycemic control among children, adolescents, and young adults with type 1 diabetes. JAMA 2017;318(14):1358–66.

33. Cardona-Hernandez R, Schwandt A, Alkandari H, et al. Glycemic outcome associated with insulin pump and glucose sensor use in children and adolescents with type 1 diabetes. Data from the international pediatric registry SWEET. Diabetes Care 2021;44(5):1176–84.

34. Noor N, Kamboj MK, Triolo T, et al. Hybrid closed-loop systems and glycemic outcomes in children and adults with type 1 diabetes: real-world evidence from a U.S.-based multicenter collaborative. Diabetes Care 2022;45(8):e118–9.

35. Abraham MB, de Bock M, Smith GJ, et al. Effect of a hybrid closed-loop system on glycemic and psychosocial outcomes in children and adolescents with type 1 diabetes: a randomized clinical trial. JAMA Pediatr 2021;175(12):1227–35.

36. Ware J, Hovorka R. Closed-loop control in very young children with type 1 diabetes. reply. N Engl J Med 2022;386(15):1482–3.
37. Wadwa RP, Reed ZW, Buckingham BA, et al. Trial of hybrid closed-loop control in young children with type 1 diabetes. N Engl J Med 2023;388(11):991–1001.
38. Gonder-Frederick L, Nyer M, Shepard JA, et al. Assessing fear of hypoglycemia in children with Type 1 diabetes and their parents. Diabetes Manag 2011;1(6): 627–39.
39. Farrington C. Psychosocial impacts of hybrid closed-loop systems in the management of diabetes: a review. Diabet Med 2018;35(4):436–49.
40. Franceschi R, Mozzillo E, Di Candia F, et al. A systematic review on the impact of commercially available hybrid closed loop systems on psychological outcomes in youths with type 1 diabetes and their parents. Diabet Med 2023;e15099.
41. Corathers S, Williford DN, Kichler J, et al. Implementation of psychosocial screening into diabetes clinics: experience from the type 1 diabetes exchange quality improvement network. Curr Diabetes Rep 2023;23(2):19–28.
42. Harrington KR, Boyle CT, Miller KM, et al. Management and family burdens endorsed by parents of youth <7 years old with type 1 diabetes. J Diabetes Sci Technol 2017;11(5):980–7.
43. Pierce JS, Kozikowski C, Lee JM, et al. Type 1 diabetes in very young children: a model of parent and child influences on management and outcomes. Pediatr Diabetes 2017;18(1):17–25.
44. Trojanowski PJ, Niehaus CE, Fischer S, et al. Parenting and psychological health in youth with type 1 diabetes: systematic review. J Pediatr Psychol 2021;46(10): 1213–37.
45. Garey CJ, Clements MA, McAuliffe-Fogarty AH, et al. The association between depression symptom endorsement and glycemic outcomes in adolescents with type 1 diabetes. Pediatr Diabetes 2022;23(2):248–57.
46. Grey M, Whittemore R, Tamborlane W. Depression in type 1 diabetes in children: natural history and correlates. J Psychosom Res 2002;53(4):907–11.
47. ElSayed NA, Aleppo G, Aroda VR, et al. Facilitating positive health behaviors and well-being to improve health outcomes: standards of care in diabetes-2023. Diabetes Care 2023;46(Supple 1):S68–96.
48. Majidi S, Ebekozien O, Noor N, et al. Inequities in health outcomes in children and adults with type 1 diabetes: data from the T1D exchange quality improvement collaborative. Clin Diabetes 2021;39(3):278–83.
49. Lipman TH, Smith JA, Patil O, et al. Racial disparities in treatment and outcomes of children with type 1 diabetes. Pediatr Diabetes 2021;22(2):241–8.
50. Ebekozien O, Agarwal S, Noor N, et al. Inequities in diabetic ketoacidosis among patients with type 1 diabetes and COVID-19: data from 52 US Clinical Centers. J Clin Endocrinol Metab 2021;106(4):e1755–62.
51. Lavik AR, Ebekozien O, Noor N, et al. Trends in Type 1 diabetic ketoacidosis during COVID-19 Surges at 7 US Centers: highest burden on non-hispanic black patients. J Clin Endocrinol Metab 2022;107(7):1948–55.
52. Addala A, Auzanneau M, Miller K, et al. A decade of disparities in diabetes technology use and HbA1c in pediatric type 1 diabetes: a transatlantic comparison. Diabetes Care 2021;44(1):133–40.
53. Willi SM, Miller KM, DiMeglio LA, et al. Racial-ethnic disparities in management and outcomes among children with type 1 diabetes. Pediatrics 2015;135(3): 424–34. https://doi.org/10.1542/peds.2014-1774.
54. Odugbesan O, Addala A, Nelson G, et al. Implicit racial-ethnic and insurance-mediated bias to recommending diabetes technology: insights from T1D

exchange multicenter pediatric and adult diabetes provider cohort. Diabetes Technol Therapeut 2022;24(9):619–27.

55. Ginnard OZB, Alonso GT, Corathers SD, et al. Quality improvement in diabetes care: a review of initiatives and outcomes in the T1D exchange quality improvement collaborative. Clin Diabetes 2021;39(3):256–63.

56. Prahalad P, Rioles N, Noor N, et al. T1D exchange quality improvement collaborative: Accelerating change through benchmarking and improvement science for people with type 1 diabetes. J Diabetes 2022;14(1):83–7.

57. Prahalad P, Ebekozien O, Alonso GT, et al. Multi-clinic quality improvement initiative increases continuous glucose monitoring use among adolescents and young adults with type 1 diabetes. Clin Diabetes 2021;39(3):264–71.

58. Lyons SK, Ebekozien O, Garrity A, et al. Increasing insulin pump use among 12- to 26-year-olds with type 1 diabetes: results from the T1D exchange quality improvement collaborative. Clin Diabetes 2021;39(3):272–7.

59. Ebekozien O, Mungmode A, Buckingham D, et al. Achieving equity in diabetes research: borrowing from the field of quality improvement using a practical framework and improvement tools. Diabetes Spectr 2022;35(3):304–12.

60. Ebekozien O, Mungmode A, Odugbesan O, et al. Addressing type 1 diabetes health inequities in the United States: Approaches from the T1D Exchange QI Collaborative. J Diabetes 2022;14(1):79–82.

Young Adults with Type 1 Diabetes

Priyanka Mathias, MD[a], Sarah D. Corathers, MD[b],
Samantha A. Carreon, PhD[c], Marisa E. Hilliard, PhD[c],
Jaclyn L. Papadakis, PhD[d], Jill Weissberg-Benchell, PhD, CDCES[d],
Jennifer K. Raymond, MD, MCR[e],
Elizabeth A. Pyatak, PhD, OTR/L, CDCES[f],
Shivani Agarwal, MD, MPH[a,g,*]

KEYWORDS

- Young adults • Type 1 diabetes • Health-care transition • Developmental challenges
- Marginalized youth • Targeted interventions

KEY POINTS

- Young adulthood is a unique phase in life with multiple developmental, social, and health-care changes that complicate type 1 diabetes self-management and can be associated with worsening of health and psychosocial outcomes.
- Young adults (YA) from marginalized groups experience negative social determinants of health, stigma, and effects of structural racism that are associated with high risk for even worse outcomes.
- We review evidence-based care approaches that improve outcomes for YA with type 1 diabetes, including health-care transition clinics, psychosocial care interventions, telehealth and mobile strategies, occupational therapy approaches, and mitigation or elimination of root causes of inequity to improve diabetes self-management.

[a] Fleischer Institute for Diabetes and Metabolism, Albert Einstein College of Medicine-Montefiore Medical Center, 1180 Morris Park Avenue, Bronx, NY 10467, USA; [b] Cincinnati Children's Hospital Medical Center, University of Cincinnati College of Medicine, 3333 Burnet Avenue, Cincinnati, OH 45229, USA; [c] Baylor College of Medicine and Texas Children's Hospital, 1102 Bates Avenue, Suite 940, Houston, TX 77030, USA; [d] Northwestern University Feinberg School of Medicine, Pritzker Department of Psychiatry and Behavioral Health, Ann and Robert H. Lurie Children's Hospital of Chicago, 225 East Chicago Avenue, Box 10, Chicago, IL 60611, USA; [e] Division of Pediatric Endocrinology, Children's Hospital Los Angeles, 4650 Sunset Boulevard. MS 61, Los Angeles, CA, USA; [f] Chan Division of Occupational Science and Occupational Therapy, Ostrow School of Dentistry, University of Southern California, 1540 Alcazar Street, CHP-133, Los Angeles, CA 90089-9003, USA; [g] NY Regional Center for Diabetes Translation Research, Albert Einstein College of Medicine, 1180 Morris Park Avenue, Bronx, NY 10467, USA
* Corresponding author. 1180 Morris Park Avenue, Bronx, NY 10467.
E-mail address: pmathias@montefiore.org

Endocrinol Metab Clin N Am 53 (2024) 39–52
https://doi.org/10.1016/j.ecl.2023.09.001
0889-8529/24/© 2023 Elsevier Inc. All rights reserved.

INTRODUCTION

Young adulthood (ages 18–30 years) is a unique developmental phase marked by multiple concurrent transitions, including physical, psychological, financial, and social changes that influence type 1 diabetes (T1D) self-management.[1,2] Coinciding with these normative transitions, young adults (YA) with T1D face unique obstacles navigating the transition from pediatric to adult medical care. During this time, high-quality care is fragmented, resulting in suboptimal glycemic control, early microvascular complications, preventable hospitalizations, and premature mortality.[3]

Data from the T1D Exchange indicate that only 14% of youth with T1D in the United States achieve target glycemic goals (HbA1c). HbA1c levels increase during late adolescence and young adulthood and have worsened over time.[4] In addition, diabetes technology use was lowest in the YA age group, with widening age disparity during the last decade.[4] The SEARCH for Diabetes in Youth study further demonstrated that approximately one-third (32%) of YA with T1D had at least 1 diabetes-related complication (retinopathy, neuropathy, or nephropathy) at a mean age of 21 years.[5] Moreover, mortality for YA with T1D was 1.5 times greater compared to YA without diabetes.[6]

There is a critical need to review and implement evidence-based strategies to improve outcomes and address care gaps for this vulnerable population.[7,8] In this narrative review, we summarize the unique health-care considerations for YA with T1D, psychosocial risk factors and outcomes, racial-ethnic disparities, and evidence-based approaches to care.

SECTION ONE: UNIQUE HEALTH-CARE CONSIDERATIONS FOR YOUNG ADULTS WITH TYPE 1 DIABETES

The Intersection of Young Adult Development and Type 1 Diabetes

Common developmental challenges of young adulthood complicate diabetes self-management and health-care transition. This intersectionality can be seen when YA have to balance typical daily activities with the demands of diabetes care. YA often report that balancing diabetes and "life" is challenging,[9] especially when related to work/school, relationships, and finances.[10] Diabetes-related tasks can also interfere with sleep, which can lead to disruptions in glycemia among YA.[11,12]

Differentiating from one's family is a key task during young adulthood[2]; yet, parental involvement is highly beneficial during this time, especially while transitioning to adult health care.[13–16] Compared to those without T1D, YA with T1D are more likely to identify as "adults," suggesting that the demands of T1D may increase perceived independence, self-sufficiency, and responsibility.[17]

Additionally, social relationships are central to YA, yet the benefits of receiving peer support related to diabetes are not always straightforward.[18,19] In certain situations, diabetes-specific support from peers is beneficial, especially when YA are satisfied with the support received.[18] However, the involvement of peers in diabetes care can also lead to negative consequences. For example, diabetes technology can be negatively influenced by romantic relationships with regard to the sensitivity of wearing technology and lack of T1D partner support.[20]

Young adulthood is also unique because it represents a peak time for the onset of mental health symptoms.[21,22] Although all people with diabetes are at an increased risk for diagnosis of psychological conditions,[23] challenges associated with living with and managing T1D may exacerbate emotional and psychological distress during young adulthood.[24] YA with T1D experience increased rates of depression, anxiety, and eating disorders compared with both YA without diabetes[25] and adolescents with diabetes.[26]

YA with T1D and depression describe their depression as negatively affecting their physical, emotional, and social well-being.[25] Depressive symptoms have also been associated with higher HbA1c and somatic symptoms (eg, lethargy, sleep difficulty), which highlights the complexity of the relationship between diabetes and depression.[27] Anxiety disorders in YA with T1D have also shown to be associated with higher HbA1c levels, rates of diabetic ketoacidosis (DKA), and hospital admissions than those without anxiety disorders.[28] In addition, anxiety symptoms are associated with less engagement in self-management behaviors, more depressive symptoms, and greater fear of hypoglycemia.[29] Female YA with T1D experience twice the risk for engaging in disordered eating behaviors and receiving eating disorder diagnoses than peers without diabetes.[30,31] Furthermore, one study quotes that up to 40% of YA women with T1D omit insulin for weight loss.[32]

Finally, diabetes distress is also highly prevalent in YA with T1D. Compared with older adults, YA with T1D experience greater diabetes distress and engage less in diabetes self-management.[33] Diabetes distress describes the stress and burden of living with and managing diabetes but may not represent depression or anxiety, although it can be considered a precursor. Diabetes distress also resulted in YA reporting feeling less ready to transfer to adult care, poorer self-management skills, and lower health-related quality of life, as well as predicting higher HbA1c levels.[34,35,36]

Disparities in Outcomes for Young Adults with Type 1 Diabetes from Minoritized Groups

YA from minoritized groups exhibit poorer health outcomes than NHW peers, which is attributed to systemic inequities.[37–41] The SEARCH for Diabetes in Youth study has shown a disproportionate increase in the prevalence and incidence of T1D among YA from minoritized groups, with the incidence among Hispanic youth increasing 3.5 times as fast as non-Hispanic White (NHW) youth.[42] Among YA in the T1D Exchange, mean HbA1c levels were 10.3% among non-Hispanic Black (NHB) and 9.2% among Hispanic YA, compared with 8.3% among NHW YA, after adjusting for insurance type and socioeconomic status (SES; $P < .001$).[43] In addition, NHB YA had higher rates of DKA, severe hypoglycemia, and the lowest rates of insulin pump and continuous glucose monitor (CGM) use compared with NHW YA. Furthermore, among 300 YA with T1D in the Young Adult Racial Disparities in Diabetes (YARDD) study, NHB YA had 2.26% points higher mean HbA1c than NHW YA, despite accounting for differences in SES, and were attributed to disparities in lower use of diabetes technology use, higher diabetes distress, and lower self-rated diabetes self-management.[38] Longitudinal studies of HbA1c trajectories have demonstrated that NHB and Hispanic youth have higher HbA1c levels at diabetes diagnosis and have the most rapidly increasing HbA1c levels, increasing the risk of diabetes-related complications in young adulthood.[41] In addition, quality of life has been shown to be lowest among minoritized youth with T1D and could be exacerbated in the YA years.[44]

Reasons for these disparities in outcomes include negative influences of social determinants of health (SDOH), lower social support, financial barriers, and inequity in health-care access and delivery.[37] SDOH are heightened in the YA period given increased independence during this life stage, which can worsen factors such as residential and financial instability, transportation challenges, and food insecurity.[45] In addition, disparate use of diabetes technology may account for some of the glycemic disparity. Stark differences in rates of technology uptake among NHB YA persist after accounting for SES, demographics, and health-care factors.[4,38,46] Even where universal coverage for technology is offered, inequities in adoption and use remain.[47] These barriers to universal adoption may reflect implicit bias in clinic processes and communication strategies at the provider and health-care system levels, such as limited shared decision-making, inadequate tailoring of therapeutics, and cumbersome insurance authorization processes,[48–50] which considered together with the care needs of YA, only exacerbate the influences of structural racism, stigma, health-care trauma, and resultant poor outcomes for minoritized YA with T1D.[49]

SECTION TWO: EVIDENCE-BASED STRATEGIES TO IMPROVE OUTCOMES FOR YOUNG ADULTS WITH TYPE 1 DIABETES
New Health-care Delivery Models

Health-care transition clinics
Overwhelming evidence shows that YA with T1D transitioning from pediatric to adult diabetes care experience higher HbA1c, psychological issues, hospitalizations, and mortality in the transfer period, when loss to follow-up care is at its highest.[3,39,51–53] Moreover, a lack of YA-centered care delivery results in poor clinic attendance and higher HbA1c levels.[54] Prolonged transfer time from pediatric to adult clinics has also been shown to be associated with higher HbA1c and increased hospitalization days after transfer to adult care.[55] The American Diabetes Association and other professional societies have published guidelines to facilitate the transition from pediatric to adult T1D care.[56] Structured transition programs have resulted in improvement in glycemic outcomes, more consistent follow-up in outpatient care, decreases in hospital admissions, and reduction in the length of stay for DKA readmission.[57–60]

Successful components and strategies of health-care transition clinics is covered more in depth in this issue by Malik and colleagues in the article titled "Incorporating the Six Core Elements of Health Care Transition in Type 1 Diabetes Care for Emerging Adults." In brief, an overview of the literature yields more high-quality studies testing transition preparation and transfer coordination versus receivership roles. One study from Australia used a diabetes educator as a transition clinic coordinator, reminder calls and rebooking missed appointments, and phone support for sick day management demonstrating reduction in HbA1c ($9.3 \pm 2.17\%$ to $8.8 \pm 1.9\%$, $P < .001$), maintenance of clinic attendance, and reduction in DKA hospital admission rates by 30%, with maintenance of effects at 30 months posttransition.[57] Another study from the United Kingdom showed that transferring care to a collaboration of combined pediatric and adult providers or transfer of care to a dedicated YA transition clinic was associated with improved clinic attendance at follow-up.[61] A multicenter randomized controlled trial in Canada testing effects of a transition coordinator showed improvement in clinic attendance (mean [SD] number of visits 4.1 [1.1] vs 3.6 [1.2], $P = .002$), patient satisfaction, and diabetes distress compared with standard care among 205 YA with T1D, but benefits were not sustained 12 months post-intervention.[60] Another study from the United States testing the LEAP (Let's Empower and Prepare) program focused on structured diabetes education and access to a transition coordinator at a YA diabetes clinic, demonstrating reduction in HbA1c levels, less hypoglycemia, and improvement in overall well-being at 12 months compared with standard care.[62] Finally, with more focus on receivership versus preparation or transfer coordination, a preliminary study of 71 YA with T1D transitioning from pediatric care to a YA T1D program in adult care demonstrated reduction in HbA1c levels, improved glucose monitoring, and program satisfaction.[63] Overall, the data demonstrate that implementing a structured transition program is overwhelmingly beneficial. More research needs to be done on the receivership side to understand the role of adult care in maintaining follow-up and mitigating long-term complications. In addition, more standardization of transition programs is needed to facilitate implementation and dissemination.

Telehealth interventions

Before the coronavirus disease 2019 (COVID-19) pandemic, telehealth and telemedicine accounted for less than 1% of health-care visits.[64] In early 2020, rapid regulatory changes necessitated by lockdowns and social distancing led to exponential growth in telehealth.[65,66] Studies conducted before and during the COVID-19 pandemic have found equivalent or superior influences on glycemia and high satisfaction levels among people with T1D receiving care via telehealth, including those from marginalized communities.[67–69] Among YA with T1D, telehealth has been used successfully for clinic visits, peer group sessions, group diabetes education, and self-management interventions, and may address known care gaps for this vulnerable group.

The CoYoT1 Clinic intervention for YA with T1D, which combines telehealth clinic visits and virtual peer groups, has shown the benefits of telehealth-delivered clinic visits and peer groups. Telehealth, as compared with in-person care clinic visits, increased visit frequency[70,71] and decreased physician-related distress.[71] In one study, these benefits were attributable to improvements among Latinx YA.[72] Telehealth visits also improved quality of life and were cost-neutral relative to in-person care.[73] Virtual peer group sessions for YA with T1D improved diabetes-related distress and problem-solving,[74] and the combined telehealth/virtual peer group intervention improved diabetes distress, self-efficacy, diabetes-related communication, and depressive symptoms.[75] A study of group telehealth transition education for YA with T1D confirmed the feasibility of such an approach.[76] Finally, a study evaluating a telehealth occupational therapy self-management intervention for YA with T1D demonstrated improvements in the performance of diabetes-related occupations (eg, meal preparation, checking glucose), with comparable engagement to in-person care.[77]

Best practices for successful implementation of telehealth care delivery models to improve outcomes for YA with T1D include flexibility in scheduling after hours and rescheduling to accommodate for frequent changes in work and school schedules; improving consistent communication with YA by leveraging technology to provide a means of contact other than phone calls to the clinic or portal messages; and ensuring that YA from socially and geographically marginalized communities are offered unique approaches with telehealth to minimize access issues that could exacerbate health inequities. Thus, when designed with YA needs and versatility in mind, telehealth can be an accessible, impactful, and transformative care model for YA with T1D. As coverage for telehealth changes since declaring the COVID-19 emergency, various influences on access to care, medical, and psychosocial outcomes should be studied, especially for YA who may be particularly vulnerable to such shifts in health care.

Psychosocial and Behavioral Care Interventions

Psychosocial care

Guidelines identify the need for psychosocial care throughout the life span of people with T1D.[78] Psychosocial care can vary in form and may include behavioral health consultation within a clinic setting, individual or family counseling, or therapy by a mental health professional, home-based intervention for individuals with higher social needs, or peer/social support groups.[79] Although such guidelines for psychosocial care across the life span are impactful, few psychosocial interventions are designed *specifically* for YA with T1D.[80] Interventions designed for this age group would ideally address key developmental issues such as assuming independent responsibility for diabetes care, promoting adaptive health behaviors, and reducing risky behaviors. Efforts have been made to identify the core outcomes that should be targeted by such interventions (eg, diabetes-related quality of life).[81] Existing interventions designed for YA include formal peer support groups[82] and informal online peer communities, both of which have led to adaptive outcomes.[83,84] A review reported that most intervention studies including YA-targeted education, self-management, transition, and general support.[85] Although no studies specifically targeted diabetes distress, participants often experienced a reduction in distress, likely due to social and emotional support. Further, one study found that YA perceptions about the consequences of diabetes and their control over it predicted various psychosocial outcomes 5 years later, but there was no association with glycemia.[86,87] This suggests that adequate psychosocial support targeting one's experience of having diabetes has the potential to improve psychosocial well-being regardless of glycemic outcomes. More psychosocial interventions are needed targeting YA. Fortunately, YA have reported interest, especially in programs emphasizing reeducation and incorporating technology.[88]

Online and mobile health interventions for peer support and diabetes self-management
Research suggests that youth and YA may benefit from online social interaction, especially when seeking to connect with others with similar developmental and/or health conditions.[89] YA often use social media to look up general health information, supplement clinical care, and obtain support from others.[89,90] Social media offers YA with T1D the opportunity to engage with and create content related to their diabetes-related experiences.[91] A qualitative study found that online activities of YA with diabetes were diverse and complex, including production and consumption of online content. This study also highlighted that social media engagement with diabetes-related resources and content varied based on YA engagement with sources of support offline.[92]

Mobile health (mHealth) interventions (eg, delivered by involving technology, including mHealth apps) have demonstrated promise in supporting diabetes self-management. In contrast to the research using mHealth apps for adolescents with T1D,[93] few studies have evaluated this approach with YA. In a cross-sectional survey assessing the use of mHealth tools to deliver self-management support to YA with T1D, engagement with mHealth apps was lower than expected, related to the lack of awareness of available apps, expectations that apps would not be helpful, and privacy concerns.[94] Participants showed strong interest in using text messaging for diabetes self-management support.[94] This study also noted that the access, frequent use of, and convenience of mobile devices in this population presents promise for using mHealth to provide information and support to YA with T1D.[94] Preliminary results from an ongoing study engaging YA users in developing an mHealth app to support diabetes self-management[95] indicated that YA had positive impressions of the app and described the intervention positively in terms of promoting self-management through peer support and sharing information with healthcare professionals.[96] Another ongoing randomized trial is currently testing an app that sends daily and weekly messages to YA about self-management goals and goal adherence, with the aim of improving glycemic outcomes.[97] Future research in this area will guide the direction of interventions to support YA using mobile and digital platforms.

Integrated Social and Medical Care Interventions
YA with T1D have a high degree of social needs and challenges influencing their care, predicting worse short-term and long-term glycemic and mental health outcomes.[37] These findings support the need to test more interventions that tailor care where SDOH and inequities in health care are targeted to reduce disease self-management challenges and improve outcomes.[59,98]

Agarwal and colleagues conducted semistructured individual interviews in a cohort of underserved YA with T1D to examine interactions with health-care providers.[49] Results revealed lack of shared decision-making and inadequate incorporation of preferences and biases of YA into conversations on treatment decisions. In addition, multistakeholder user-centered design workshops identified that key elements needed for deciding on T1D technology included social needs management and linkage, peer and family support, and visual and hands-on education.[48]

Several interventions are ongoing to address unmet social and health-care needs for YA with T1D to target root causes of inequity; however, more are needed. One study found that clinical practice transformations, such as social needs management, CGM device trials, and provider bias training resulted in a 4-fold increase in CGM prescriptions for YA with T1D, with no differences among Hispanic, NHB, and NHW YA.[99] Additionally, an ongoing randomized controlled trial is testing whether a T1D-specific community health worker model offering social needs screening and management, peer support, and navigation to T1D technology, will improve T1D technology uptake, HbA1c levels, and consistency of outpatient care utilization for minoritized YA with T1D.[100] More studies are urgently needed to understand whether co-management of social and health needs will improve outcomes effectively for minoritized YA with T1D.

SECTION THREE: SUMMARY AND FUTURE DIRECTIONS

YA with T1D require tailored interventions to meet their unique developmental, diabetes-related, and health-care transition needs. Furthermore, there is a critical need to accelerate the study of adaptable practices that specifically address diabetes self-management, care engagement, and psychosocial care in this vulnerable population, to optimize the dose of clinical intervention planned.

Future directions should include more focus and testing of YA-specific evidence-based care strategies that leverage the unique aspects and preferences of YA with T1D. Dissemination, implementation, and cost-effectiveness of care models need to be studied to successfully generalize and disseminate high-quality care approaches. Finally, medical education needs to be modified to teach health-care providers on care approaches that foster trust and rapport with YA, that demonstrates how trust influences outpatient follow-up, self-management, medical outcomes, and mental health for YA with T1D. Prioritizing intervention in young adulthood can significantly and positively alter the trajectory of adulthood, and reduce cost and mortality across the adult life span.

CLINICS CARE POINTS

- YA with T1D need tailored care approaches that incorporate the competing personal and social constraints of young adulthood. Emphasis on creating new habits to solidify diabetes self-management, HbA1c, and treatment of mental health conditions to prevent diabetes complications during this vulnerable period is recommended.

- For minoritized YA with T1D, unmet social needs must be addressed and incorporated into diabetes care plans, with referrals to appropriate community resources if available.

- Screening YA with T1D for diabetes distress, depression, anxiety, disordered eating, and other mental health conditions is integral to care. Planning for early intervention with referrals to a mental health provider trained in diabetes is also advised.

- Transition from pediatric to adult health care should be a planned organized process, which includes transition preparation, transfer completion, and long-term maintenance in adult care.

- Telehealth and mobile health strategies may be particularly effective in YA with T1D, offering new care access and peer support opportunities that are not otherwise possible for in-person care.

DISCLOSURE

M.E. Hilliard receives support from 1R01DK119246. S.Carreon. receives support from 3R01DK119246-03S1. S. Agarwal is a health disparities advisor to Medtronic, Inc. and Beta Bionics, and receives CGM devices for research from Dexcom Inc. S. Agarwal receives support from the NIDDK (1R01DK111022) and JDRF (4-SRA-2022-1187-M-B and 4-SRA-2021-1071-M-B). No other potential conflicts of interest relevant to this article were reported.

REFERENCES

1. Arnett J. Emerging Adulthood: The Winding Road from the Late Teens Through the Twenties (2nd edition)2019.
2. Arnett JJ. Emerging adulthood. A theory of development from the late teens through the twenties. Am Psychol 2000;55(5):469–80.
3. Bryden KS, Dunger DB, Mayou RA, et al. Poor prognosis of young adults with type 1 diabetes: a longitudinal study. Diabetes Care 2003;26(4):1052–7.
4. Foster NC, Beck RW, Miller KM, et al. State of Type 1 Diabetes Management and Outcomes from the T1D Exchange in 2016-2018. Diabetes Technol Therapeut 2019;21(2):66–72.
5. Dabelea D, Stafford JM, Mayer-Davis EJ, et al, SEARCH for Diabetes in Youth Research Group. Association of Type 1 Diabetes vs Type 2 Diabetes Diagnosed During Childhood and Adolescence With Complications During Teenage Years and Young Adulthood. JAMA 2017;317(8):825–35.
6. Lawrence JM, Reynolds K, Saydah SH, et al, SEARCH for Diabetes in Youth Study Group, SEARCH for Diabetes in Youth Study Group:. Demographic Correlates of Short-Term Mortality Among Youth and Young Adults With Youth-Onset Diabetes Diagnosed From 2002 to 2015: The SEARCH for Diabetes in Youth Study. Diabetes Care 2021;44(12):2691–8.
7. Rachas A, Lefeuvre D, Meyer L, et al. Evaluating Continuity During Transfer to Adult Care: A Systematic Review. Pediatrics 2016;138(1).
8. Buschur EO, Glick B, Kamboj MK. Transition of care for patients with type 1 diabetes mellitus from pediatric to adult health care systems. Transl Pediatr 2017; 6(4):373–82.
9. Ramchandani N, Way N, Melkus GD, et al. Challenges to Diabetes Self-Management in Emerging Adults With Type 1 Diabetes. Diabetes Educ 2019; 45(5):484–97.
10. Joiner KL, Holland ML, Grey M. Stressful Life Events in Young Adults With Type 1 Diabetes in the U.S. T1D Exchange Clinic Registry. J Nurs Scholarsh 2018; 50(6):676–86.
11. Griggs S, Redeker NS, Crawford SL, et al. Sleep, self-management, neurocognitive function, and glycemia in emerging adults with Type 1 diabetes mellitus: A research protocol. Res Nurs Health 2020;43(4):317–28.
12. Griggs S, Whittemore R, Redeker NS, et al. Facilitators and Barriers of Sleep in Young Adults With Type 1 Diabetes. Diabetes Educ 2020;46(3):242–51.
13. Baker AC, Wiebe DJ, Kelly CS, et al. Structural model of patient-centered communication and diabetes management in early emerging adults at the transfer to adult care. J Behav Med 2019;42(5):831–41.
14. Helgeson VS, Vaughn AK, Seltman H, et al. Relation of parent knowledge to glycemic control among emerging adults with type 1 diabetes: a mediational model. J Behav Med 2018;41(2):186–94.

15. Kelly CS, Berg CA, Lansing AH, et al. Keeping parents connected in early emerging adulthood: Diabetes-related disclosure and solicitation. J Fam Psychol 2019;33(7):809–18.
16. Simms M, Baumann K, Monaghan M. Health Communication Experiences of Emerging Adults with Type 1 Diabetes. Clin Pract Pediatr Psychol 2017;5(4):415–25.
17. Luyckx K, Moons P, Weets I. Self-classification as an adult in patients with type 1 diabetes: relationships with glycemic control and illness coping. Patient Educ Couns 2011;85(2):245–50.
18. Raymaekers K, Helgeson VS, Prikken S, et al. Diabetes-specific friend support in emerging adults with type 1 diabetes: Does satisfaction with support matter? J Behav Med 2021;44(3):402–11.
19. Saylor J, Lee S, Ness M, et al. Positive Health Benefits of Peer Support and Connections for College Students With Type 1 Diabetes Mellitus. Diabetes Educ 2018;44(4):340–7.
20. Jeremy B, Yorgason JS, Ness Michelle, et al. Emerging ideas. health technology use and perceptions of romantic relationships by emerging adults with type 1 diabetes. Fam Relat 2021;70(2).
21. Solmi M, Radua J, Olivola M, et al. Age at onset of mental disorders worldwide: large-scale meta-analysis of 192 epidemiological studies. Mol Psychiatry 2022;27(1):281–95.
22. Kessler RC, Berglund P, Demler O, et al. Lifetime prevalence and age-of-onset distributions of DSM-IV disorders in the National Comorbidity Survey Replication. Arch Gen Psychiatr 2005;62(6):593–602.
23. Ducat L, Rubenstein A, Philipson LH, et al. A review of the mental health issues of diabetes conference. Diabetes Care 2015;38(2):333–8.
24. Balfe M, Doyle F, Smith D, et al. What's distressing about having type 1 diabetes? A qualitative study of young adults' perspectives. BMC Endocr Disord 2013;13:25.
25. Hillege S, Beale B, McMaster R. Enhancing management of depression and type 1 diabetes in adolescents and young adults. Arch Psychiatr Nurs 2011;25(6):e57–67.
26. Gutierrez-Colina AM, Corathers S, Beal S, et al. Young Adults With Type 1 Diabetes Preparing to Transition to Adult Care: Psychosocial Functioning and Associations With Self-Management and Health Outcomes. Diabetes Spectr 2020;33(3):255–63.
27. Bächle C, Lange K, Stahl-Pehe A, et al. Associations between HbA1c and depressive symptoms in young adults with early-onset type 1 diabetes. Psychoneuroendocrinology 2015;55:48–58.
28. Galler A, Tittel SR, Baumeister H, et al. Worse glycemic control, higher rates of diabetic ketoacidosis, and more hospitalizations in children, adolescents, and young adults with type 1 diabetes and anxiety disorders. Pediatr Diabetes 2021;22(3):519–28.
29. Rechenberg K, Whittemore R, Grey M. Anxiety in Youth With Type 1 Diabetes. J Pediatr Nurs 2017;32:64–71.
30. Hanlan ME, Griffith J, Patel N, et al. Eating disorders and disordered eating in type 1 diabetes: prevalence, screening, and treatment options. Curr Diabetes Rep 2013;13:909–16.
31. Jones JM, Lawson ML, Daneman D, et al. Eating disorders in adolescent females with and without type 1 diabetes: cross sectional study. BMJ 2000;320(7249):1563–6.

32. Pinhas-Hamiel O, Hamiel U, Levy-Shraga Y. Eating disorders in adolescents with type 1 diabetes: Challenges in diagnosis and treatment. World J Diabetes 2015;6(3):517–26.

33. Vallis M, Willaing I, Holt RIG. Emerging adulthood and Type 1 diabetes: insights from the DAWN2 Study. Diabet Med 2018;35(2):203–13.

34. Sattoe J, Peeters M, Bronner M, et al. Transfer in care and diabetes distress in young adults with type 1 diabetes mellitus. BMJ Open Diabetes Res Care 2021;9(2).

35. Hislop AL, Fegan PG, Schlaeppi MJ, et al. Prevalence and associations of psychological distress in young adults with Type 1 diabetes. Diabet Med 2008; 25(1):91–6.

36. Hagger V, Hendrieckx C, Cameron F, et al. Diabetes distress is more strongly associated with HbA1c than depressive symptoms in adolescents with type 1 diabetes: Results from Diabetes MILES Youth-Australia. Pediatr Diabetes 2018;19(4):840–7.

37. Agarwal S, Hilliard M, Butler A. Disparities in Care Delivery and Outcomes in Young Adults With Diabetes. Curr Diabetes Rep 2018;18(9):65.

38. Agarwal S, Kanapka LG, Raymond JK, et al. Racial-Ethnic Inequity in Young Adults With Type 1 Diabetes. J Clin Endocrinol Metab 2020;105(8):e2960–9.

39. Clements MA, Foster NC, Maahs DM, et al, T1D Exchange Clinic Network. Hemoglobin A1c (HbA1c) changes over time among adolescent and young adult participants in the T1D exchange clinic registry. Pediatr Diabetes 2016;17(5): 327–36.

40. Clements MA, Schwandt A, Donaghue KC, et al, Australasian Diabetes Data Network ADDN Study Group, the T1D Exchange Clinic Network T1DX, and the German/Austrian/Luxembourgian Diabetes-Patienten-Verlaufsdokumentation DPV initiative. Five heterogeneous HbA1c trajectories from childhood to adulthood in youth with type 1 diabetes from three different continents: A group-based modeling approach. Pediatr Diabetes 2019;20(7):920–31.

41. Kahkoska AR, Shay CM, Crandell J, et al. Association of Race and Ethnicity With Glycemic Control and Hemoglobin A(1c) Levels in Youth With Type 1 Diabetes. JAMA Netw Open 2018;1(5).

42. Mayer-Davis EJ, Lawrence JM, Dabelea D, et al, SEARCH for Diabetes in Youth Study. Incidence Trends of Type 1 and Type 2 Diabetes among Youths, 2002-2012. N Engl J Med 2017;376(15):1419–29.

43. Majidi S, Ebekozien O, Noor N, et al, T1D Exchange Quality Improvement Collaborative Study Group. Inequities in Health Outcomes in Children and Adults With Type 1 Diabetes: Data From the T1D Exchange Quality Improvement Collaborative. Clin Diabetes 2021;39(3):278–83.

44. Naughton MJ, Ruggiero AM, Lawrence JM, et al, SEARCH for Diabetes in Youth Study Group. Health-related quality of life of children and adolescents with type 1 or type 2 diabetes mellitus: SEARCH for Diabetes in Youth Study. Arch Pediatr Adolesc Med 2008;162(7):649–57.

45. Odugbesan O, Addala A, Nelson G, et al. Implicit Racial-Ethnic and Insurance-Mediated Bias to Recommending Diabetes Technology: Insights from T1D Exchange Multicenter Pediatric and Adult Diabetes Provider Cohort. Diabetes Technol Therapeut 2022;24(9):619–27.

46. Ebekozien O, Agarwal S, Noor N, et al. Inequities in Diabetic Ketoacidosis Among Patients With Type 1 Diabetes and COVID-19: Data From 52 US Clinical Centers. J Clin Endocrinol Metab 2021;106(4):e1755–62.

47. McKergow E, Parkin L, Barson DJ, et al. Demographic and regional disparities in insulin pump utilization in a setting of universal funding: a New Zealand nationwide study. Acta Diabetol 2017;54(1):63–71.

48. Agarwal S, Crespo-Ramos G, Leung SL, et al. Solutions to Address Inequity in Diabetes Technology Use in Type 1 Diabetes: Results from Multidisciplinary Stakeholder Co-creation Workshops. Diabetes Technol Therapeut 2022;24(6): 381–9.

49. Agarwal S, Crespo-Ramos G, Long JA, et al. "I Didn't Really Have a Choice": Qualitative Analysis of Racial-Ethnic Disparities in Diabetes Technology Use Among Young Adults with Type 1 Diabetes. Diabetes Technol Therapeut 2021;23(9):616–22.

50. Lawton J, Kimbell B, Rankin D, et al, CLOuD Consortium. Health professionals' views about who would benefit from using a closed-loop system: a qualitative study. Diabet Med 2020;37(6):1030–7.

51. Pinhas-Hamiel O, Hamiel U, Boyko V, et al. Trajectories of HbA1c levels in children and youth with type 1 diabetes. PLoS One 2014;9(10):e109109.

52. Nip ASY, Lodish M. Trend of Diabetes-Related Hospital Admissions During the Transition Period From Adolescence to Adulthood in the State of California. Diabetes Care 2021;44(12):2723–8.

53. Lyons SK, Libman IM, Sperling MA. Clinical review: Diabetes in the adolescent: transitional issues. J Clin Endocrinol Metab 2013;98(12):4639–45.

54. Morrissey EC, Dinneen SF, Lowry M, et al. Reimagining care for young adults living with type 1 diabetes. J Diabetes Investig 2022;13(8):1294–9.

55. Tilden DR, French B, Shoemaker AH, et al. Prolonged lapses between pediatric and adult care are associated with rise in HbA1c and inpatient days among patients with type 1 diabetes. Diabetes Res Clin Pract 2022;192:110113.

56. Peters A, Laffel L, American Diabetes Association Transitions Working Group. Diabetes care for emerging adults: recommendations for transition from pediatric to adult diabetes care systems: a position statement of the American Diabetes Association, with representation by the American College of Osteopathic Family Physicians, the American Academy of Pediatrics, the American Association of Clinical Endocrinologists, the American Osteopathic Association, the Centers for Disease Control and Prevention, Children with Diabetes, The Endocrine Society, the International Society for Pediatric and Adolescent Diabetes, Juvenile Diabetes Research Foundation International, the National Diabetes Education Program, and the Pediatric Endocrine Society (formerly Lawson Wilkins Pediatric Endocrine Society). Diabetes Care 2011;34(11): 2477–85.

57. Farrell K, Fernandez R, Salamonson Y, et al. Health outcomes for youth with type 1 diabetes at 18 months and 30 months post transition from pediatric to adult care. Diabetes Res Clin Pract 2018;139:163–9.

58. Holmes-Walker DJ, Llewellyn AC, Farrell K. A transition care programme which improves diabetes control and reduces hospital admission rates in young adults with Type 1 diabetes aged 15-25 years. Diabet Med 2007;24(7):764–9.

59. O'Hara MC, Hynes L, O'Donnell M, et al, Irish Type 1 Diabetes Young Adult Study Group. A systematic review of interventions to improve outcomes for young adults with Type 1 diabetes. Diabet Med 2017;34(6):753–69.

60. Spaic T, Robinson T, Goldbloom E, et al, JDRF Canadian Clinical Trial CCTN1102 Study Group. Closing the Gap: Results of the Multicenter Canadian Randomized Controlled Trial of Structured Transition in Young Adults With Type 1 Diabetes. Diabetes Care 2019;42(6):1018–26.

61. Sparud-Lundin C, Ohrn I, Danielson E, et al. Glycaemic control and diabetes care utilization in young adults with Type 1 diabetes. Diabet Med 2008;25(8): 968–73.

62. Sequeira PA, Pyatak EA, Weigensberg MJ, et al. Let's Empower and Prepare (LEAP): Evaluation of a Structured Transition Program for Young Adults With Type 1 Diabetes. Diabetes Care 2015;38(8):1412–9.

63. Agarwal S, Raymond JK, Schutta MH, et al. An Adult Health Care-Based Pediatric to Adult Transition Program for Emerging Adults With Type 1 Diabetes. Diabetes Educ 2017;43(1):87–96.

64. Shaver J. The State of Telehealth Before and After the COVID-19 Pandemic. Prim Care 2022;49(4):517–30.

65. Patel SY, Mehrotra A, Huskamp HA, et al. Variation In Telemedicine Use And Outpatient Care During The COVID-19 Pandemic In The United States. Health Aff 2021;40(2):349–58.

66. Bestsennyy OGG, Harris A, Rost J. Telehealth: a quarter trillion-dollar post-COVID-19 reality? McKinsey & Company; 2021. Available at: https://connectwithcare.org/wp-content/uploads/2021/07/telehealth-a-quarter-trillion-dollar-post-covid-19-reality.pdf.

67. Crossen SS, Wagner DV. Narrowing the Divide: The Role of Telehealth in Type 1 Diabetes Care for Marginalized Communities. J Diabetes Sci Technol 2023; 17(4):901–8.

68. Eiland LA, Drincic A. Rural Telehealth Visits in the Management of Type 1 Diabetes. J Diabetes Sci Technol 2022;16(4):852–7.

69. Kompala T, Neinstein AB. Telehealth in type 1 diabetes. Curr Opin Endocrinol Diabetes Obes 2021;28(1):21–9.

70. Reid MW, Krishnan S, Berget C, et al. CoYoT1 Clinic: Home Telemedicine Increases Young Adult Engagement in Diabetes Care. Diabetes Technol Therapeut 2018;20(5):370–9.

71. Garcia JF, Faye E, Reid MW, et al. Greater Telehealth Use Results in Increased Visit Frequency and Lower Physician Related-Distress in Adolescents and Young Adults With Type 1 Diabetes. J Diabetes Sci Technol 2023;17(4):878–86.

72. Garcia JJRM, Pyatak E, Fogel JL, et al. 1021-P: Telehealth Benefits among Latinx Adolescents and Young Adults (AYA) with Type 1 Diabetes (T1D). Diabetes 2022;71(Supplement_1):2022.

73. Wan W, Nathan AG, Skandari MR, et al. Cost-effectiveness of Shared Telemedicine Appointments in Young Adults With T1D: CoYoT1 Trial. Diabetes Care 2019;42(8):1589–92.

74. Bisno DI, Reid MW, Fogel JL, et al. Virtual Group Appointments Reduce Distress and Improve Care Management in Young Adults with Type 1 Diabetes. J Diabetes Sci Technol 2022;16(6):1419–27.

75. Bakhach M, Reid MW, Pyatak EA, et al. Home Telemedicine (CoYoT1 Clinic): A Novel Approach to Improve Psychosocial Outcomes in Young Adults With Diabetes. Diabetes Educ 2019;45(4):420–30.

76. Albanese-O'Neill A, Beauchamp G, Thomas N, et al. Transition Education for Young Adults With Type 1 Diabetes: Pilot Feasibility Study for a Group Telehealth Intervention. JMIR Diabetes 2018;3(4):e10909.

77. Mitchell S, Sideris J, Blanchard J, et al. Telehealth Lifestyle Redesign Occupational Therapy for Diabetes: Preliminary Effectiveness, Satisfaction, and Engagement. OTJR (Thorofare N J). 2023;43(3):426–34.

78. Young-Hyman D, de Groot M, Hill-Briggs F, et al. Psychosocial Care for People With Diabetes: A Position Statement of the American Diabetes Association. Diabetes Care 2016;39(12):2126–40.

79. de Wit M, Gajewska KA, Goethals ER, et al. ISPAD Clinical Practice Consensus Guidelines 2022: Psychological care of children, adolescents and young adults with diabetes. Pediatr Diabetes 2022;23(8):1373–89.

80. Monaghan M, Helgeson V, Wiebe D. Type 1 diabetes in young adulthood. Curr Diabetes Rev 2015;11(4):239–50.

81. Byrne M, O'Connell A, Egan AM, et al. A core outcomes set for clinical trials of interventions for young adults with type 1 diabetes: an international, multi-perspective Delphi consensus study. Trials 2017;18(1):602.

82. Markowitz JT, Laffel LM. Transitions in care: support group for young adults with Type 1 diabetes. Diabet Med 2012;29(4):522–5.

83. Rasmussen B, Ward G, Jenkins A, et al. Young adults' management of Type 1 diabetes during life transitions. J Clin Nurs 2011;20(13–14):1981–92.

84. Sparud-Lundin C, Ohrn I, Danielson E. Redefining relationships and identity in young adults with type 1 diabetes. J Adv Nurs 2010;66(1):128–38.

85. Wentzell K, Vessey JA, Laffel LMB. How Do the Challenges of Emerging Adulthood Inform our Understanding of Diabetes Distress? An Integrative Review. Curr Diabetes Rep 2020;20(6):21.

86. Rassart J, Luyckx K, Berg CA, et al. Psychosocial functioning and glycemic control in emerging adults with Type 1 diabetes: A 5-year follow-up study. Health Psychol 2015;34(11):1058–65.

87. Rassart J, Luyckx K, Oris L, et al. Coping with type 1 diabetes through emerging adulthood: Longitudinal associations with perceived control and haemoglobin A1c. Psychol Health 2016;31(5):622–35.

88. Wiley J, Westbrook M, Long J, et al. Diabetes education: the experiences of young adults with type 1 diabetes. Diabetes Ther 2014;5(1):299–321.

89. Psihogios AM, Ahmed AM, McKelvey ER, et al. Social media to promote treatment adherence among adolescents and young adults with chronic health conditions: A topical review and TikTok application. Clin Pract Pediatr Psychol 2022; 10(4):440–51.

90. Litchman ML, Walker HR, Ng AH, et al. State of the Science: A Scoping Review and Gap Analysis of Diabetes Online Communities. J Diabetes Sci Technol 2019;13(3):466–92.

91. Hilliard ME, Sparling KM, Hitchcock J, et al. The emerging diabetes online community. Curr Diabetes Rev 2015;11(4):261–72.

92. Fergie G, Hunt K, Hilton S. Social media as a space for support: Young adults' perspectives on producing and consuming user-generated content about diabetes and mental health. Soc Sci Med 2016;170:46–54.

93. Holtz BE, Murray KM, Hershey DD, et al. Developing a Patient-Centered mHealth App: A Tool for Adolescents With Type 1 Diabetes and Their Parents. JMIR Mhealth Uhealth 2017;5(4):e53.

94. Dobson R, Whittaker R, Murphy R, et al. The Use of Mobile Health to Deliver Self-Management Support to Young People With Type 1 Diabetes: A Cross-Sectional Survey. JMIR Diabetes 2017;2(1):e4.

95. Castensøe-Seidenfaden P, Reventlov Husted G, Teilmann G, et al. Designing a Self-Management App for Young People With Type 1 Diabetes: Methodological Challenges, Experiences, and Recommendations. JMIR Mhealth Uhealth 2017; 5(10):e124.

96. Husted GR, Weis J, Teilmann G, et al. Exploring the Influence of a Smartphone App (Young with Diabetes) on Young People's Self-Management: Qualitative Study. JMIR Mhealth Uhealth 2018;6(2):e43.

97. Stanger C, Kowatsch T, Xie H, et al. A Digital Health Intervention (SweetGoals) for Young Adults With Type 1 Diabetes: Protocol for a Factorial Randomized Trial. JMIR Res Protoc 2021;10(2):e27109.

98. Redondo MJ, Libman I, Cheng P, et al, Pediatric Diabetes Consortium. Racial/ethnic minority youth with recent-onset type 1 diabetes have poor prognostic factors. Diabetes Care 2018;41(5):1017–24.

99. Mathias P, Mahali LP, Agarwal S. Targeting technology in underserved adults with type 1 diabetes: effect of diabetes practice transformations on improving equity in CGM prescribing behaviors. Diabetes Care 2022;45(10):2231–7.

100. Agarwal S. T1DTechCHW: enhancing the community health worker model to promote diabetes technology use in young adults from underrepresented minority groups (T1DTechCHW). ClinicalTrials.gov Identifier; 2022.

Incorporating the Six Core Elements of Health Care Transition in Type 1 Diabetes Care for Emerging Adults

Faisal S. Malik, MD, MSHS[a,b,]*, Kathryn W. Weaver, MD[c],
Sarah D. Corathers, MD[d], Patience H. White, MD, MA[e]

KEYWORDS

- Type 1 diabetes • Adolescents • Young adults • Health care transition

KEY POINTS

- Implementation of a structured transition process can support improved patient health and societal outcomes for emerging adults with type 1 diabetes.
- Pediatric diabetes providers play a critical role in supporting health care transition planning and successful transfer to adult diabetes care.
- Effective transition to adult care requires active involvement from adult diabetes providers to plan for incorporation of emerging adults into their practice.

INTRODUCTION

Health care transition (HCT) is the purposeful, planned movement of adolescents and young adults with and without chronic physical, behavioral, and developmental conditions from child-centered to adult-oriented health care systems.[1] HCT not only represents the passage from one developmental stage to another (dependence to independence to interdependence) but also represents the transition from family-centered pediatric care to patient-centered adult care. Youth with type 1 diabetes (T1D) typically require an expanded process of transition planning and integration

---

[a] Department of Pediatrics, University of Washington School of Medicine, Seattle, WA, USA; [b] Development, Seattle Children's Research Institute, Center for Child Health, Behavior, 1920 Terry Avenue, CURE-3, Seattle, WA 98101, USA; [c] Department of Medicine, University of Washington School of Medicine, 325 Ninth Avenue, Seattle, WA 98104, USA; [d] Cincinnati Children's Hospital Department of Pediatrics, University of Cincinnati College of Medicine, 3333 Burnet Avenue, MLC 7012, Cincinnati, OH 45229, USA; [e] Department of Medicine and Pediatrics, George Washington University School of Medicine, 5335 Wisconsin Avenue NW, Suite 440, Washington, DC 20015, USA
* Corresponding author. 1920 Terry Avenue, CURE-3, Seattle, WA 98101.
E-mail address: faisal.malik@seattlechildrens.org

Endocrinol Metab Clin N Am 53 (2024) 53–65
https://doi.org/10.1016/j.ecl.2023.09.003
0889-8529/24/© 2023 Elsevier Inc. All rights reserved.

into adult health care to address the exchange of more complex health information, competencies around diabetes self-management, and often the change to a different health care setting.[2]

Clinical guidelines and the research literature recognize the significance of a structured transition process for emerging adults with T1D.[2,3] Yet, a growing body of literature finds persistent problems in the provision of recommended HCT services, as well as adverse outcomes associated with the lack of these services.[3] The most recent National Survey of Children's Health asking parents if their 12 to 17-year-olds received transition preparation showed that only 23% of youth with special health care needs (eg, T1D) reported receiving HCT preparation.[4]

Systematic reviews demonstrate that a structured transition process can improve the public health quadruple aim outcomes including (1) higher emerging adult and caregiver satisfaction, (2) improved overall health outcomes such as better treatment regimen adherence, (3) improved health care utilization, including reduced time between the last pediatric visit and the first adult visit and lower rates of hospitalization, and (4) positive clinician experience.[5] Diabetes transition programs that offer a structured transition process for emerging adults have demonstrated improved health outcomes such as decreased HbA_{1c}, as well as improved health care utilization including increased ambulatory diabetes clinic attendance and reduced hospitalizations for diabetic ketoacidosis.[6,7] Taking a structured approach to planning for HCT, creating a smooth handoff during transfer, and introducing the emerging adult to adult practice is central to helping adolescents and young adults with T1D learn diabetes self-management and advocacy skills.

The American Academy of Pediatrics, the American Academy of Family Physicians, and the American College of Physicians joined together and published the 2018 Clinical Report[3] that presented guiding principles around HCT. The Clinical Report outlines a structured process called the Six Core Elements of HCT, tested in several learning collaboratives using quality improvement methodologies.[8] This article reviews the Six Core Elements of HCT and outlines practical approaches on how the Six Core Elements can be incorporated into ambulatory diabetes care to support successful HCT of emerging adults with T1D.

DISCUSSION
Six Core Elements of Health Care Transition

The Six Core Elements is not a model of care but rather a pathway or approach that can be customized to improve the structured approach to HCT in many different types of primary or specialty care practices and should be customized to the complexity of emerging adults involved and practice resources. The Six Core Elements has been adapted for use in various models of care and practice settings, such as HCT clinics, HCT consult services, and school-based health and mental health clinics. They have also been used for a broad population of youth and young adults with and without special health care needs, including those with medically complex conditions, intellectual and developmental disability, and mental health conditions.[9–15]

The Six Core Elements were developed with extensive input from emerging adults, families, and clinicians including physicians, nurses, social workers, and clinic staff who are experts in HCT. The Six Core Elements for a pediatric diabetes practice include: (1) *transition and care policy/guide* for emerging adults and families that describes the HCT process and what to expect; (2) *tracking and monitoring* to be sure the emerging adult is receiving the HCT services in the Six Core Elements; (3) *transition readiness assessment* repeated throughout the HCT process to learn what skills the emerging adult with T1D needs to address to better prepare them for managing their own health; (4) *transition planning* with a plan of care that summarizes their medical care and details the needed steps to attain the goals that the emerging adults identifies; (5) *transfer of care* activities include a transfer package, with a transfer letter including the adherence history of coming to clinic to give the adult provider an idea of the likelihood the emerging adult will come to the first adult appointment, the final transition readiness assessment, plan of care, medical summary and emergency care plan, and, if needed, legal documents and other clinical records that will be shared with the new adult clinician; and (6) *transfer completion* that includes the confirmation of attendance at the initial adult visit, as well as feedback to the pediatric practice by the emerging adult and family about the HCT process and if they felt prepared to transition to adult care. Recognizing the importance of adult providers in the HCT process, the Six Core Elements also are available for adult clinicians who are integrating emerging adults with diabetes into their practice. In addition to the transition and care policy/guide and tracking and monitoring core elements, the remaining 4 core elements for adult diabetes practice focus on orientation and integration into adult practice, as well as supporting successful initial adult practice visits and ongoing care for emerging adults. **Fig. 1** outlines the delineation of health care transition activities and tools for both pediatric and adult practices.

Currently, there are 3 Six Core Element packages[16] available with tools and implementation guides[17] for (1) pediatric practices where the youth is moving to an adult health care clinician, (2) family medicine and med-peds practices that will care for the youth through the life span, and (3) internal medicine/family medicine/med-peds clinicians to assist in integrating the emerging adult into their adult medical practice. Each package outlines in 6 steps what clinicians can do to create a structured approach, with sample tools in English and Spanish that can be customized.

Incorporating the Six Core Elements in Pediatric Diabetes Care

A key to implementing a structured HCT approach is developing an invested team motivated to implement a framework to support HCT. Using quality improvement and implementation science methodology is a proven strategy to iteratively design reliable and sustainable processes in a clinic or system to improve process outcomes.[10] It is essential that emerging adults with T1D and families are equal partners[18] on the team throughout the process, along with both pediatric and adult clinicians and staff, as well as information technology experts.

Transition care and policy for a pediatric practice

The first step in creating a structured HCT process is to develop a transition care and policy that formalizes your diabetes practice's approach to HCT. Key considerations include specific content to incorporate in the policy (eg, at what age will your practice start the HCT planning process, when are youth expected to leave practice), as well as the process to develop and implement the policy (eg, whose job will it be to share and discuss the HCT policy with the youth and caregiver, how will you inform all staff about the practice's approach to HCT). In the HCT policy, the changes in privacy and consent that happen at age 18 should be emphasized. Ideally, it should align with your own institutional approach, so that there is consistency of policy across sites of care within an organization.

It is best practice to ensure that the policy is at an appropriate reading level, offered in languages common among your clinic population, and is concise. The involvement of key stakeholders in the development of a transition and care policy/guide is critical. It is now increasingly expected that individuals or groups involved in or affected by

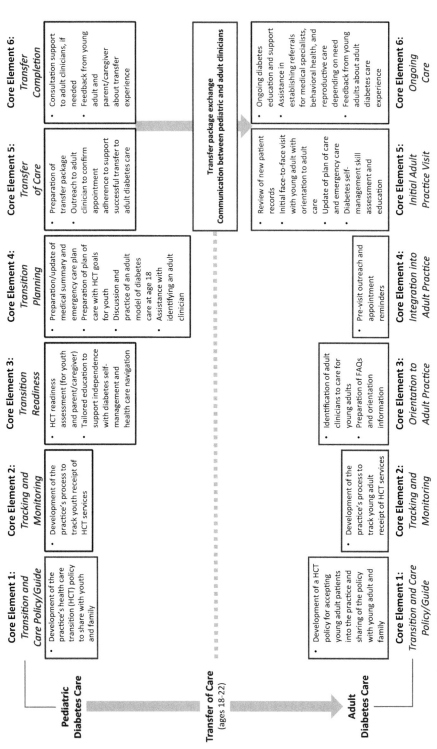

Fig. 1. Six Core Elements of health care transition for pediatric and adult diabetes practices. (*The Six Core Elements of Health Care Transition™ are the copyright of Got Transition®. This version of the Six Core Elements has been modified and is used with permission.*)

health-related and health care-related decisions, programs, or policies should have a say in the planning, conduct, dissemination, uptake, and evaluation of health care policy.[19] The development of a policy also provides an opportunity to align practices across both pediatric and adult institutions if there is a planned change in clinicians. For example, the joint University of Washington Medicine Diabetes Institute and Seattle Children's Hospital HCT policy for emerging adults with diabetes was developed with input from emerging adults with diabetes, caregivers of emerging adults, pediatric and adult diabetes providers nurses, social workers, psychologists, adolescent medicine physicians, and diabetes advocacy group representatives. Stakeholder involvement can help to ensure a guideline's acceptability and feasibility to the end users.[19]

Tracking and monitoring emerging adults with diabetes in pediatric care

Documenting progress in the process of HCT is essential for identifying emerging adults in need of HCT interventions. Tracking may begin as a manually updated list on a routine basis. However, as processes and programs grow, there are significant advantages to using discrete data fields within the electronic medical record. Standard and shared documentation fields for an interdisciplinary team facilitate longitudinal, asynchronous, transition planning that can be seen by members of the care team. Routinely documenting in a standardized format enables clinics to generate reports in preparation for upcoming visits (previsit planning), track clinic attendance, monitor progress on transition preparation pathway, and identify time between visits to mitigate loss to follow-up. Some data elements that are useful include the following: (1) dates of transition readiness assessments, (2) transition plan discussion, (3) name of adult provider(s) when identified, and (4) anticipated dates of adult care visits. Ideally, transition tracking includes or easily references documentation to education and self-management skills relevant to transition planning so that team members can easily see what has previously been done and update information as indicated.

In addition to facilitating clinical care, tracking discrete data elements enables improvement initiatives that rely on the ability to measure a metric over time to define specific goals. For example, the Cincinnati Children's Transition Quality Improvement Program set goals based on proximity to transfer to increase the proportion of emerging adults with diabetes aged 19 years or older with a documented transition of care plan by 40% from baseline each year over 2 years and to increase the proportion of emerging adults aged 15 to 18 years with a transition of care plan in place by 20% per year during a 5-year period.

Transition readiness assessment

Skill development is essential for successful HCT and includes, "cognitive and social skills to communicate and articulate health needs and preferences."[20] General transition readiness assessment tools, including the Transition Readiness Assessment Questionnaire (TRAQ),[21] have been validated and used clinically with heterogeneous samples of emerging adults with chronic health conditions, including T1D.[22] The TRAQ assesses 5 domains: managing medications, appointment keeping, tracking health issues, talking with providers, and managing daily activities. It includes 20 items, which patients answer on a Likert scale: 1 = "No, I do not know how"; 2 = "No, but I want to learn"; 3 = "No, but I am learning to do this"; 4 = "Yes, I have started doing this"; and 5 = "Yes, I always do this when I need to." Another general transition planning questionnaires that has undergone pilot feasibility testing for integration into the organizational electronic health record is the UNC TRxANSITION tool.[23] In Canada, clinicians who developed the diabetes-specific "On TRAck" transition readiness scale are beginning to assess its reliability and validity compared with TRANSITION-Q, a generic transition readiness questionnaire.[24]

Although general transition tools may be useful, particularly when applied at an organizational level across multiple conditions, specific self-management and skill acquisition for a particular type of chronic condition may not be captured in a general assessment tool.[25,26] There is growing consensus that condition-specific transition readiness assessments that address the medical, psychological, and cognitive needs of unique populations are useful.[25,26] A transition preparation tool with the purpose to assess readiness for independent self-management as a precursor to establishing readiness for transfer from pediatric to adult health care includes emerging adults self-report and parent proxy questionnaires assessing readiness for independent diabetes self-management (20-item RISQ-T and 15-item RISQ-P).[27] Furthermore, the evaluation of additional psychosocial domains, such as screening for diabetes distress or depression symptoms, risk behaviors, self-efficacy, barriers to diabetes self-management, and areas of diabetes strengths and resilience could be an important element of transition preparation.[2,28]

The Readiness for Emerging Adults with Diabetes Diagnosed in Youth (READDY) was developed[29] to assess self-reported confidence levels on diabetes-specific health knowledge and skills in 4 topic areas (Diabetes Knowledge, Health System Navigation, Insulin Self-Management, and Health Behaviors). In this framework, higher confidence in one's ability to perform health-related skills indicates a higher level of readiness for transition. A Likert reporting scale enables clinicians to identify priority topics for educational interventions and follow changes in responses over time. READDY is now in use in more than 30 diabetes centers and is available in 4 languages. The authors maintain a creative commons license and share the tool freely but ask centers who are interested in using READDY for clinical care to sign an agreement allowing the authors to track its use. An innovative aspect of the READDY tool is the model for care delivery that integrates a transition readiness assessment with opportunities for ongoing longitudinal interventions based on patient-directed responses. Specifically, READDY answer responses include both a present and future intention (ie, "I plan to start") that provides insights into topics patients want to explore. There is not a total score but rather a score for each domain so practices can identify priority topics for intervention and pace transition preparation over time.

Several factors can influence selection of the most appropriate tool for the assessment of transition preparation. Similar to other patient-reported outcomes administered in clinical care settings, the measure should be relevant to patient experience with response options that guide meaningful interactions and identify symptoms or topics for real-time intervention without undue burden to complete.[30] Practical implementation considerations include number of items, ease of completion, parent versus self-report, and availability (permission and potential cost of proprietary measures). Additional considerations could include the use of the same measure either across an organization or across other diabetes clinics to allow for future cross comparison at a population level.[31]

Transition planning
Survey of pediatric groups show there is a wide variation in the information sent to receiving providers.[32] Ideally, Got Transition recommends that a transfer summary from the pediatric office communicate transition readiness, a medical summary, emergency care plan, and HCT goals. There are also advocacy tools to guide patients and families to create succinct medical history documents in preparation for transition to adult care. The transfer summary document should include information about duration

of diabetes, current treatment regimen (eg, diabetes technology use, insulin doses), additional conditions and medications, recent screening and prevention results (eg, last eye examination), known complications related to diabetes, challenges in diabetes management, primary language and preferred communication methods, social history including living situation, guardianship status if relevant, school or employment, and support system.[33] An example of a clinical summary form is available from the Endocrine Society, which also includes a useful delineation for both the pediatric clinician and patient/family to sign to endorse a jointly produced summary.

Transfer of care to adult diabetes provider and transfer completion

It is best practice for pediatric providers to confirm with the adult practice that the transfer has been completed. Interruptions in care should be avoided with the goal of maintaining the same frequency of visits that the patient was receiving in pediatric care. Implementation of a formal transition coordinator to track clinic patients to prevent lost to follow up should be considered because this intervention has consistently been shown to improve follow-up.[34,35] Furthermore, to improve the practice's HCT approach, feedback should be elicited from all stakeholders involved in the HCT process.

Incorporating the Six Core Elements in Adult Diabetes Care

There are differences between pediatric and adult diabetes care models that influence all parties involved in HCT. Once readiness to transition has been established, several critical elements should be met by the adult care team to ensure the transfer of care to an adult care model is successful.

Transition care and policy for an adult practice

Adult providers report that emerging adults are not well prepared to transition to adult diabetes care.[36] Similar to pediatric clinics, adult practices accepting young adult patients with diabetes into their practice should draft a transition policy that describes the practice's approach to transition in order to alleviate confusion and frustration about the HCT process. This is a patient-facing document and is meant to describe the practice's approach to care.

Many of the aspects will be similar to the transition policy described above for pediatric practices. The adult policy should emphasize the development of a plan for emergency medical care. After transitioning to an adult care model, this aspect of care can be especially confusing for emerging adults with diabetes and may lead to delays in life-saving care in the event of diabetic ketoacidosis. Additionally, there should be a description of anticipated changes in health insurance coverage that will inevitably happen for most young adults and how the practice plans to support young adults through that change. Finally, the transition policy should outline the best method of contacting the clinic and how to access the patient portal. These 3 described elements represent common issues that often complicate the care of emerging adults with diabetes immediately after transition to an adult care model.

Tracking and monitoring emerging adults with diabetes in adult care

As discussed previously, the receipt of HCT-related care should be tracked and recorded. When possible, this is most effective when integrated into the electronic medical record in a standard format, which will allow the care team to generate reports and monitor progress. Metrics specific to care of the emerging adult in an adult care setting include documentation of the date of the first visit, date the clinic transition policy was discussed with the patient specifically including a discussion around privacy and consent, tracking of ongoing self-care assessment and education, monitoring of referrals to and appointments with subspeciality providers, glycemic data, and visit history. A record of emerging adult patients seen in practice can identify those who are lost to follow-up or may be experiencing other barriers to care.

Orientation to adult practice

In addition to offering an orientation to the adult practice and providing young adult-friendly welcome materials that describe confidentiality, services offered, and the logistics of obtaining care, this core element also recommends identifying providers that are comfortable with emerging adult diabetes care.

Emerging adults report a desire to have a point person to serve as a bridge between pediatric and adult care[37] and engage in developmentally appropriate conversations,[38] including a visit with a provider who is knowledgeable in issues specific to emerging with diabetes[39] such as issues specific to the college years. The entire team—from the front office to the clinical team—should receive education on the intersection of diabetes and emerging adulthood and should be prepared to care for this population. To support successful HCT, adult endocrinology clinics with an interest in caring for the emerging adult should identify themselves to their pediatric colleagues.

Integration into adult practice

Despite the use of a transfer summary being a key recommendation of the American Diabetes Association,[2] adult providers who receive emerging adults with diabetes note that it is rare for adult providers to receive a transition summary.[36,40,41] Before an emerging adult's first visit, it is important to ensure receipt of transfer package, including final transition readiness assessment, plan of care with transition goals and prioritized actions, medical summary, current emergency care plan, as well as legal documents, condition fact sheet, and additional clinical records if needed.

This core element also recommends communication by the adult provider office with the young adult to remind them of the appointment and identify any special needs or preference. This intentional contact is critical because prolonged lapses in care are associated with higher HbA$_{1c}$ and more hospitalizations.[42] Similar to pediatric practices, adult practices should consider employing a point person (eg, transition coordinator) to ensure emerging adults are not lost in the transfer process moving from pediatric to adult diabetes care.

Initial visits with adult providers

Similar to pediatric and adult providers, emerging adults with diabetes also find the transition process difficult. They report the transition from pediatric to adult care as jarring and poorly planned with a lack of focus on issues that are specifically relevant to the emerging adult, such as sexuality and alcohol use.[39] These needs are not often met, leading to dissatisfaction with care. Adult clinicians also feel unprepared to deal with issues such as substance use disorders, disordered eating, and depression[36] and their influence on diabetes management, and many are not familiar with recommended guidelines on diabetes HCT care.[41]

Specific measures should be taken at the emerging adult's first visit to the adult provider's office. The initial visit should address concerns the young adult may have about the care transition and include a description of differences between pediatric care and adult care. Receiving adult providers must walk the fine line between establishing rapport with patients and emphasizing the importance of ongoing glycemic management. Emerging adults have highlighted the importance of a good fit with an adult care provider.[38] Adult clinicians should plan for ongoing diabetes education needs after the transition to adult care and should be prepared to objectively assess diabetes knowledge with a self-management assessment. This assessment and education are especially important for emerging adults who were diagnosed with diabetes at a very young age because their guardians likely received the bulk of diabetes education at diagnosis and subsequent clinic visits. This intervention may require additional support from diabetes educators that will go beyond the standard of care for typical adult endocrinology or primary care practices.

Ongoing care for emerging adult with diabetes

To support successful integration of emerging adults into practice, receiving adult endocrinologists can implement several interventions.[17,43] Adult endocrinologists should improve their understanding of pivotal guidelines around transition to adult care for people with diabetes[2] and be familiar with transition resources from Got Transition, the American Diabetes Association, and The Endocrine Society.

For emerging adults with diabetes, a critical piece of ongoing care is connecting patients with mental health professionals and peer support. Mental health comorbidities play a major role in the lives of emerging adults with diabetes[44] and those with more mental health concerns trend toward higher HbA_{1c} levels.[45] Adult providers who care for emerging adults with T1D should, therefore, be prepared to screen for depression, anxiety, and diabetes distress and offer support when these conditions are identified. Finally, approximately 1 in 5 youth and young adults with T1D develop disordered eating behaviors.[46] Thus, screening and referral to a treatment program that is willing to work with emerging adults with diabetes is essential.

Using a team-based approach to address common issues in emerging adulthood should be considered.[43] A social worker or nurse care manager, for example, can address the anticipated complexities of health insurance changes that influence this group. Young adults are 2 times more likely to be uninsured than any other group.[47] A certified diabetes educator knowledgeable in issues specific to the emerging adult can ensure young adult patients have a medical point of contact when diabetes-related questions arise in between visits. Of course, a noted challenge in the adult care setting is the availability of fewer resources as compared with pediatric context to address important psychosocial needs.[31]

SUMMARY

HCT from pediatric to adult health care refers to a set of actions designed to ensure continuity of care between pediatric and adult health care settings. HCT should take place over time, beginning in adolescence in a pediatric approach to care and continuing into adulthood in an adult approach to care. Even if an emerging adult with diabetes remains with the same provider into adulthood, preparation for adult-focused care is necessary. Because of the mobility of emerging adults and the continued specialization of diabetes care, the likelihood that they will change providers is almost certain. Thus, there is commonly a need to establish a structured transition process consistently available to support emerging adults with their diabetes care.

Got Transition's Six Core Elements of HCT offer a structured approach to the phases of HCT support for emerging adults with T1D for both pediatric and adult practices. Measurement tools are available to be used to measure implementation of the Six Core Elements such as the Current Assessment of HCT Activities and the HCT Process Measurement Tool. The Six Core Elements also have companion Implementation Guides available.[17] The Implementation Guides are intended to help clinicians, practices, and systems to support HCT improvements using the Six Core Elements of

HCT for their youth and young adults transitioning to adult-centered care with or without changing their clinician.

The transition from pediatric to adult diabetes care should incorporate the life course approach and all emerging adult clinicians during this transition have a key part in the process that includes planning, transfer, and integration into the adult practice. Each clinician assists the emerging adult to gain health literacy, be able to care for their health, and know how to use the different health systems where they receive their care. The implementation of a structured transition process can support improved patient health and societal outcomes for emerging adults with T1D.

CLINICS CARE POINTS

- The development of a HCT policy, which formalizes a pediatric or adult diabetes practice's approach to HCT, is an important first step to supporting effective HCT.
- Pediatric diabetes providers should assess transition readiness prior to transfer to adult diabetes care and support diabetes self-management and health care navigation skill development.
- A transfer summary document co-created with the emerging adult with T1D and their family, as well as handoff communication between the current pediatric diabetes and future adult diabetes provider of an emerging adult, is critical for successful transfer of care.
- Adult diabetes practices should offer an orientation to emerging adults at initial visits, review differences between pediatric and adult diabetes care, and plan to provide tailored ongoing care that meets the unique needs of emerging adults with T1D.

DISCLOSURE

No disclosures to report.

REFERENCES

1. Cooley WC, Sagerman PJ, American Academy of Pediatrics, American Academy of Family Physicians, American College of Physicians, Transitions Clinical Report Authoring Group. Supporting the health care transition from adolescence to adulthood in the medical home. Pediatrics 2011;128(1):182–200.
2. Peters A, Laffel L, American Diabetes Association Transitions Working Group. Diabetes care for emerging adults: recommendations for transition from pediatric to adult diabetes care systems: a position statement of the American Diabetes Association, with representation by the American College of Osteopathic Family Physicians, the American Academy of Pediatrics, the American Association of Clinical Endocrinologists, the American Osteopathic Association, the Centers for Disease Control and Prevention, Children with Diabetes, The Endocrine Society, the International Society for Pediatric and Adolescent Diabetes, Juvenile Diabetes Research Foundation International, the National Diabetes Education Program, and the Pediatric Endocrine Society (formerly Lawson Wilkins Pediatric Endocrine Society). Diabetes Care 2011;34(11):2477–85.
3. White PH, Cooley WC. Transitions Clinical Report Authoring Group, American Academy Of Pediatrics, American Academy Of Family Physicians, American College Of Physicians. Supporting the Health Care Transition From Adolescence to Adulthood in the Medical Home. Pediatrics 2018;142(5). https://doi.org/10.1542/peds.2018-2587.

4. Child and Adolescent Health Measurement Initiative. 2022 National Survey of Children's Health data query. Data Resource Center for Child and Adolescent Health supported by the U.S. Department of Health and Human Services, Health Resources and Services Administration, Maternal and Child Health Bureau. Available at: www.childhealthdata.org. Accessed October 15, 2023.

5. Schmidt A, Ilango SM, McManus MA, et al. Outcomes of Pediatric to Adult Health Care Transition Interventions: An Updated Systematic Review. J Pediatr Nurs 2020;51:92–107.

6. Holmes-Walker DJ, Llewellyn AC, Farrell K. A transition care programme which improves diabetes control and reduces hospital admission rates in young adults with Type 1 diabetes aged 15-25 years. Diabet Med 2007;24(7):764–9.

7. Farrell K, Fernandez R, Salamonson Y, et al. Health outcomes for youth with type 1 diabetes at 18 months and 30 months post transition from pediatric to adult care. Diabetes Res Clin Pract 2018;139:163–9.

8. McManus M, White P, Barbour A, et al. Pediatric to adult transition: a quality improvement model for primary care. J Adolesc Health 2015;56(1):73–8.

9. McManus M, White P. Transition to Adult Health Care Services for Young Adults with Chronic Medical Illness and Psychiatric Comorbidity. Child Adolesc Psychiatr Clin N Am 2017;26(2):367–80.

10. Ayers LR, Beyea SC, Godfrey MM, et al. Quality improvement learning collaboratives. Qual Manag Health Care 2005;14(4):234–47.

11. Jones MR, Robbins BW, Augustine M, et al. Transfer from pediatric to adult endocrinology. Endocr Pract 2017;23(7):822–30.

12. Lestishock L, Nova S, Disabato J. Improving Adolescent and Young Adult Engagement in the Process of Transitioning to Adult Care. J Adolesc Health 2021;69(3):424–31.

13. Ames JL, Massolo ML, Davignon MN, et al. Transitioning youth with autism spectrum disorders and other special health care needs into adult primary care: A provider survey. Autism 2021;25(3):731–43.

14. Fremion E, Cowley R, Berens J, et al. Improved health care transition for young adults with developmental disabilities referred from designated transition clinics. J Pediatr Nurs 2022;67:27–33.

15. Jones MR, Hooper TJ, Cuomo C, et al. Evaluation of a Health Care Transition Improvement Process in Seven Large Health Care Systems. J Pediatr Nurs 2019;47:44–50.

16. White P, Schmidt A, Shorr J, et al. Six core elements of health care transition™ 3.0. Washington, DC: Got Transition, The National Alliance to Advance Adolescent Health; 2020.

17. White P, Schmidt A, Ilango S, et al. How to implement the six core elements of health care transition 3.0. Washington, DC: Got Transition, The National Alliance to Advance Adolescent Health; 2020.

18. Batalden M, Batalden P, Margolis P, et al. Coproduction of healthcare service. BMJ Qual Saf 2016;25(7):509–17.

19. Petkovic J, Riddle A, Akl EA, et al. Protocol for the development of guidance for stakeholder engagement in health and healthcare guideline development and implementation. Syst Rev 2020;9(1):21.

20. Massey PM, Prelip M, Calimlim BM, et al. Contextualizing an expanded definition of health literacy among adolescents in the health care setting. Health Educ Res 2012;27(6):961–74.

21. Wood DL, Sawicki GS, Miller MD, et al. The Transition Readiness Assessment Questionnaire (TRAQ): its factor structure, reliability, and validity. Acad Pediatr 2014;14(4):415–22.
22. Chan JT, Soni J, Sahni D, et al. Measuring the Transition Readiness of Adolescents With Type 1 Diabetes Using the Transition Readiness Assessment Questionnaire. Clin Diabetes 2019;37(4):347–52.
23. Gray WN, Partain L, Benekos E, et al. Integrating transition readiness assessment into clinical practice: Adaptation of the UNC TRXANSITION index into the cerner electronic medical record. J Pediatr Nurs 2022. https://doi.org/10.1016/j.pedn.2022.11.032.
24. Al Khalifah RA, McConnell M, Al Nahari AA, et al. Development and Validation of the Transition Readiness Assessment Instrument in Type 1 Diabetes "On TRAck". Can J Diabetes 2022;46(5):510–7.
25. Beal SJ, Riddle IK, Kichler JC, et al. The Associations of Chronic Condition Type and Individual Characteristics With Transition Readiness. Acad Pediatr 2016;16(7):660–7.
26. Schwartz LA, Tuchman LK, Hobbie WL, et al. A social-ecological model of readiness for transition to adult-oriented care for adolescents and young adults with chronic health conditions. Research Support, Non-U.S. Gov't Review. Child: care, health and development 2011;37(6):883–95.
27. Goethals ER, Commissariat PV, Volkening LK, et al. Assessing readiness for independent self-care in adolescents with type 1 diabetes: Introducing the RISQ. Diabetes Res Clin Pract 2020;162:108110.
28. Gutierrez-Colina AM, Corathers S, Beal S, et al. Young Adults With Type 1 Diabetes Preparing to Transition to Adult Care: Psychosocial Functioning and Associations With Self-Management and Health Outcomes. Diabetes Spectr 2020;33(3):255–63.
29. Corathers SD, Yi-Frazier JP, Kichler JC, et al. Development and Implementation of the Readiness Assessment of Emerging Adults With Type 1 Diabetes Diagnosed in Youth (READDY) Tool. Diabetes Spectr 2020;33(1):99–103.
30. Corathers SD, Mara CA, Chundi PK, et al. Psychosocial Patient-Reported Outcomes in Pediatric and Adolescent Diabetes: a Review and Case Example. Curr Diabetes Rep 2017;17(7):45.
31. Corathers S, Williford DN, Kichler J, et al. Implementation of Psychosocial Screening into Diabetes Clinics: Experience from the Type 1 Diabetes Exchange Quality Improvement Network. Curr Diabetes Rep 2023;23(2):19–28.
32. Agarwal S, Garvey KC, Raymond JK, et al. Perspectives on care for young adults with type 1 diabetes transitioning from pediatric to adult health systems: A national survey of pediatric endocrinologists. Pediatr Diabetes 2017;18(7):524–31.
33. Benchimol EI, Afif W, Plamondon S, et al. Medical Summary Template for the Transfer of Patients with Inflammatory Bowel Disease from Pediatric to Adult Care. J Can Assoc Gastroenterol 2022;5(1):3–11.
34. Butalia S, Crawford SG, McGuire KA, et al. Improved transition to adult care in youth with type 1 diabetes: a pragmatic clinical trial. Diabetologia 2021;64(4):758–66.
35. Spaic T, Robinson T, Goldbloom E, et al. Closing the Gap: Results of the Multicenter Canadian Randomized Controlled Trial of Structured Transition in Young Adults With Type 1 Diabetes. Diabetes Care 2019;42(6):1018–26.
36. Garvey KC, Telo GH, Needleman JS, et al. Health Care Transition in Young Adults With Type 1 Diabetes: Perspectives of Adult Endocrinologists in the U.S. Diabetes Care 2016;39(2):190–7.

37. Cassidy M, Doucet S, Luke A, et al. Improving the transition from paediatric to adult healthcare: a scoping review on the recommendations of young adults with lived experience. BMJ Open 2022;12(12):e051314.

38. Hilliard ME, Perlus JG, Clark LM, et al. Perspectives from before and after the pediatric to adult care transition: a mixed-methods study in type 1 diabetes. Diabetes Care 2014;37(2):346–54.

39. Garvey KC, Beste MG, Luff D, et al. Experiences of health care transition voiced by young adults with type 1 diabetes: a qualitative study. Adolesc Health Med Ther 2014;5:191–8.

40. Gray W, Dorriz P, Kim H, et al. Adult Provider Perspectives on Transition and Transfer to Adult Care: A Multi-Specialty, Multi-Institutional Exploration. J Pediatr Nurs 2021;59:173–80.

41. Michaud S, Dasgupta K, Bell L, et al. Adult care providers' perspectives on the transition to adult care for emerging adults with Type 1 diabetes: a cross-sectional survey. Diabet Med 2018;35(7):846–54.

42. Tilden DR, French B, Shoemaker AH, et al. Prolonged lapses between pediatric and adult care are associated with rise in HbA1c and inpatient days among patients with type 1 diabetes. Diabetes Res Clin Pract 2022;192:110113.

43. Iyengar J, Thomas IH, Soleimanpour SA. Transition from pediatric to adult care in emerging adults with type 1 diabetes: a blueprint for effective receivership. Clin Diabetes Endocrinol 2019;5:3.

44. Cooper MN, Lin A, Alvares GA, et al. Psychiatric disorders during early adulthood in those with childhood onset type 1 diabetes: Rates and clinical risk factors from population-based follow-up. Pediatr Diabetes 2017;18(7):599–606.

45. Bernstein CM, Stockwell MS, Gallagher MP, et al. Mental health issues in adolescents and young adults with type 1 diabetes: prevalence and impact on glycemic control. Clin Pediatr (Phila) 2013;52(1):10–5.

46. Nip ASY, Reboussin BA, Dabelea D, et al. Disordered Eating Behaviors in Youth and Young Adults With Type 1 or Type 2 Diabetes Receiving Insulin Therapy: The SEARCH for Diabetes in Youth Study. Diabetes Care 2019;42(5):859–66.

47. Buschur EO, Glick B, Kamboj MK. Transition of care for patients with type 1 diabetes mellitus from pediatric to adult health care systems. Transl Pediatr 2017; 6(4):373–82.

Optimizing Glycemic Outcomes for Minoritized and Medically Underserved Adults Living with Type 1 Diabetes

Devin W. Steenkamp, MD[a],*, Kathryn L. Fantasia, MD, MSc[a,b],
Howard A. Wolpert, MD[a]

KEYWORDS

- Type 1 diabetes • Outcomes • Minority • Underserved • Social risk factors

KEY POINTS

- The American Diabetes Association Professional Practice Committee recommends that continuous glucose monitoring and automated insulin delivery systems be offered to adults with type 1 diabetes (T1D) who can use the devices safely.
- Individuals living with T1D from minoritized and lower income communities have poorer health outcomes and lower use of diabetes technologies. Some of the reasons for the disparities include limited health literacy, barriers to access to care, inadequate health insurance coverage, provider implicit bias, and broad exclusion from many of the trials evaluating diabetes technologies.
- Educational and specialty referral initiatives can be effective in overcoming clinical inertia and increasing the use of advanced technologies.
- Social risk factors and barriers that can compete with diabetes self-care need to be considered in the formulation of treatment plans and collaborative goal setting.
- Advanced diabetes technologies can be successfully introduced in adult medically underserved populations living with T1D.

INTRODUCTION

Type 1 diabetes (T1D) is a chronic condition characterized by autoimmune destruction of pancreatic beta cells, resulting in near-absolute insulin deficiency and reliance on life-long exogenous insulin therapy.[1] In recent years, advances in diabetes technology, including increasingly sophisticated continuous glucose monitors (CGM) and

[a] Section of Endocrinology, Diabetes and Nutrition, Department of Medicine, Boston University Chobanian & Avedisian School of Medicine and Boston Medical Center, 72 East Concord Street, C3, Boston, MA 02118, USA; [b] Department of Medicine, Evans Center for Implementation and Improvement Sciences (CIIS), Boston University Chobanian & Avedisian School of Medicine, Boston, MA, USA
* Corresponding author.
E-mail address: desteenk@bu.edu

Endocrinol Metab Clin N Am 53 (2024) 67–80
https://doi.org/10.1016/j.ecl.2023.07.001
0889-8529/24/© 2023 Elsevier Inc. All rights reserved.
endo.theclinics.com

automated insulin delivery (AID) systems, have transformed the management of T1D, leading to improvements in glycemic control and quality of life.[2] Consistent use of these technologies has become part of the standard of care. However, to date, most of the randomized controlled trials evaluating use of technologies in T1D have been in more socially advantaged and predominantly non-Hispanic White patients followed at specialized diabetes care centers.[3–6] Furthermore, these efficacy studies have excluded patients with T1D who have markedly elevated A1c levels. Consistent with the American Diabetes Association Professional Practice Committee recommendations that CGM and AID systems should be offered for diabetes management for youth and adults with T1D who can use the devices safely,[2] the aim of this review is to broadly review factors that underly successful technology implementation in populations who have traditionally been excluded from benefit.

BACKGROUND

It is well established that individuals living with T1D from minoritized and lower income communities have poorer health outcomes and use of diabetes technologies in these populations remains low.[7–11] Some of the more common reasons for these disparities include well-recognized social determinants of health, including barriers to access to care and health insurance coverage limitations, limited health literacy, and the fact that minoritized populations have largely been excluded from many of the randomized controlled trials evaluating diabetes technologies. Recently, clinician implicit bias has been identified as an important contributor to poor device uptake.[12] Health care providers who prescribe diabetes technologies are highly influential and act as "gatekeepers" for their patients, making specific device recommendations, supporting device initiation and training, and providing ongoing longitudinal support.[13] However, many adult endocrinology fellow trainees feel under-prepared in terms of critical aspects of technology use, creating an additional potential barrier to this important gatekeeper role.[14] Technology also advances quickly, which may result in clinician discomfort with recommending devices that they have limited familiarity with. Moreover, even in health care systems with universal insurance coverage for insulin pumps and CGM, this has not necessarily resolved these disparities.[15,16]

Finally, many underserved patients entering diabetes management programs or seeking primary care have limited diabetes self-management skills, nutritional literacy, and high levels of diabetes distress, creating a potential bias where clinicians may feel that the technology is too complex for implementation.[17,18]

APPROACH
Emphasis on Team-Based Diabetes Care

It is well established that people living with T1D[19] benefit from multidisciplinary care teams that include clinicians with expertise in behavioral, nutritional, medical, and other relevant services.[20–22] However, minoritized and medically underserved people with diabetes (PWD) are often unable to access many of these critical clinical resources, or resources are not appropriately or are insufficiently developed to address the issues that are most relevant to underserved PWD.[23] For example, standard nutritional resources often fail to sufficiently address culturally appropriate food choices.[24] Furthermore, important social determinants of health[25] that directly affect glycemic outcomes are often incompletely addressed in busy medical appointments and clinician familiarity with family, inter-personal, employment, and community dynamics that may contribute to diabetes distress are often amplified in underserved PWD.[25] As a result of the frequently increased care complexity, care teams often need to be larger and particularly attentive to patient concerns that fall outside the scope of typical biomedical model office appointments. For example, a PWD who works a part-time job or in a transitory role may need to navigate changing health insurance benefits (public vs commercial insurance benefits) that may necessitate transitions between "in-network" providers, different versions of insulin, or challenges obtaining consistent CGM or insulin pump supplies.[26] Oftentimes, these challenges result in unnecessary hospitalizations or emergency department visits and periods where patients are required to navigate transitions between multiple dose injection therapy and insulin pump therapy. In addition, many medical centers and medical practices are ill-equipped and under-resourced to support PWD who are expected to navigate these challenges.[27] Therefore, it is perhaps even more critical that clinicians caring for minoritized and medically underserved PWD work together to provide "wrap-around" care structures that can act as both a safety net and provide structured longitudinal care that allows PWD to thrive.[28] **Box 1** provides a recommended list of health care roles that may support underserved PWDs. Dedicated Quality Improvement (QI) teams are also invaluable to provide real-world data insights as they work together within institutions as well as within larger collaborative learning networks and broader health equity advisory committees to plan and study interventions that are aimed to reduce inequities in care.[29,30]

Recognition of Provider Implicit Bias in Diabetes Technology Adoption

It is important to recognize that socioeconomic, demographic factors, health literacy, and health care location are not solely responsible for decreased adoption of diabetes technology in underserved PWD. Minoritized adults living with T1D report that they have never been offered the option of engaging in a shared decision-making process in terms of beginning on a CGM or insulin pump.[31] Oftentimes, health care providers have an unconscious bias, whereby they fail to raise the availability of technologies or recognize the potential for more advanced diabetes self-management capacity in an individual patient,[12] PWD with limited English proficiency are at risk for lower quality patient-clinician communication, decreased shared decision-making, and may be particularly at risk of this implicit bias. Because of cultural differences and socioeconomic and educational imbalances, the relationship between clinician and patient can become paternalistic and prescriptive, distracting from the model of collaborative coaching and decision-making required to foster engagement in diabetes self-care. Clinicians should receive training in implicit bias reduction and communication skills and need to maintain self-awareness about these behavioral

---

Box 1
Recommended health care system roles to support underserved people living with T1D

- Endocrinologists/Primary Care Physicians
- Licensed Clinical Social Worker/Psychologist
- Registered Dietitians
- Certified Diabetes Care and Education Specialists
- Clinical Pharmacists
- Diabetes Technology Navigators/Durable Medical Equipment and Pharmacy liaisons
- Implementation Scientists/QI Teams
- Patient Advocates/Community Advisory Groups

dynamics and biases, and guard against therapeutic clinical inertia. It is important to create an environment where modern technologies and therapeutics are discussed with patients at all clinic visits and where patients are encouraged to explore their options in a non-judgmental, linguistically, and culturally sensitive manner.[32]

Clinician and Patient Education in Diabetes Technology Adoption

In order to increase clinician comfort and familiarity with the various devices and latest advances in technologies and care delivery, we suggest prioritization of educational resources or conference time where clinicians can review relevant academic publications that are of interest and relevance to the outcomes they seek to improve (eg, journal club). This may include review of literature that encourages a person-centered approach to care, the latest technology advancements, and articles that address relevant social determinants of health. Similarly, it is often helpful to develop patient-directed, linguistic, and socioculturally-adapted educational materials that address the specific needs of minoritized PWDs.

Adapting existing evidence-based treatment strategies such as patient facing education, as opposed to creating interventions de novo, can enhance acceptability, facilitate efficient dissemination to broader audiences, and better meet the needs of minoritized and medically underserved adults with T1D. Adapting interventions for context and with respect to linguistic and sociocultural background has been recommended as a method to reduce inequities.[33,34] Stakeholder involvement and codesign serve as helpful methods by which to adapt interventions in an acceptable and appropriate fashion for specific populations of patients.[35,36] Data to support adapting interventions to enhance cultural appropriateness exist within chronic disease management, including in type 2 diabetes prevention[37,38] and treatment[39,40] and for adapting interventions for those with T1D to cultural context in international[41,42] and US settings[43,44] though a majority are focused on the care of youth with T1D. The potential benefits of culturally-adapted education and behavioral interventions in the management of adults with T1D warrant further investigation.

At the level of the clinic or diabetes program itself, we highly encourage implementation of structured education and device referral, and training processes while working to ensure timely access to clinic-based diabetes technology trainers. Specialized care pathways focused on training patients in more advanced diabetes self-management skills and the use of diabetes technology help facilitate patient increased referrals and ensure that patients access clinicians with appropriate expertise. Alternatively, given that many practices lack internal skilled Certified Diabetes Care and Education Specialist (CDCES) staff clinicians, we suggest taking steps to develop a strong working relationship with industry-based device manufacturer trainers or external CDCES who can onboard patients onto appropriate devices while working to ensure appropriate and safe transitions of care.

Importance of Behavior Change as a Central Focus of Diabetes Self-Management

Optimization of patient behavior is central to achieving desired glycemic outcomes. However, reaching and maintaining a desired glycemic outcome is facilitated through increasing patient self-efficacy, strengthening patient-clinician relationships, and fostering an increased comfort in living with diabetes.[45] Behavioral goals need to be individualized, and most importantly, attainable so that patients feel rewarded for their efforts and develop a sense of self-efficacy that promotes further engagement in self-care. Clinicians caring for patients with chronic illness have a unique opportunity to exert a positive influence and foster a strong working relationship with their patients. The clinician role becomes a "coaching" role, where over time, mutual trust and partnerships develop that creates further opportunities for clinicians to support behavior change, yielding increased engagement and incremental, progressive successes. Clinicians caring for PWD play a critical role to influence lifelong healthful habits. In the context of underserved PWD, these concepts become even more relevant. Even though glycemic targets may not change, behavior is influenced by personal as well as broader sociocultural and socioeconomic factors and life stressors that may not align with a traditional biomedical model approach to care. For example, a PWD experiencing homelessness, unemployment, and with food insecurity has unmet basic needs for food and shelter and any treatment approach needs to consider the patient's perspective, challenges, and goals within the context of their individual lived experiences. Furthermore, providers need to guard against making premature judgements whereby advanced diabetes concepts or technologies are deemed to be too complex to consider. The practical benefits of diabetes technology— including, for example, reduction in the need for fingerstick blood glucose measurements and risk for hypoglycemia in the workplace, the ability to take insulin boluses discretely while on the go in a busy service job, and improved sleep quality (both from reduced hypoglycemia and hyperglycemia-induced nocturia)—relieve the daily burdens of managing diabetes and improve quality of life. Framing the advantages in terms of these immediate benefits can trigger patient interest in exploring potential use of technology. Who is an ideal CGM or AID system candidate? Just because it may take more time and require increased resource utilization, is this sufficient justification to dismiss a particular patient in terms of potential device candidacy? If these types of issues and biases are neglected, clinicians risk alienating and frustrating patients, given that diabetes is a self-managed condition, and all treatment strategies are successful only if the patient is cared for in a way that supports self-implementation and improvement over time. There are several considerations in preparing patients to successfully start on advanced diabetes technology, in particular pump therapy and AID systems. Consider competing life demands that may limit the time that can be committed to mastering new skills; schedule the pump start when there are not other distracting priorities, such as starting a new job or searching for new living accommodations. Set realistic expectations about the benefit/burden trade-offs with technology and providing a "road map" for how this evolves over time as their self-mastery advances. In this regard, it can be helpful to prepare patients by pointing out that it is normal for many of the tasks related to use of diabetes technology— such as inserting infusion catheters, loading insulin pumps, trouble-shooting insulin non-delivery—to initially feel burdensome; however, in time, these additional self-management tasks become routine.

Increasing Implementation of Diabetes Technologies into Routine Clinical Care

Most adults with T1D in the United States are treated by primary care providers with the nationwide shortage of specialist endocrinologists already well documented.[46] Primary care providers have reported low confidence in delivering T1D care, and are frequently uncomfortable with management of traditional insulin pumps, resulting in a lack of access to the expert clinical guidance required for successful use of advanced diabetes technologies.[47,48] Furthermore, primary care providers caring for underserved and minoritized populations may be less likely to have extensive clinical experience in the use of advanced diabetes technologies, largely resulting from significantly lower use in this population. There are also widespread, complex, and time-consuming logistical challenges to overcome obtaining durable medical equipment supplies that stymy efforts to onboard technology at scale.[26] Nonetheless, in a recent survey, over 75% of primary care providers reported willingness to prescribe artificial pancreas technology (AID) to individuals living with T1D.[48] While CGM alone often improves glycemic control, AID systems, that combine an insulin pump, CGM and control algorithm that modulates insulin delivery based on CGM glucose inputs, provides additional benefits—including more effective hypoglycemia mitigation and increased time in range (TIR 70–180 mg/dL).[3,49] Real world data indicate that individuals using CGM who have poor glycemic control can benefit significantly from AID systems.[50] Efforts should prioritize development of interdisciplinary QI and implementation science (IS) teams that are tasked to increase clinician familiarity with the available devices, support necessary infrastructure development, focus on clinician team-building, and develop educational materials that are aimed toward improved uptake of devices. Given logistical challenges, it is often very valuable to solicit institutional support for an administrative role to manage the extensive paperwork required to obtain insurance approval for devices, assist patients in ensuring timely delivery of device supplies as well as replacement of failed devices, along with providing general patient facing support. This role is critical to support the clinicians in a diabetes program caring for underserved populations. Furthermore, it is imperative that successful implementation strategies and real-world outcome data are widely disseminated.

The Value of Physical Activity in Optimizing Glycemic Outcomes

The value of consistent physical activity in improving overall health and wellbeing in individuals living with diabetes is well established.[51] However, exercise, particularly aerobic and interval exercise, increases the risk of hypoglycemia in insulin users, which may result in undesirable exercise avoidance.[52,53] Furthermore, PWD who work in industries or jobs that involve physical labor may deliberately keep their glucose levels elevated during working hours to avoid exercise-induced hypoglycemia, which can disrupt work performance. The tension between recognizing the benefit of exercise while balancing the risk of hypoglycemia at the jobsite and the perceived risk of losing gainful employment because of recurrent hypoglycemia is a challenge that many PWD struggle with. Nonetheless, PWD should be encouraged and supported to incorporate structured physical activity into their daily routines,[52] with the largest drop in glucose expected during and after aerobic activity. Time should be devoted to coaching patients to understand the effects of various types of exercise on their glucose dynamics and how to anticipate, recognize, and respond to potential hypoglycemia.[52] Even though resistance training results in less hypoglycemia and has lower glucose lowering capability, in comparison to aerobic and interval training, time in range (TIR 70–180 mg/dL) is modestly increased in the 24-h period after all forms of structured exercise.[54] However, the challenge for the clinician is allowing space to encourage specific dialogue with regards to a PWD desire to exercise. Addressing patient concerns, including possible hypoglycemia aversion, frustration with unexplained glucose excursions around exercise, and insulin dosing strategies are all integral to successful efforts to support safe and enjoyable exercise.

FUTURE RESEARCH CONSIDERATIONS

In the future, as the focus in research moves from efficacy trials, primarily focused on regulatory approval, to effectiveness studies to support the practical and safe implementation of advanced technologies in the broader diabetes population and community-based clinics, trial design will need to evolve. All the pivotal trials examining the potential benefits of advanced technology versus the "standard-of-care" diabetes therapies have been designed to assure internal validity, with careful matching of study arms for visit frequency and attention, and selected study subjects. In contrast, trials to evaluate real-world use of these technologies will need to be designed with a view to ensuring that the study protocol and findings have high generalizability and external validity; accordingly, matching study arms for visit frequency and clinical encounter time will not be a study design imperative. As the inclusion criteria for trials are broadened and there are fewer restrictions on enrollment, it is possible that dropouts and non-adherence will be higher than in previous efficacy trials of advanced diabetes technology. Because of this Intention to Treat (ITT) analysis—which estimates the effect of being assigned to a treatment, not the effect of the treatment itself—would under-estimate the magnitude of the potential benefits derived by those study patients who used the technology. In keeping with the recommendations of Hernán and colleagues regarding the analysis of effectiveness research, both ITT and per-protocol (PP) analyses will need to be performed to get a meaningful measure of the potential benefits of the technology in users.[55,56]

DISCUSSION

Active approaches to mitigate disparities in care and advance health equity are required to optimize glycemic outcomes for broad populations of adults with T1D, including those from minoritized communities who carry increased burden of acute and chronic diabetes-related complications.[57,58] Though evidence-based interventions to improve glycemic control in T1D exist, racial and ethnic inequities in care are now well documented, with Black, Latino, and individuals with low socioeconomic status less likely to access routine endocrine subspecialty care[59] and use diabetes technologies that are now considered standard of care.[8,60,61] Disparities in care stem partly from policy and community level determinants, including restrictive insurance coverage and adverse social determinants of health. Approaches from the fields of IS and QI can offer focused methods to improve adoption of evidence-based interventions.

IS is the study of methods to promote and increase the uptake of evidence-based practices into routine care.[62] QI focuses on identifying and remediating systems issues driving outcomes through continuous processes of testing change ideas.[63] While both share a common goal of improving the quality of health care services and improving patient outcomes, IS focuses on how to implement evidence-based interventions and why efforts may or may not be successful through consideration of multiple contextual factors.[62] Multiple IS frameworks have been modified to address contextual determinants influencing equity in adoption of evidence-based practices and are a useful lens to examine and design interventions to both avoid increasing and work toward ameliorating these inequities.[64–66] While a discussion of the similarities and differences between IS and QI and their methods is beyond the scope of this review, both serve as disciplines to examine gaps and inequities in care and to work actively to improve patient outcomes. Both clinicians and PWD are benefitted by the creation of multidisciplinary teams involving IS and QI scientists who can examine the impact of implementation strategies, such as those outlined here, including educational meetings and outreach and creating new clinical teams and care pathways, and repeated tests of change in improving health care delivery.[67] Collaboration between IS and QI scientists can allow for rapid and rigorous evaluation and dissemination of strategies to improve care across health systems that can benefit PWD more broadly.[68]

Ensuring attention to strategies that promote equity in health care and outcomes along the continuum from research to provision of clinical care is imperative. The importance of recruiting diverse populations into clinical trials to ensure generalizability of interventions to racially and ethnically diverse populations has recently been acknowledged by the US Food and Drug Administration guidance on diversity requirements for clinical trials. Additionally, earlier focus on increasing the speed of innovation uptake is required as it is estimated that it takes nearly 17 years from demonstration of innovation efficacy to uptake into routine clinical practice.[69] As it has been suggested that evaluation of both effectiveness and implementation in clinical research helps to speed translational gains and uptake of interventions into clinical practice, it has been argued that such integration of ISshould occur earlier in the translational pipeline.[70,71]

SUMMARY

Minoritized and medically underserved adults living with T1D frequently encounter multiple obstacles to successful diabetes self-management that directly impact on their ability to thrive while living with diabetes. Clinicians who care for these patients have the opportunity to shift the narrative and significantly improve clinical outcomes. Modern diabetes therapeutics—most importantly CGM and AID systems—are highly effective at helping PWD increase the likelihood of meeting glycemic outcomes. Clinicians should work together in local clinical teams and in larger collaborative networks to dismantle bias, increase internal self-awareness, address misconceptions, and endeavor to reduce barriers to successful diabetes care.

CLINICS CARE POINTS – *BULLETED LIST OF EVIDENCE-BASED PEARLS AND PITFALLS RELEVANT TO THE POINT OF CARE*

- Prioritize development of an interdisciplinary team that is supported to learn, iterate, and implement changes together. (QI Framework)
- Solicit institutional support for an administrative role to manage the extensive paperwork required to obtain insurance approval for devices, assist patients in ensuring timely delivery of device supplies as well as replacement of failed devices, along with providing general patient facing support is critical to support a diabetes program caring for underserved populations.
- Prioritize educational/conference time where clinicians can review relevant academic publications that are of interest and relevance to improving outcomes.
- Develop patient-directed, linguistic, and socioculturally adapted educational materials that address the specific needs of minoritized patients with T1D.
- Devote educational resources to improve clinician and patient familiarity with the various devices, referral, and training processes.
- Ensure timely access to clinic-based diabetes technology trainers or alternatively develop a strong working relationship with industry-based device manufacturer trainers that ensures appropriate and safe transitions of care.

CASE STUDY

A 35-year-old man, living with T1D for 7 years, presents to the refugee health clinic at the Boston Medical Center, a safety net academic medical center, that cares for a large medically underserved and minoritized population. Six months prior to presentation, he relocated as an asylee, with his wife and 2 young children, from Ethiopia to the United States, and is unemployed and living in a local shelter with his family. He has no other medical comorbidities but suffers from post-traumatic stress disorder (PTSD) and depression. His A1c is 9.5% and he is injecting multidose insulin (insulin glargine at bedtime and insulin lispro before meals) via a syringe filled from vials. He checks his glucose consistently 4 times daily using a glucometer and struggles with frequent hypoglycemia whenever he is physically active, so avoids structured exercise, even though he was an avid runner prior to his diabetes diagnosis. Before relocating to the United States, he worked overnight stocking shelves in a large department store in Africa. His primary priority is the well-being of his family and food and housing insecurity is his major concern. He plans to establish primary care at a local urban community health center, nearby to his shelter. He has no prior experience with diabetes technology or formal diabetes education and is unfamiliar with the US health care system.

How would you approach the multifaceted needs of this patient? Our approach to his care is summarized in the section below.

The Refugee Clinic, located within the internal medicine department, is specifically resourced to address many of his needs. He was connected to social work services, which began to help him obtain Medicaid health insurance, social security, and complete housing and childcare support applications. He was also referred to the onsite therapeutic food pantry, which is integrated with the Boston Medical Center Rooftop Garden and Teaching Kitchen, where nutrition education, cooking skills, and access to registered dieticians are provided to all patients within the health system.[72] The teaching kitchen is also integrated into the specialty diabetes education program, which is staffed by members of the endocrinology department. Evening group educational sessions are scheduled where PWD meet with each other, along with CDCES, chefs, registered dieticians, and clinical pharmacists. A portion of each session is devoted to demonstrating culinary skills and a portion is devoted to basic diabetes and nutritional educational content. After connecting with diabetes care services through his referral to the teaching kitchen, he established a working relationship with a registered dietician/CDCES, with particular expertise in T1D and diabetes technology, who is based in the specialty diabetes clinic and works closely with an endocrinologist who is part of the T1D QI team in the department. Soon after establishing care in the endocrinology department, he was offered the opportunity to begin on CGM and was connected with our diabetes technology administrative navigator who worked with his Medicaid insurance plan and durable medical equipment providers to support initiation of CGM. He was also connected with an integrated behavioral health clinician working in the refugee health clinic to help manage his PTSD and depression while he established primary care at a local internal medicine practice within the medical center. At this practice, he was referred to work with a clinical pharmacist/CDCES with a strong focus on diabetes care. The group of pharmacists in this practice routinely meets every 1 to 2 weeks with a specialist diabetologist in the academic medical center for an hour-long zoom-based tele-mentoring session where patient cases are discussed and specialty input is sought. During one of these sessions, his case and pertinent Dexcom G6 CGM data were presented, and recommendations were relayed for implementation into his care plan. Despite an improvement in his A1c to 8.3%, he was noted to have recurrent post-prandial hypoglycemia with hypoglycemic unawareness and was encouraged to enroll in the AID/insulin pump education program by his care team. Despite initial hesitancy, he entered the educational program, which is staffed by specialty diabetes clinic RD/CDCES clinicians and spent 16 hours in direct one-on-one education sessions over a period of 8 months learning the specific skills to succeed on the Tandem T-slim X2 pump with Control IQ. His educational process was not smooth. His education progress was interrupted numerous times to attend to ill health in his family, failed efforts to secure a steady job, immigration and legal challenges, and mental health struggles. However, with the support of the numerous clinicians, administrators, educators, food services, and the safety net system at large, he currently is doing well on the Tandem AID system and has an A1c of 7.8% with time in range (70–180 mg/dL) of 50% to 65%, time below range consistently less than 2%, has secured stable housing and has started to take up running again.

DISCLOSURE

The authors do not have any significant disclosures that are relevant to this work.

REFERENCES

1. Association AD. 2. Classification and Diagnosis of Diabetes. Diabetes Care 2021; 44(Suppl 1):S15–33.
2. Association AD. 7. Diabetes Technology. Diabetes Care 2021;44(Suppl 1): S85–99.
3. Brown SA, Kovatchev BP, Raghinaru D, et al. Six-Month Randomized, Multicenter Trial of Closed-Loop Control in Type 1 Diabetes. N Engl J Med 2019;381(18): 1707–17.
4. Bergenstal RM, Garg S, Weinzimer SA, et al. Safety of a Hybrid Closed-Loop Insulin Delivery System in Patients With Type 1 Diabetes. JAMA 2016;316(13): 1407–8.
5. Beck RW, Riddlesworth T, Ruedy K, et al. Effect of Continuous Glucose Monitoring on Glycemic Control in Adults With Type 1 Diabetes Using Insulin Injections: The DIAMOND Randomized Clinical Trial. JAMA 2017;317(4):371–8.
6. Tamborlane WV, Beck RW, Bode BW, et al. Continuous glucose monitoring and intensive treatment of type 1 diabetes. N Engl J Med 2008;359(14):1464–76.
7. Miller KM, Beck RW, Foster NC, et al. HbA1c Levels in Type 1 Diabetes from Early Childhood to Older Adults: A Deeper Dive into the Influence of Technology and Socioeconomic Status on HbA1c in the T1D Exchange Clinic Registry Findings. Diabetes Technol Therapeut 2020;22(9):645–50.
8. Fantasia KL, Wirunsawanya K, Lee C, et al. Racial Disparities in Diabetes Technology Use and Outcomes in Type 1 Diabetes in a Safety-Net Hospital. J Diabetes Sci Technol 2021;15(5):1010–7.
9. Agarwal S, Hilliard M, Butler A. Disparities in Care Delivery and Outcomes in Young Adults With Diabetes. Curr Diabetes Rep 2018;18(9):65.
10. Agarwal S, Schechter C, Gonzalez J, et al. Racial-Ethnic Disparities in Diabetes Technology use Among Young Adults with Type 1 Diabetes. Diabetes Technol Therapeut 2021;23(4):306–13.
11. Ju Z, Piarulli A, Bielick L, et al. Advanced Diabetes Technology Remains Underutilized in Underserved Populations: Early Hybrid Closed-Loop System Experience at an Academic Safety Net Hospital. Diabetes Technol Therapeut 2021.
12. Odugbesan O, Addala A, Nelson G, et al. Implicit Racial-Ethnic and Insurance-Mediated Bias to Recommending Diabetes Technology: Insights from T1D Exchange Multicenter Pediatric and Adult Diabetes Provider Cohort. Diabetes Technol Ther 2022;24(9):619–27.
13. Addala A, Hanes S, Naranjo D, et al. Provider Implicit Bias Impacts Pediatric Type 1 Diabetes Technology Recommendations in the United States: Findings from The Gatekeeper Study. J Diabetes Sci Technol 2021;15(5):1027–33.
14. Fantasia KL, Demers LB, Steenkamp DW, et al. An Opportunity for Improvement: Evaluation of Diabetes Technology Education Among Adult Endocrinology Training Programs. J Diabetes Sci Technol 2022. https://doi.org/10.1177/ 19322968221077132. 19322968221077132.

15. Ladd JM, Sharma A, Rahme E, et al. Comparison of Socioeconomic Disparities in Pump Uptake Among Children With Type 1 Diabetes in 2 Canadian Provinces With Different Payment Models. JAMA Netw Open 2022;5(5):e2210464.
16. McKergow E, Parkin L, Barson DJ, et al. Demographic and regional disparities in insulin pump utilization in a setting of universal funding: a New Zealand nationwide study. Acta Diabetol 2017;54(1):63–71.
17. Eakin EG, Bull SS, Glasgow RE, et al. Reaching those most in need: a review of diabetes self-management interventions in disadvantaged populations. Diabetes Metab Res Rev 2002;18(1):26–35.
18. Fegan-Bohm K, Minard CG, Anderson BJ, et al. Diabetes distress and HbA1c in racially/ethnically and socioeconomically diverse youth with type 1 diabetes. Pediatr Diabetes 2020;21(7):1362–9.
19. Kesavadev J, Srinivasan S, Saboo B, et al. The Do-It-Yourself Artificial Pancreas: A Comprehensive Review. Diabetes Ther 2020;11(6):1217–35.
20. Powers MA, Bardsley JK, Cypress M, et al. Diabetes Self-management Education and Support in Adults With Type 2 Diabetes: A Consensus Report of the American Diabetes Association, the Association of Diabetes Care and Education Specialists, the Academy of Nutrition and Dietetics, the American Academy of Family Physicians, the American Academy of PAs, the American Association of Nurse Practitioners, and the American Pharmacists Association. Diabetes Care 2020.
21. Duncan I, Ahmed T, Li QE, et al. Assessing the value of the diabetes educator. Diabetes Educat 2011;37(5):638–57.
22. EH W. The role of patient care teams in chronic disease management. Br Med J 2000;569–72.
23. Davidson MB. Effect of nurse-directed diabetes care in a minority population. Diabetes Care 2003;26(8):2281–7.
24. Satia JA. Diet-related disparities: understanding the problem and accelerating solutions. J Am Diet Assoc 2009;109(4):610–5.
25. Golden SH, Joseph JJ, Hill-Briggs F. Casting a Health Equity Lens on Endocrinology and Diabetes. J Clin Endocrinol Metab 2021;106(4):e1909–16.
26. Modzelewski KL, Murati J, Charoenngam N, et al. Delays in Continuous Glucose Monitoring Device Initiation: A Single Center Experience and a Call to Change. Diabetes Technol Therapeut 2022;24(6):390–5.
27. Kelley AT, Nocon RS, O'Brien MJ. Diabetes Management in Community Health Centers: a Review of Policies and Programs. Curr Diabetes Rep 2020;20(2):8.
28. Pottie K, Hadi A, Chen J, et al. Realist review to understand the efficacy of culturally appropriate diabetes education programmes. Diabet Med 2013;30(9):1017–25.
29. Ebekozien O, Mungmode A, Buckingham D, et al. Achieving Equity in Diabetes Research: Borrowing From the Field of Quality Improvement Using a Practical Framework and Improvement Tools. Diabetes Spectr 2022;35(3):304–12.
30. Ebekozien O, Mungmode A, Odugbesan O, et al. Addressing type 1 diabetes health inequities in the United States: Approaches from the T1D Exchange QI Collaborative. J Diabetes 2022;14(1):79–82.
31. Agarwal S, Crespo-Ramos G, Long JA, et al. "I Didn't Really Have a Choice": Qualitative Analysis of Racial-Ethnic Disparities in Diabetes Technology Use Among Young Adults with Type 1 Diabetes. Diabetes Technol Therapeut 2021;23(9):616–22.
32. Ndjaboue R, Chipenda Dansokho S, Boudreault B, et al. Patients' perspectives on how to improve diabetes care and self-management: qualitative study. BMJ Open 2020;10(4):e032762.

33. Torres-Ruiz M, Robinson-Ector K, Attinson D, et al. A Portfolio Analysis of Culturally Tailored Trials to Address Health and Healthcare Disparities. Int J Environ Res Public Health 2018;15(9).

34. Moore G, Campbell M, Copeland L, et al. Adapting interventions to new contexts-the ADAPT guidance. BMJ 2021;374:n1679.

35. Sheridan S, Schrandt S, Forsythe L, et al. The PCORI Engagement Rubric: Promising Practices for Partnering in Research. Ann Fam Med 2017;15(2):165–70.

36. Robert G, Cornwell J, Locock L, et al. Patients and staff as codesigners of healthcare services. BMJ 2015;350:g7714.

37. AuYoung M, Moin T, Richardson CR, et al. The Diabetes Prevention Program for Underserved Populations: A Brief Review of Strategies in the Real World. Diabetes Spectr 2019;32(4):312–7.

38. Williams JH, Auslander WF, de Groot M, et al. Cultural relevancy of a diabetes prevention nutrition program for African American women. Health Promot Pract 2006;7(1):56–67.

39. Singh H, Fulton J, Mirzazada S, et al. Community-Based Culturally Tailored Education Programs for Black Communities with Cardiovascular Disease, Diabetes, Hypertension, and Stroke: Systematic Review Findings. J Racial Ethn Health Disparities 2022. https://doi.org/10.1007/s40615-022-01474-5.

40. Peek ME, Harmon SA, Scott SJ, et al. Culturally tailoring patient education and communication skills training to empower African-Americans with diabetes. Transl Behav Med 2012;2(3):296–308.

41. Guo J, Luo J, Huang L, et al. Adaptation and Feasibility Testing of a Coping Skills Training Program for Chinese Youth with Type 1 Diabetes. J Pediatr Nurs 2020;54: e78–83.

42. Rouf S, Rbiai N, Baibai K, et al. Feasibility and Efficiency of a Novel Bolus Calculator (IF-DIABETE) for Patients With Type 1 Diabetes: A Nonrandomized Single-Arm Pilot Study. Cureus 2021;13(1):e12646.

43. Berlin KS, Klages KL, Banks GG, et al. Toward the Development of a Culturally Humble Intervention to Improve Glycemic Control and Quality of Life among Adolescents with Type-1 Diabetes and Their Families. Behav Med 2021;47(2): 99–110.

44. Rose M, Aronow L, Breen S, et al. Considering Culture: A Review of Pediatric Behavioral Intervention Research in Type 1 Diabetes. Curr Diabetes Rep 2018; 18(4):16.

45. Wolpert HA, Anderson BJ. Management of diabetes: are doctors framing the benefits from the wrong perspective? BMJ 2001;323(7319):994–6.

46. Vigersky RA, Fish L, Hogan P, et al. The clinical endocrinology workforce: current status and future projections of supply and demand. J Clin Endocrinol Metab 2014;99(9):3112–21.

47. Lal RA, Cuttriss N, Haller MJ, et al. Primary Care Providers in California and Florida Report Low Confidence in Providing Type 1 Diabetes Care. Clin Diabetes 2020;38(2):159–65.

48. O'Donovan A, Oser SM, Parascando J, et al. Determining the Perception and Willingness of Primary Care Providers to Prescribe Advanced Diabetes Technologies. J Patient Cent Res Rev 2021;8(3):272–6.

49. Bergenstal RM, Nimri R, Beck RW, et al. A comparison of two hybrid closed-loop systems in adolescents and young adults with type 1 diabetes (FLAIR): a multicentre, randomised, crossover trial. Lancet 2021;397(10270):208–19.

50. Forlenza GP, Breton MD, Kovatchev BP. Candidate Selection for Hybrid Closed Loop Systems. Diabetes Technol Ther 2021;23(11):760–2.

51. Riddell MC, Davis EA, Mayer-Davis EJ, et al. Advances in Exercise and Nutrition as Therapy in Diabetes. Diabetes Technol Therapeut 2021;23(S2):S131–42.
52. Riddell MC, Gallen IW, Smart CE, et al. Exercise management in type 1 diabetes: a consensus statement. Lancet Diabetes Endocrinol 2017;5(5):377–90.
53. Morrison D, Paldus B, Zaharieva DP, et al. Late Afternoon Vigorous Exercise Increases Postmeal but Not Overnight Hypoglycemia in Adults with Type 1 Diabetes Managed with Automated Insulin Delivery. Diabetes Technol Therapeut 2022;24(12):873–80.
54. Riddell MC, Li Z, Gal RL, et al. Examining the Acute Glycemic Effects of Different Types of Structured Exercise Sessions in Type 1 Diabetes in a Real-World Setting: The Type 1 Diabetes and Exercise Initiative (T1DEXI). Diabetes Care 2023;46(4):704–13.
55. Hernán MA, Hernández-Díaz S. Beyond the intention-to-treat in comparative effectiveness research. Clin Trials 2012;9(1):48–55.
56. Hernán MA, Robins JM. Per-Protocol Analyses of Pragmatic Trials. N Engl J Med 2017;377(14):1391–8.
57. Spanakis EK, Golden SH. Race/ethnic difference in diabetes and diabetic complications. Curr Diabetes Rep 2013;13(6):814–23.
58. McCoy RG, Galindo RJ, Swarna KS, et al. Sociodemographic, Clinical, and Treatment-Related Factors Associated With Hyperglycemic Crises Among Adults With Type 1 or Type 2 Diabetes in the US From 2014 to 2020. JAMA Netw Open 2021;4(9):e2123471.
59. Walker AF, Hood KK, Gurka MJ, et al. Barriers to Technology Use and Endocrinology Care for Underserved Communities With Type 1 Diabetes. Diabetes Care 2021;44(7):1480–90.
60. Kanbour S, Jones M, Abusamaan MS, et al. Racial Disparities in Access and Use of Diabetes Technology Among Adult Patients With Type 1 Diabetes in a U.S. Academic Medical Center. Diabetes Care 2023;46(1):56–64.
61. Foster NC, Beck RW, Miller KM, et al. State of Type 1 Diabetes Management and Outcomes from the T1D Exchange in 2016-2018. Diabetes Technol Therapeut 2019;21(2):66–72.
62. Bauer MS, Damschroder L, Hagedorn H, et al. An introduction to implementation science for the non-specialist. BMC Psychol 2015;3(1):32.
63. Backhouse A, Ogunlayi F. Quality improvement into practice. BMJ 2020;368:m865.
64. Shelton RC, Chambers DA, Glasgow RE. An Extension of RE-AIM to Enhance Sustainability: Addressing Dynamic Context and Promoting Health Equity Over Time. Front Public Health 2020;8:134.
65. Woodward EN, Matthieu MM, Uchendu US, et al. The health equity implementation framework: proposal and preliminary study of hepatitis C virus treatment. Implement Sci 2019;14(1):26.
66. Eslava-Schmalbach J, Garzón-Orjuela N, Elias V, et al. Conceptual framework of equity-focused implementation research for health programs (EquIR). Int J Equity Health 2019;18(1):80.
67. Powell BJ, Waltz TJ, Chinman MJ, et al. A refined compilation of implementation strategies: results from the Expert Recommendations for Implementing Change (ERIC) project. Implement Sci 2015;10:21.
68. Tyler A, Glasgow RE. Implementing Improvements: Opportunities to Integrate Quality Improvement and Implementation Science. Hosp Pediatr 2021;11(5):536–45.

69. America IoMUCoQoHCi. Crossing the Quality Chasm: A New Health System for the 21st Century. 2001.
70. Curran GM, Bauer M, Mittman B, et al. Effectiveness-implementation hybrid designs: combining elements of clinical effectiveness and implementation research to enhance public health impact. Med Care 2012;50(3):217–26.
71. Leppin AL, Mahoney JE, Stevens KR, et al. Situating dissemination and implementation sciences within and across the translational research spectrum - ADDENDUM. J Clin Transl Sci 2020;4(4):371.
72. Weinstein O, Donovan K, McCarthy AC, et al. Nourishing Underserved Populations Despite Scarcer Resources: Adaptations of an Urban Safety Net Hospital During the COVID-19 Pandemic. Am J Public Health 2021;111(4):663–6.

Emerging Technologies and Therapeutics for Type 1 Diabetes

Halis Kaan Akturk, MD[a],*, Alexis M. McKee, MD[b]

KEYWORDS

- Type 1 diabetes • Continuous glucose monitoring • Hybrid closed loop
- Smart insulin pens

KEY POINTS

- Diabetes technologies are evolving, and new generation continuous glucose monitors and hybrid-closed loop systems are changing lives of the people with type 1 diabetes.
- The efforts for a cure have been moving forward with stem cell research and gene editing.
- New adjunctive therapies in type 1 diabetes are ready for phase 3 clinical trials.
- Digital technologies and smart pen sleeves and caps are helping day-to-day diabetes management and decreasing the burden of type 1 diabetes.

INTRODUCTION

Advancements in diabetes technologies in recent years changed the landscape of type 1 diabetes (T1D) management.[1] Increasing the use of continuous glucose monitors (CGM) and hybrid closed loop (HCL) insulin pumps decrease A1c and hypoglycemia while improving time in range and quality of life.[1-3] A recent study investigated the changes in diabetes technology use from 2016 to 2020 in 1455 patients with T1D.[4] CGM use increased from 32.9% to 75.3%, and HCL use increased from 0.3% to 27.9%. Overall, A1C decreased from 8.9% to 8.6% ($P < .0001$).[4] Early initiation of the diabetes technologies have better outcomes, such as initiation of CGM in the first year of T1D diagnosis has been shown to be associated with significantly lower A1c in 7 years.[5] However, access to these technologies are still a problem in the United States for some, especially for minorities, due to many reasons including implicit bias, insurance, lack of endocrinologists, and lack of knowledge about these technologies.[6]

[a] Barbara Davis Center for Diabetes, University of Colorado, 1775 Aurora Court, Room 1319, Aurora, CO 80045, USA; [b] Division of Endocrinology, Metabolism & Lipid Research, Washington University in St. Louis School of Medicine, St Louis, MO, USA
* Corresponding author.
E-mail address: halis.akturk@cuanschutz.edu

Endocrinol Metab Clin N Am 53 (2024) 81–91
https://doi.org/10.1016/j.ecl.2023.07.002
0889-8529/24/© 2023 Elsevier Inc. All rights reserved.

CONTINUOUS GLUCOSE MONITORING SYSTEMS

CGM use has been increasing in the United States in the last decade with the improvements in the systems. New generation CGMs are smaller, have better accuracy as measured with a mean absolute relative difference (MARD), and integrate with HCL systems.[7] New generation FDA-approved CGMs include Dexcom G7, Libre 3, and Eversense E3.

The FreeStyle Libre 3 is a single-use, disposable sensor that is applied to the back of the upper arm and can be worn for 14 days.[8] It is the smallest CGM to date and is a real-time CGM with 1 piece applicator unlike the 1st and 2nd generation Libre series. It has vitamin C interference over 500 mg, similar to Libre 2. Recently, the FDA approved a reader device that displays real-time glucose readings. The US FDA cleared Free-Style Libre 2 and FreeStyle Libre 3 sensors for integration with automated insulin delivery systems. The modified sensors were also cleared for use by children as young as 2 years old and for wear time up to 15 days. Current FreeStyle Libre 2 and FreeStyle Libre 3 sensors available today in the United States are approved for people of 4 years and older and have a wear time of up to 14 days. Additionally, the clearance allows for FreeStyle Libre 2 and FreeStyle Libre 3 sensors—both those available today and the modified sensors available in the future—to be used by women with all types of diabetes (type 1, type 2, and gestational) who are pregnant.

Dexcom G7 is 60% smaller than the 6th generation and it has a simplified applicator. Unlike Dexcom G6's 2 hour warm up, the G7 is functional after 30 minutes.[9] Additionally, the sensor and transmitter are combined into one piece with an additional 12 hours of CGM use in between sensor changes.[9] Dexcom G7 users can delay the first alert for high sensor glucose until the sensor reading is at or past the alert setting. It is also FDA-approved to be used in pregnancy. In 316 adults, for arm- and abdomen-placed sensors, overall MARDs were 8.2% and 9.1%, respectively.[10] Overall %15/15, %20/20, and %30/30 agreement rates were 89.6%, 95.3%, and 98.8% for arm-placed sensors and 85.5%, 93.2%, and 98.1% for abdomen-placed sensors.[10] In 127 children, for arm-placed sensors, the overall MARD was 8.1% and overall %15/15, %20/20, and %30/30 agreement rates were 88.8%, 95.3%, and 98.7%, respectively.[11] For abdomen-placed sensors, the overall MARD was 9.0% and overall %15/15, %20/20, and %30/30 agreement rates were 86.0%, 92.9%, and 97.7%, respectively.[11] Not surprisingly based on the studies, the FDA-approved Dexcom G7 for only used in the arm.

The Eversense E3 by Senseonics is a 6 month implantable CGM. To date, it is the only FDA-approved implantable CGM in the United States. It is approved to be used in adults with diabetes and should be calibrated 2 times a day in the first 21 days and then once a day rest of 6 month use. It has a 24 hours warm-up time and it is the only CGM with vibration alerts with a wearable transmitter.[12] In a study with 90 adults with diabetes, using the current version of the sensor, modified (sacrificial boronic acid) sensor, the percent CGM readings within 20%/20% of yellow springs instruments (YSI) values was 93.9%; overall MARD was 8.5%.[12] The confirmed alert detection rate at 70 mg/dL was 94% and 180 mg/dL was 99%. The median percentage of time for one calibration per day was 63%.[12] About 90% of the sacrificial boronic acid (SBA) sensors survived 180 days.[12]

The use of digital apps may improve diabetes care and quality of life in T1D. One study showed that increased engagement with a CGM app can increase time in range, decrease hypoglycemia rate, and help remote monitoring of loved ones with T1D.[13] More research is necessary to determine their benefits in long term in T1D care.

HYBRID CLOSED LOOPS

Currently, the FDA-approved HCL systems in the United States are Medtronic 670/770/780G series, Tandem Control IQ, Omnipod 5, and iLet Bionic Pancreas.

Medtronic 780G is the latest HCL from Medtronic that has been in use in Europe since 2020 and was recently FDA approved in April 2023 for T1D patients aged 7 years or older. Compared with 770G, the main differences include an adjustable glucose target for "SmartGuard," that is called auto mode in this system. Glucose targets can be 100, 110, and 120 mg/dL.[14] Of note, 100 mg/dL is the lowest target in any FDA-approved HCL system to date. The new autocorrect feature delivers small auto boluses for high glucose that can be turned on and off independently. The 780G can be used in patients requiring between 8 and 250 units of insulin per day and can be used with Medtronic Guardian 3 or 4 CGM.[14] The Guardian 4 sensor does not require any fingerstick calibrations, and users reported fewer requirements for fingerstick confirmation when going to automation mode with the new system.[15] There is smartwatch access with a mobile app. Users can also use FDA-approved extended infusion set up to 7 days with this system.

As the 780G was recently approved by the FDA in the United States, most of the literature is from Europe and other parts of the world. A recent study with 109 children aged 7 to 17 years and 67 adults with T1D showed that 3 month use of 780G with Guardian 4 CGM was safe and effective.[15] Pediatric and adult A1C were 7.2% ± 0.7% and 6.8% ± 0.7%, respectively, and there were no serious adverse events.[15] Smartguard exits averaged 0.1/d, and there were few blood glucose measurements (0.8/day–1.0/d).[15] Another multicenter observational real-world study investigated the first 6 month of 780G use in 111 children and adolescents aged 7 to 18 years.[16] International Consensus targets for a time in the range were met by 72.1% of the participants.[16] A shorter duration of active insulin time and a lower target of sensor glucose were significant predictors for optimal glycemic control.[16]

A randomized parallel group study evaluated the 780G in insulin pump and CGM naïve adults with T1D transitioning from multiple daily injection (MDI) and self-monitoring blood glucose (SMBG) to 780G.[17] Participants from the 780G group had significant improvements in A1c levels (treatment effect, −0.6% [95% CI −0.9, −0.2]; $P = .005$) and in quality of life compared with MDI + SMBG group.[17] Time spent in the target range (70–180 mg/dL) increased from 69.3% ± 12.3% at baseline to 85.0% ± 6.3% at 3 months in the 780G group, while remaining unchanged in the control group (treatment effect, 21.5% [95% CI 15.7, 27.3]; $P < .001$).[17] The time below range (<70 mg/dL) decreased from 8.7% ± 7.3% to 2.1% ± 1.7% in the HCL group and remained unchanged in the MDI + SMBG group (treatment effect, −4.4% [95% CI −7.4, −2.1]; $P < .001$).[17] On the basis of the data and clinical experience, it seems most useful to use a glucose target of 100 mg/dL and a 2 hour active insulin time with the 780G system.

The Omnipod 5 is an HCL system that uses a patch insulin pump which is controlled with a smartphone app or a controller device.[18,19] It is the only system that considers CGM trends in decision making in the algorithm. The target can be customized from 110 to 150 mg/dL in 10 mg/dL increments.[18] In a study including 111 children and 124 adults with T1D in 3 months, A_{1c} was significantly reduced in children by 0.71% (mean ± SD: 7.67% ± 0.95% to 6.99% ± 0.63%, $P < .0001$) and in adults by 0.38% (7.16% ± 0.86% to 6.78% ± 0.68%, $P < .0001$).[18] Time in range was improved from standard therapy by 15.6% ± 11.5% or 3.7 hour/day in children and 9.3% ± 11.8% or 2.2 hour/day in adults (both $P < .0001$).[18]

iLet Bionic Pancreas is the newest FDA-approved HCL system. The system is programed using the user's weight and can be alerted to meal announcements by the individual, but it does not require carb counting. In a 13 week clinical trial of 219 participants of 6 to 79 years of age with T1D assigned to the bionic pancreas or standard of care,[20] the A1c decreased from 7.9% to 7.3% in the bionic-pancreas group and remained unchanged in the standard-care group (mean adjusted difference at 13 weeks, −0.5% points; 95% confidence interval [CI], −0.6 to −0.3; P < .001).[20] Of note, the minorities (all non-White participants) decreased A1c more than Whites. In Whites (n = 240), the mean baseline-adjusted difference in 13 week A1c between the bionic pancreas group and standard of care group was −0.45% (95% CI −0.61 to −0.29; P < .001), while this difference among Minorities (n = 84) was −0.53% (−0.83 to −0.24; P < .001).[21]

The Tandem Control IQ system works by automatically increasing the programed basal insulin delivery rate when glucose levels are predicted to exceed 160 mg/dL.[22] In addition to modulating the basal rates, the system can also deliver an automatic correction bolus dose of insulin if glucose levels are predicted to increase above 180 mg/dL. This occurs up to once per hour during normal operation and delivers 60% of the dose calculated based on the user's insulin sensitivity (ISF) factor.[12] In a real-world use study with 9451 users, at baseline, the median percent time in range was 63.6 (interquartile range [IQR]: 49.9%–75.6%) and increased to 73.6% (IQR: 64.4%–81.8%) for the 12 months of Control IQ technology use with no significant changes over time.[23] A study with 4243 Medicare and 1332 Medicaid users of Control IQ showed that after starting Control IQ, the Medicare group had significant improvement in TIR (64% vs 74%; P < .0001), and the Medicaid group also had significant improvement in TIR (46% vs 60%; P < .0001).[24]

The auto bolus feature in the newer HCL systems has the ability to compensate for missed boluses, which is advantageous for busy professionals, adolescents, those facing challenges with carbohydrate counting, adolescents, and older adults with T1D. A recent study with 780G with 34 adolescents with T1D compared the fix group (simplified meal announcement by preset of 3 personalized fixed carbohydrate amounts) or the flex group (precise carbohydrate counting) and followed for 12 weeks.[25] The TIR was 73.5% ± 6.7% in the fix and 80.3% ± 7.4% in the flex group, with a between-group difference of 6.8% in favor of flex (P = .043).[25] Time greater than 250 mg/dL was better in the flex group (P = .012), whereas A1c (P = .168), time below range (P = .283), and time between 180 and 250 mg/dL (P = .114) did not differ.[25] Another study evaluated Tandem Control IQ in 30 adults with groups (n = 10) with minimal or no user-initiated boluses (auto >90%) compared with age, gender, and diabetes duration-matched adults with T1D with intermediate (auto 50%–90%) and high bolusing behavior (auto 10%–49%).[22] Compared with baseline, there was a significant decrease in A1c by 1.6%% ± 0.8% and an increase in time in range by 19.3% ± 6.4% (P < .001 for both) over 12 months of Tandem Control IQ use in auto greater than 90% use group without increasing time below range.[22] While it is not advised to miss boluses or bolus late with these HCL systems, newer generation HCL systems can compensate which opens the door for individuals who are not strict carbohydrate counters to still be candidates for HCL systems.

HCL systems have been reported to be used successfully in special situations such as pregnancy, diabetic gastroparesis, and cystic fibrosis-related diabetes; however, their safety and efficacy should be investigated in larger clinical trials.[26–29]

SMART INSULIN PENS, PEN CAPS

The development of new smart insulin pens with connectivity is a promising approach for improving and simplifying the management of T1D. The published literature on smart insulin pens with connectivity is limited.[30] However, they may offer the potential for increased adherence to quality of life and monitoring with the documentation of insulin administrations and mimicking an insulin pump use with some features for bolusing.[30]

Smart Insulin Pens

Smart insulin pens are devices that assist individuals with T1D in insulin dosing calculations. Currently, there are 2 smart insulin pens available in the United States: InPen and NovoPen Echo. The InPen device connects with the users with compatible Android or iOS smartphones to an app that can be programed by their diabetes provider. The InPen app can store fixed doses of mealtime insulin, provide meal-estimated insulin doses or operate on insulin-to-carbohydrate and ISF inputs. The InPen allows for connectivity to the Medtronic Guardian 3 sensor and to Dexcom G6 CGM. It has other features that allow for reminders to be set for insulin administration and tracking of the expiration of insulin in the cartridge and insulin on board.[31] Reports can be generated for providers to review and discuss with the patient. The InPen is compatible with Lispro, Aspart, and faster Aspart cartridges. The pen injector allows the user to dial the desired dose from 0.5 to 30 units in one-half unit increments.[31]

The NovoPen Echo stores both the timing and the amount of insulin delivered which can later be downloaded for review.[32] This pen works with Aspart 100 unit/mL cartridges containing a total of 300 units and can deliver in 0.5 unit increments up to 30 units. The digital display shows how many units of insulin are injected in hourly segments and tracks battery life.[32]

Pen Caps

The Bigfoot Unity Diabetes Management System, approved in August 2021, uses a smart insulin pen cap that is compatible with the typical disposable insulin pens. It works by scanning the FreeStyle Libre 2 sensor with the pen cap.[33] On basis of settings, the recommended insulin dose is displayed along with the CGM glucose and glucose trend arrow. The BigFoot Unity system includes 2 types of pen caps: one for rapid-acting bolus insulin and one for long-acting basal insulin.[33] The timing of the insulin is recorded. Two real-time glucose alarms are available, including a mandatory alarm for glucose at 55 mg/dL or lower and an optional glucose alarm at 70 mg/dL. If the basal insulin dose is missed over a 24 hour period, the patient is also alerted. The pen cap itself lasts 2 years and is rechargeable.

Tempo pen cap with its app from Eli Lilly, works with all Eli Lilly insulins, bolus, and basal. The app can combine the data with readings from Tempo Blood Glucose Meter and/or Dexcom G6 CGM and provides personalized progress reports to assist with the self-management of diabetes.[34]

DISPARITIES IN THE USE OF DIABETES TECHNOLOGY IN TYPE 1 DIABETES

Despite major advances in diabetes technology over the last 2 decades, it is clear that there are substantial disparities in their utilization.[35] Much of the data to date on disparities in technology utilization are generated by the T1D Exchange QI Collaborative, a network of adult and pediatric diabetes centers in the United States. Overall, the T1D data show that technology utilization is low in individuals from minority and lower socioeconomic backgrounds in both pediatric and adult populations.[36-39]

Outside of the T1D registry, disparities in insulin pump utilization have been demonstrated by studies examining large electronic health databases in the United States. In a retrospective cohort analysis of young adult patients with T1D, low insulin pump utilization was shown, particularly in Black and Hispanic minorities, males and individuals with governmental insurance despite insulin pump showing superior HbA1c control without an increase in DKA events.[40] This study also noted that it was unclear why Black and Hispanic subjects had lower odds of receiving insulin pump therapy but wrote that it may, in part, be due to the provider's unconscious or conscious bias.[40]

Overall, there is a movement to have greater racial/ethnic diversity in diabetes technology trials to overcome these barriers and move toward more equitable prescribing of these life-changing technologies.

INPATIENT USE OF CONTINUE GLUCOSE MONITORING

Few areas of medicine have advanced as quickly as the landscape of diabetes technology including major leaps forward in insulin pumps, CGM, and automated insulin delivery systems. As the utilization of these devices expands in the outpatient setting, invariably, they have made their way into the hospital. Before coronavirus-19 (COVID-19), CGM was studied with a vision for glucose telemetry by Spanakis.[41] In March 2020, the World Health Organization declared COVID-19 a pandemic and subsequently the FDA issued emergency authorization of inpatient use of CGM to preserve personal protective equipment (PPE) which was in short supply.[42] After these measures, several observational studies aimed to establish the feasibility and accuracy of inpatient CGM were published demonstrating the utility of inpatient CGM to reduce both hypo and hyper glycemia. Additional benefits included decreased frequency of point-of-care (POC) glucose checks and decreased utilization of PPE.

In a retrospective study analyzing 218 patients with matched-pair CGM (Dexcom G6) and capillary POC glucose data from 3 inpatient CGM studies of noncritically ill hospitalized patients, the overall MARD was 12.8%.[43] The results of the Clarke error grid analyses showed 98.7% of values where in zones A and B indicating that discrepancies between CGM and POC glucose data would have little-to-no effect on the clinical outcome. Overall, these findings are reassuring that in noncritically ill hospitalized patients, CGM is a reliable tool for monitoring glucose values.

In terms of clinical outcomes, inpatient CGM-guided (Dexcom G6) insulin administration in hospitalized patients with diabetes has been shown in a randomized clinical trial to produce similar glycemic control but a significant reduction in hypoglycemic events when compared with usual care POC-guided insulin adjustment.[44]

According to an Endocrine Society Clinical Practice Guideline, adults with insulin-treated diabetes hospitalized for noncritical illness who are at high risk of hypoglycemia, CGM with adjunctive POC glucose monitoring is recommended.[45]

STEM CELL THERAPIES

The history of islet cell transplantation brought to light the ability of β cells to engraft and function after transplantation, giving rise to an arm of regenerative therapies for T1D.[46] A promising technique currently under study is the ability to transplant human stem cell (SC)-derived β cells, which has advantages over traditional islet transplantation which is limited by pancreatic tissue availability and the need for immunosuppression.[47] Human pluripotent SCs, both embryonic and induced pluripotent, garner the most enthusiasm for creating functional β cells that will be able to divide and differentiate.[48,49]

Recently, ViaCyte created a SC-derived pancreatic endoderm cell population, referred to as PEC-01, which matured into insulin-producing endocrine cells in rodent models.[50] The first iteration of this technology in 2014 was flawed by a foreign body response to the device encapsulation component, which led to fibrosis and loss of insulin secretion.[50] In the second iteration in 2017, the PEC-direct device was engineered to allow for an opening where vasculature could penetrate allowing for nutrient exchange.[50] This technique was overall successful, and the grafts showed measurable c-peptide. However, the vasculature allowed for interaction between the host cells and the device, which led to the need for immunosuppression.

Interestingly, in addition to demonstrating β cell function, many of the cells stained positive for α cells secreting glucagon.[50]

To overcome the issues of graft fibrosis and the need for immunosuppression, the Vertex Pharmaceuticals began a human clinical trial with T1D patients in 2021 where a SC-derived product, VX-880, was transplanted without an immune-protective device. Initial findings seem promising and await peer review.[50]

In March 2023, Vertex announced FDA Clearance of Investigational New Drug Application for VX-264, a novel encapsulated cell therapy for the treatment of T1D.[51] VX-264, an allogeneic human SC-derived islets are encapsulated in a channel array device designed to shield the cells from the body's immune system and to be surgically implanted. Vertex initiates a Phase 1/2 clinical trial to study the safety, tolerability, and efficacy of VX-264 in patients with T1D. The company previously received approval from Health Canada on the Clinical Trial Application for VX-264, and the Phase 1/2 trial is ongoing in Canada. The clinical trial is a Phase 1/2, single-arm, open-label study in patients who have T1D. Approximately 17 patients will be enrolled in the global clinical trial.

Challenges in the regenerative SC therapies for T1D remain, particularly in terms of the ability to generate a highly functional, uniform cell-based product for transplantation that does not require immunosuppression.[50]

ADJUNCTIVE THERAPIES IN TYPE 1 DIABETES

Despite advanced diabetes technologies and therapeutics, many people with T1D do not achieve target A1c levels and have problems with high postprandial blood glucose, weight gain, and increased insulin resistance.[52] A need exists for adjunctive therapies to insulin in the management of T1D to prevent long-term complications and achieve better glycemic profiles. In the last decade, many medications used in the treatment of type 2 diabetes have been tried in T1D such as metformin, glucagon-like peptide-1 receptor agonists, and sodium-glucose cotransporter 2 inhibitors (SGLT2i).[53] The use of SGLT2i in T1D as an adjunctive therapy has been approved in Europe and Japan with some limitations; however, the US FDA denied its use in T1D due to an increased risk of diabetic ketoacidosis.[54] Since then, new molecules have been developed as an adjunct therapy in T1D.

Volagidemab, an antagonistic monoclonal glucagon receptor antibody, was evaluated in a phase 2 placebo-controlled randomized trial in 13 weeks as an adjunctive therapy to T1D.[55] Eligible participants ($n = 79$) were randomized to receive weekly subcutaneous injections of placebo, 35 mg volagidemab, or 70 mg volagidemab.[55] At week 13, the placebo-corrected reduction in A1c percentage was −0.53 (95% CI = −0.89 to −0.17, nominal $P = .004$) in the 35 mg volagidemab group and −0.49 (95% CI = −0.85 to −0.12, nominal $P = .010$) in the 70 mg volagidemab group.[55] There was no change in weight or increase in hypoglycemia. However, there was an increase in liver transaminase levels, blood pressure, and LDL cholesterol.

TTP399, a novel hepatoselective glucokinase activator, was investigated in a phase 1b/2 study in people with T1D.[56] The SimpliciT1 was a placebo-controlled randomized study that used 800 mg TTP399 or matched placebo for 12 weeks.[56] The difference in change in A_{1c} from baseline to week 12 between TTP399 and placebo was −0.7% in CGM and insulin pump users.[56] There was no increase in hypoglycemia frequency.

SUMMARY

Diabetes technologies and therapeutics for the management of T1D rapidly evolved in the last decade. CGM, HCL, smart insulin pens, digital apps, and newer rapid and long-acting insulins are the mainstay of current T1D management. Emerging therapies for a cure in T1D are ongoing, and they are more promising than ever, while newer adjunctive therapies are likely to be approved to decrease insulin requirements, weight, and A1c. Future focus areas for diabetes technology include decreasing disparities in T1D care and increasing utilization of these devices in inpatient settings and pregnancy. As new developments materialize, the hope is to reach the lowest rates of complications in diabetes in history and decrease the burden of diabetes for those living with this disease.

CLINICS CARE POINTS

- Diabetes technologies should be used in all people with T1D with a motivation, a follow plan, and a good comprehension.
- Providers should discuss diabetes technologies with all people with T1D to find a good fit for their lives.
- Providers should focus on decreasing disparities in diabetes technology use and encourage minorities to be involved in clinical trials.

DISCLOSURES

H.K. Akturk reports receiving research funding through University of Colorado from Medtronic, Tandem Diabetes, Eli Lilly & Co, United States, Dexcom, United States, Senseonics, Mannkind, Jaeb Center, IAFNS, United States; consulting fees through University of Colorado from Dexcom, Medtronic, Tandem Diabetes. A.M. McKee has participated on advisory boards for Medtronic Inc. and Novo Nordisk.

REFERENCES

1. Akturk HK, Garg S. Technological advances shaping diabetes care. Curr Opin Endocrinol Diabetes Obes 2019;26:84–9.
2. Berget C, Akturk HK, Messer LH, et al. Real-world performance of hybrid closed loop in youth, young adults, adults and older adults with type 1 diabetes: Identifying a clinical target for hybrid closed-loop use. Diabetes Obes Metabol 2021; 23:2048–57.
3. Akturk HK, Giordano D, Champakanath A, et al. Long-term real-life glycaemic outcomes with a hybrid closed-loop system compared with sensor-augmented pump therapy in patients with type 1 diabetes. Diabetes Obes Metabol 2020; 22:583–9.
4. Alonso GT, Triolo TM, Akturk HK, et al. Increased Technology Use Associated With Lower A1C in a Large Pediatric Clinical Population. Diabetes Care 2023; 46:1218–22.
5. Champakanath A, Akturk HK, Alonso GT, et al. Continuous Glucose Monitoring Initiation Within First Year of Type 1 Diabetes Diagnosis Is Associated With Improved Glycemic Outcomes: 7-Year Follow-Up Study. Diabetes Care 2022;45:750–3.
6. Akturk HK, Rompicherla S, Rioles N, et al. Factors Associated With Improved A1C Among Adults With Type 1 Diabetes in the United States. Clin Diabetes 2022;41: 76–80.
7. Garg SK, Akturk HK. A New Era in Continuous Glucose Monitoring: Food and Drug Administration Creates a New Category of Factory-Calibrated Nonadjunctive, Interoperable Class II Medical Devices. Diabetes Technol Therapeut 2018;20:391–4.

8. Nguyen A, White JR. FreeStyle Libre 3. Clin Diabetes 2022;41:127–8.
9. Welsh JB, Psavko S, Zhang X, et al. Comparisons of Fifth-, Sixth-, and Seventh-Generation Continuous Glucose Monitoring Systems. J diabetes science and technology 2022. 19322968221099879.
10. Garg SK, Kipnes M, Castorino K, et al. Accuracy and Safety of Dexcom G7 Continuous Glucose Monitoring in Adults with Diabetes. Diabetes Technol Therapeut 2022;24:373–80.
11. Laffel LM, Bailey TS, Christiansen MP, et al. Accuracy of a Seventh-Generation Continuous Glucose Monitoring System in Children and Adolescents With Type 1 Diabetes. J Diabetes Sci Technol 2022. 19322968221091816.
12. Garg SK, Liljenquist D, Bode B, et al. Evaluation of Accuracy and Safety of the Next-Generation Up to 180-Day Long-Term Implantable Eversense Continuous Glucose Monitoring System: The PROMISE Study. Diabetes Technol Therapeut 2022;24:84–92.
13. Akturk HK, Dowd R, Shankar K, et al. Real-World Evidence and Glycemic Improvement Using Dexcom G6 Features. Diabetes Technol Therapeut 2021; 23. S21-s6.
14. Silva JD, Lepore G, Battelino T, et al. Real-World Performance of the MiniMed™ 780G System: First Report of Outcomes from 4120 Users. Diabetes Technol Therapeut 2022;24:113–9.
15. Cordero TL, Dai Z, Arrieta A, et al. Glycemic Outcomes During Early Use of the MiniMed™ 780G Advanced Hybrid Closed-Loop System with Guardian™ 4 Sensor. Diabetes technol ther 2023. https://doi.org/10.1089/dia.2023.0123.
16. Lombardo F, Passanisi S, Alibrandi A, et al. MiniMed 780G Six-Month Use in Children and Adolescents with Type 1 Diabetes: Clinical Targets and Predictors of Optimal Glucose Control. Diabetes Technol Therapeut 2023;25:404–13.
17. Matejko B, Juza A, Kieć-Wilk B, et al. Transitioning of People With Type 1 Diabetes From Multiple Daily Injections and Self-Monitoring of Blood Glucose Directly to MiniMed 780G Advanced Hybrid Closed-Loop System: A Two-Center, Randomized, Controlled Study. Diabetes Care 2022;45:2628–35.
18. Brown SA, Forlenza GP, Bode BW, et al. Multicenter Trial of a Tubeless, On-Body Automated Insulin Delivery System With Customizable Glycemic Targets in Pediatric and Adult Participants With Type 1 Diabetes. Diabetes Care 2021;44: 1630–40.
19. Cobry EC, Berget C, Messer LH, et al. Review of the Omnipod(®) 5 Automated Glucose Control System Powered by Horizon™ for the treatment of Type 1 diabetes. Ther Deliv 2020;11:507–19.
20. Russell SJ, Beck RW, Damiano ER, et al. Multicenter, Randomized Trial of a Bionic Pancreas in Type 1 Diabetes. N Engl J Med 2022;387:1161–72.
21. Castellanos LE, Russell SJ, Damiano ER, et al. The Insulin-Only Bionic Pancreas Improves Glycemic Control in Non-Hispanic White and Minority Adults and Children With Type 1 Diabetes. Diabetes Care 2023;46:1185–90.
22. Akturk HK, Snell-Bergeon J, Shah VN. Efficacy and Safety of Tandem Control IQ Without User-Initiated Boluses in Adults with Uncontrolled Type 1 Diabetes. Diabetes Technol Therapeut 2022;24:779–83.
23. Breton MD, Kovatchev BP. One Year Real-World Use of the Control-IQ Advanced Hybrid Closed-Loop Technology. Diabetes Technol Therapeut 2021;23:601–8.
24. Forlenza GP, Carlson AL, Galindo RJ, et al. Real-World Evidence Supporting Tandem Control-IQ Hybrid Closed-Loop Success in the Medicare and Medicaid Type 1 and Type 2 Diabetes Populations. Diabetes Technol Therapeut 2022;24:814–23.

25. Petrovski G, Campbell J, Pasha M, et al. Simplified Meal Announcement Versus Precise Carbohydrate Counting in Adolescents With Type 1 Diabetes Using the MiniMed 780G Advanced Hybrid Closed Loop System: A Randomized Controlled Trial Comparing Glucose Control. Diabetes Care 2023;46:544–50.
26. Kaur H, Schneider N, Pyle L, et al. Efficacy of Hybrid Closed-Loop System in Adults with Type 1 Diabetes and Gastroparesis. Diabetes Technol Therapeut 2019;21:736–9.
27. Daly A, Hartnell S, Boughton CK, et al. Hybrid Closed-loop to Manage Gastroparesis in People With Type 1 Diabetes: a Case Series. J Diabetes Sci Technol 2021; 15:1216–23.
28. Polsky S, Akturk HK. Case series of a hybrid closed-loop system used in pregnancies in clinical practice. Diabetes/metabolism research and reviews 2020; 36:e3248.
29. Scully KJ, Palani G, Zheng H, et al. The Effect of Control IQ Hybrid Closed Loop Technology on Glycemic Control in Adolescents and Adults with Cystic Fibrosis-Related Diabetes. Diabetes Technol Therapeut 2022;24:446–52.
30. Heinemann L, Schnell O, Gehr B, et al. Digital Diabetes Management: A Literature Review of Smart Insulin Pens. J Diabetes Sci Technol 2022;16:587–95.
31. Gildon BW. InPen Smart Insulin Pen System: Product Review and User Experience. Diabetes Spectr 2018;31:354–8.
32. Klonoff DC, Nayberg I, Stauder U, et al. Half-Unit Insulin Pens: Disease Management in Patients With Diabetes Who Are Sensitive to Insulin. J Diabetes Sci Technol 2017;11:623–30.
33. Bigfoot Unity System Features. 2023. at https://www.diabeteseducator.org/dana tech/insulin-medicine-delivery/find-compare-delivery-devices/product-detail/big foot-unity#:~:text=Bigfoot%20Unity%20System%20includes%3A%20long, readings%20on%20demand%20without%20fingersticks.
34. Lilly Tempo pen features. 2023. Available at https://www.lillytempo.com/how-tempo-works/temposmart-app.
35. Akturk HK, Agarwal S, Hoffecker L, et al. Inequity in Racial-Ethnic Representation in Randomized Controlled Trials of Diabetes Technologies in Type 1 Diabetes: Critical Need for New Standards. Diabetes Care 2021;44:e121–3.
36. Agarwal S, Hilliard M, Butler A. Disparities in Care Delivery and Outcomes in Young Adults With Diabetes. Curr Diabetes Rep 2018;18:65.
37. Agarwal S, Kanapka LG, Raymond JK, et al. Racial-Ethnic Inequity in Young Adults With Type 1 Diabetes. J Clin Endocrinol Metabol 2020;105:e2960–9.
38. Lai CW, Lipman TH, Willi SM, et al. Racial and Ethnic Disparities in Rates of Continuous Glucose Monitor Initiation and Continued Use in Children With Type 1 Diabetes. Diabetes Care 2021;44:255–7.
39. Addala A, Auzanneau M, Miller K, et al. A Decade of Disparities in Diabetes Technology Use and HbA(1c) in Pediatric Type 1 Diabetes: A Transatlantic Comparison. Diabetes Care 2021;44:133–40.
40. McKee AM, Al-Hammadi N, Hinyard LJ. Disparities in Utilization and Outcomes With Continuous Subcutaneous Insulin Infusion in Young Adults With Type 1 Diabetes. Endocr Pract 2021;27:769–75.
41. Levitt DL, Silver KD, Spanakis EK. Inpatient Continuous Glucose Monitoring and Glycemic Outcomes. J Diabetes Sci Technol 2017;11:1028–35.
42. Gothong C, Singh LG, Satyarengga M, et al. Continuous glucose monitoring in the hospital: an update in the era of COVID-19. Curr Opin Endocrinol Diabetes Obes 2022;29:1–9.

43. Davis GM, Spanakis EK, Migdal AL, et al. Accuracy of Dexcom G6 Continuous Glucose Monitoring in Non-Critically Ill Hospitalized Patients With Diabetes. Diabetes Care 2021;44:1641–6.
44. Spanakis EK, Urrutia A, Galindo RJ, et al. Continuous Glucose Monitoring-Guided Insulin Administration in Hospitalized Patients With Diabetes: A Randomized Clinical Trial. Diabetes Care 2022;45:2369–75.
45. Korytkowski MT, Muniyappa R, Antinori-Lent K, et al. Management of Hyperglycemia in Hospitalized Adult Patients in Non-Critical Care Settings: An Endocrine Society Clinical Practice Guideline. J Clin Endocrinol Metab 2022;107:2101–28.
46. Sordi V, Monaco L, Piemonti L. Cell Therapy for Type 1 Diabetes: From Islet Transplantation to Stem Cells. Horm Res Paediatr 2022;1–12.
47. Velazco-Cruz L, Goedegebuure MM, Millman JR. Advances Toward Engineering Functionally Mature Human Pluripotent Stem Cell-Derived β Cells. Front Bioeng Biotechnol 2020;8:786.
48. Pellegrini S, Piemonti L, Sordi V. Pluripotent stem cell replacement approaches to treat type 1 diabetes. Curr Opin Pharmacol 2018;43:20–6.
49. Migliorini A, Nostro MC, Sneddon JB. Human pluripotent stem cell-derived insulin-producing cells: A regenerative medicine perspective. Cell Metabol 2021;33:721–31.
50. Hogrebe NJ, Ishahak M, Millman JR. Developments in stem cell-derived islet replacement therapy for treating type 1 diabetes. Cell Stem Cell 2023;30:530–48.
51. Vertex FDA clearance for VX-264 new drug application. 2023. Available at: https://investors.vrtx.com/news-releases/news-release-details/vertex-announces-fda-clearance-investigational-new-drug.
52. Akturk HK, Rewers A, Joseph H, et al. Possible Ways to Improve Postprandial Glucose Control in Type 1 Diabetes. Diabetes Technol Therapeut 2018;20. S224-s32.
53. Garg SK, Rewers AH, Akturk HK. Ever-Increasing Insulin-Requiring Patients Globally. Diabetes Technol Therapeut 2018;20. S21-s4.
54. Akturk HK, Rewers A, Garg SK. SGLT inhibition: a possible adjunctive treatment for type 1 diabetes. Curr Opin Endocrinol Diabetes Obes 2018;25:246–50.
55. Pettus J, Boeder SC, Christiansen MP, et al. Glucagon receptor antagonist volagidemab in type 1 diabetes: a 12-week, randomized, double-blind, phase 2 trial. Nat Med 2022;28:2092–9.
56. Klein KR, Freeman JLR, Dunn I, et al. The SimpliciT1 Study: A Randomized, Double-Blind, Placebo-Controlled Phase 1b/2 Adaptive Study of TTP399, a Hepatoselective Glucokinase Activator, for Adjunctive Treatment of Type 1 Diabetes. Diabetes Care 2021;44:960–8.

Social Determinants of Health Screening in Type 1 Diabetes Management

Nana-Hawa Yayah Jones, MD[a],*, India Cole[b],
Kelsey J. Hart, DNP, RN[b], Sarah Corathers, MD[a],
Shivani Agarwal, MD, MPH[c], Ori Odugbesan, MD, MPH[d],
Osagie Ebekozien, MD, MPH[d], Manmohan K. Kamboj, MD[e],
Michael A. Harris, PhD[f], Kathryn L. Fantasia, MD, MSc[g],
Mona Mansour, MD, MS[a,h]

KEYWORDS

- Social determinants of health • Disparities • Health equity • Type 1 diabetes
- Screening

KEY POINTS

- Socioeconomic factors influence access and care: Social determinants of health, including socioeconomic status, education level, and income, significantly impact the management and outcomes of type 1 diabetes.

Continued

[a] Division of Pediatric Endocrinology, Cincinnati Children's Hospital Medical Center, University of Cincinnati, 3333 Burnet Avenue, MLC 7012, Cincinnati, OH 45229-3039, USA; [b] James M. Anderson Center for Health Systems Excellence, Cincinnati Children's Hospital Medical Center, 3333 Burnet Avenue, MLC 15018, Cincinnati, OH 45229-3039, USA; [c] Fleischer Institute for Diabetes and Metabolism, New York Regional Center for Diabetes Translation Research, Albert Einstein College of Medicine, 1180 Morris Park Avenue, Bronx, NY 10467, USA; [d] T1D Exchange, QI & Population Health Department, 101 Federal Street Suite 440, Boston, MA 02110, USA; [e] The Ohio State University College of Medicine, Section of Endocrinology, Quality Improvement for Endocrinology, Nationwide Children's Hospital, 700 Children's Drive, Columbus, OH 43205, USA; [f] Oregon Health & Science University, Harold Schnitzer Diabetes Health Center, 707 SW Gaines Street, Portland, OR 97239, USA; [g] Section of Endocrinology, Diabetes, and Nutrition, Department of Medicine, Boston University Chobanian & Avedisian School of Medicine, 72 E Concord, C3, Boston, MA 02118, USA; [h] University of Cincinnati College of Medicine, Department of Pediatrics, Population Health- CCHMC, Division of General and Community Pediatrics, Community Engagement- HealthVine, CCHMC Coordinated School Strategy, Cincinnati Children's Hospital Medical Center, University of Cincinnati, 3333 Burnet Avenue, MLC 15018, Cincinnati, OH 45229-3039, USA
* Corresponding author. Division of Pediatric Endocrinology, Cincinnati Children's Hospital Medical Center and the University of Cincinnati, 3333 Burnet Avenue, MLC 7012, Cincinnati, OH 45229-3039.
E-mail address: Nana.jones@cchmc.org

Endocrinol Metab Clin N Am 53 (2024) 93–106
https://doi.org/10.1016/j.ecl.2023.09.006
0889-8529/24/© 2023 Elsevier Inc. All rights reserved.

Continued

- Health disparities and vulnerable populations: Disadvantaged populations, such as racial and ethnic minorities, may experience higher rates of type 1 diabetes and related complications due to unequal access to health care resources, cultural barriers, and systemic biases.
- Social determinants of health screening: Screening for social determinants of health is paramount to reduce disparities and improve overall health outcomes.

INTRODUCTION

Social determinants of health (SDOH), often referred to as social influences of health, are those nonmedical factors that impact health outcomes. Factors such as access to food, clothing, shelter, and transportation play a mitigating role in both acute and chronic disease management. Protective factors are highly influenced by where we are born, live, learn, work, eat, and play. As such, many health care disparities arise from SDOH; less social risk factors correlate to less disease burden and more protection against disease onset and exacerbation. It has been widely observed that health inequities, fueled by SDOH, are divided by race, class, and income; disproportionately affecting minority races, the working class and those with no to low income.[1]

Diabetes is one of the most common chronic diseases, impacting millions of lives worldwide, and thus is most affected by health inequities.[2] Children are no strangers to health inequities, and this was made more evident by the COVID-19 pandemic. Although the greatest rise in diabetes among children is type 2 diabetes,[3] type 1 diabetes (T1D) is more prevalent among pediatric patients.[4] Despite minority races, working class and low-income families being least likely to have T1D, they are the most likely to experience negative social influences of health; especially with T1D prevalence rising within these populations.[4] As such the American Diabetes Association, the nation's leading establishment for all people living with diabetes, published a scientific review relating to SDOH and diabetes.[1]

Here, we aim to

1. provide a succinct review of history, context, and impact of SDOH and
2. share practice implementation guidelines to effectively screen for SDOH for those caring for patients with T1D, although practices can be spread to all populations with chronic disease.

DEFINITIONS

SDOH, health disparities, and health equity are closely related. Incongruities in disease burden based on environmental factors must be identified and targeted to deliver and receive diabetes treatments equitably. Once care is equitably distributed, disease outcomes improve. The World Health Organization has clearly defined the terminology used to focus on the social influences of health.[5]

Social Determinants of Health

SDOH are the nonmedical factors that influence health outcomes. They are the conditions in which people are born, grow, work, live, and age and the wider set of forces and systems shaping the conditions of daily life. As defined by the World Health

Organization, these forces include racism, climate economic policies and systems, development agendas, social norms, and policies, as well as political systems.

Health Disparities

Health disparities are preventable differences in the burden of disease, injury, violence, or opportunities to achieve optimal health, which are experienced by socially disadvantaged populations.

Health Equity

Health equity is the state in which everyone has a fair and just opportunity to attain their highest level of health.

HISTORICAL PERSPECTIVES

To understand how risk factors negatively affect health outcomes, one needs to be aware of the historical context in which these disparities arose. Decades of research demonstrate the legacy of slavery, and colonialism imparts its most negative effect on the Black race, although continued discrimination, prejudice, and bias plague all minoritized persons.[6–9] As participants in the cultural constructs of the United States, one must understand how slavery, social injustice, and racism play a leading role in reinforcing SDOH.

Slavery

The legal institution of human bondage, primarily of Africans, prevailed in the United States for nearly four centuries starting in the 1700s as the 13 colonies, which would form the United States was established.[10] Currently, the way in which social risk factors are tied to race, particularly the Black race, has been largely influenced by US enslavement, institutionalizing the racial caste system. Ancestors of African descent were matriculated into a social stratification system of servitude. Just as health behaviors inform health outcomes, past systemic structures (behaviors) foundational to modern day living (outcomes) inform much of our class system today. Higher rates of poverty, disease, employment instability, food insecurity, and housing destabilization are all indicators of poor health or negative SDOH and more greatly affect African Americans and marginalized communities. The economic gap created by slavery and perpetuated today cannot be understated and reinforces the segregation of the have and have nots—similar to those who are more likely to achieve diabetes glycemic targets versus those who are more likely to suffer diabetes complications.[11,12]

Social Justice

The attrition of wealth, economic opportunity, and societal privilege is also tied to the historical context in which good health has been unequally distributed in the United States. Social justice includes the opportunity for everyone to achieve good health.[13] Systems that reinforce health inequities are a manifestation of social injustice. These inequities are the result of government policies and practices that unfairly disadvantage some people but not others, often most negatively impacting disadvantaged communities and their youth. The mechanisms linking social injustice to wealth gap creation and socioeconomic status (SES) is well understood.

Racism

Prejudice and discrimination based on race (racism) further misalign attainment of good health.[14] Across all genres of racism, including internalized, interpersonal, structural, and systemic, racism's significant effects on health outcomes, especially in diabetes care, cannot be understated. In a large cross-sectional study across 52 institutions, non-Hispanic (NH) Black patients with T1D were more likely to present in diabetic ketoacidosis (DKA) compared with NH White patients with T1D. Black patients with T1D faced a significantly higher frequency of DKA during the pandemic, particularly during surges of COVID-19. However, a higher proportion of NH Black patients experienced DKA versus White patients *pre*-COVID-19 pandemic as well.[15] Even before the pandemic crisis, evidence highlights that racial inequities in diabetes care were present, raising concern that factors based on race likely affect access to health care, trust in the health care system, and reduced recognition of disease, especially because T1D has higher prevalence in the majority population.[16] Environmental determinants have long been proposed as a trigger for autoimmunity in T1D.[17] The racist institution of redlining, a discriminatory practice in which suburban homeownership was withheld from people of color, places racial and ethnic minorities at greater exposure to urban areas and environmental hazards, such as polluted air and water, which can increase the risk of diabetes and other chronic diseases. Communities of color are more likely to be located near industrial sites, waste facilities, and areas with poor environmental quality, a probable theory on the rising incidence of T1D in Black children.[18]

Social Determinants of Health in Health Care

SDOH are key contributors to the unjust and avoidable differences in health outcomes between different population groups. These influences affect all components of health care and all SDOHs infer an impact on diabetes in one way or another. Studies have consistently proven that diabetes affects racial and ethnic minorities, low-income adults and their children, and the public and underinsured populations more negatively when compared with others.[1,19,20] From socioeconomic position to food and environment, T1D outcomes are worse for those suffering from the social influences of health.[21]

Access

More than 78 million Americans do not have adequate health insurance, and millions more are at risk of losing coverage. The 24% of Americans who do not have adequate insurance include individuals who are entirely uninsured and those for whom out-of-pocket costs and deductibles are disproportionately high relative to their incomes. Those uninsured and underinsured are less likely to seek preventable health care and more likely to present in worse stages of disease.[22,23] Youth with T1D living in high-poverty areas and on public insurance are significantly more likely to be admitted for DKA, and adults with T1D are more likely to ration insulin and avoid preventative health maintenance.[24] Preventative health care mitigates the severity of many diseases, especially diabetes. Accessibility of medical services deters most common T1D complications such as retinopathy, neuropathy, nephropathy, and especially cardiovascular disease, the number one cause of mortality in patients living with T1D.[25] Access is not only limited to preventative medicine but also relates to other social factors such as food environment (access to food = food security), access to safe neighborhoods, and access to education. In addition to reduced access to preventive care, limited access to diabetes technology for un-/underinsured further narrows the benefits of these devices to the privileged-widening disparity gaps in diabetes outcomes even more.[26]

Education

Higher educational attainment of caregivers of youth with T1D correlates to better glycemic control.[27] In fact, no matter the type of diabetes, diabetes-related complications demonstrate a linear relationship from highest to lowest education level. Compared with adults with college degrees, attaining less than a high school education infers a twofold risk of mortality from diabetes, and if you are a person living with T1D, not going to college is associated with a threefold risk of mortality.[1] A linear relationship between educational level and hemoglobin A1c (HgbA1c), the primary outcome of interest in diabetes management exists; lower educational level pairing with higher HbA1c. In fact, in a meta-analysis by Bijlsma-Rutte, the pooled mean difference in A1c was 0.26% (95% CI 0.09–0.43) between people with low and high educational levels.[28] Studies show that reducing the HbA1c level by 0.2% could lower the mortality by 10%.[29] Although HbA1c has its limitations, and in the landscape of T1D, time in range is becoming a more valuable marker of glycemic control, it remains clinically significant that HbA1c levels are an independent prognostic marker of both short- and long-term complications.[25] Educational status is directly linked to SES and economic mobility.[2] Patients living with diabetes who attain higher educational degrees are more likely to be healthier by the shear fact that knowledge infers improved self-management, and highly educated T1D patients are more likely to be economically stable.

Economic Stability

Inequalities in health are almost always to the disadvantage of the poor. The poor tends to die earlier and to have higher levels of morbidity than those who have wealth.[30] Also, inequalities tend to be more pronounced for objective indicators of diabetes, such as HgbA1c, hypoglycemia, microvascular, and macrovascular complications. It has been consistently reported that SES is a stronger determinant of diabetes status and outcomes than race/ethnicity.[21,31] After adjusting for age and gender, Black and Hispanic patients have statistically significantly increased odds of having diabetes, but when adjusted for SES, these odds are reduced in both races. Adjusting for age, gender, weight, blood pressure, physical activity, financial strain, insurance, and family history of diabetes, SES plays a more significant role in diabetes prevalence than race/ethnicity. SES is multifaceted in its ability to class an individual or group. It is not just measured by income but also by education and occupation.[32] In the SEARCH Food Insecurity Study in South Carolina and Washington between the years 2013 and 2015, optimal glycemic control, as categorized by HbA1c, was associated with parental education, household income, health insurance status, food assistance, and household food insecurity status. Most of these patients belonged to a demographic designated to higher household income/parental education class. Suboptimal glycemic control was more likely to be experienced by those who received government-funded health insurance or food assistance and those who were food insecure.[33]

Implicit Bias (Provider-Specific)

The wealth gap, disparities in access to care, and failures in the school system to equitably educate citizens are often deemed non-modifiable. However, provider bias is a modifiable factor known to impact health outcomes. Implicit bias is a form of bias occurring subconsciously and unintentionally, which affects judgments, decisions, and behaviors.[34] Provider bias explicitly targets health care providers' automatic assumptions about patients and their families. The inherent danger in provider bias is its implication on health outcomes.[8] Prescriptions for diabetes technology are an exemplar of the inherent dangers of provider bias. Diabetes technology, including continuous glucose monitors (CGMs) and insulin pumps, is known to improve glucose time in range.[35] Provider implicit bias to recommend diabetes technology has been observed based on insurance and race/ethnicity in both pediatric and adult diabetes provider cohorts. In fact, despite having the same disease, White patients with T1D are more likely to be offered insulin pumps and be started on CGMs than non-White patients.[26] The attitudes and perceptions of providers play a significant role in the promotion of technology utilization. In fact, providers who were "tech savvy" or had personality characteristics lending toward a more positive attitude about innovative technology, offered it more. These factors readily lead to provider-driven barriers in access to improved glycemic outcomes when provider personas are more cautious or "not yet ready" to tailor their care toward pump or CGM technology.[36]

IMPACT OF SOCIAL DETERMINANTS OF HEALTH: COST BURDEN

Not only does diabetes disproportionately burden patients in low-poverty quintiles, leading to insulin rationing and delays in seeking medical care, diabetes is one of the costliest diagnoses, and in fact, diabetes is the most expensive chronic condition in the United States. A quarter of the nation's wealth is spent on caring for people with diabetes: $237 billion in direct medical costs and another $90 billion on reduced productivity.[37] It becomes a national imperative to address the SDOH not just to do no harm but also to maintain economic stability. Significant correlations have been found between hospitalizations and deprivation indices. Patients living in deprived areas are more likely to use the emergency department and be admitted for diabetes complications, driving up health care costs. The movement toward value-based payment models is structured around health outcomes rather than processes.[38] Under these models, providers are compensated based on those health outcomes. Providers must assess SDOH to provide a framework to discuss behaviors and social factors that influence those health outcomes. SDOH often acts upstream of an individual's health over time. By identifying social needs early, health care providers can intervene proactively, providing preventive care and appropriate support services. Addressing these determinants before they escalate can help prevent the development or exacerbation of chronic conditions and reduce health care costs in the long run.

SOCIAL DETERMINANTS OF HEALTH SCREENING: IMPLEMENTATION

As noted by the Institute for Healthcare Improvement, "the Model for Improvement, developed by Associates in Process Improvement, is a simple, yet powerful tool for accelerating improvement." The Chronic Care Model identifies the essential elements of a health care system that encourage high-quality chronic disease care.[39] Pairing the two models is an effective methodology for implementing SDOH screening at health care institutions.[40]

Social Determinants of Health Screening

Implementation of SDOH screening in diabetes clinics can be standardized and effective in identifying barriers to health care needs of patients with diabetes.[41] Effectively implementing screening to identify and mediate these social factors depends on the specific needs of a clinics' patient population, ability of the center to assess these needs, breadth of clinic, as well as community resources. This section describes strategies for effective SDOH screening and response in the clinic setting.

At a minimum, we recommend screening for food security, financial resources, caregiver mental health, housing, and transportation. Others to consider are caregiver health literacy, given how relevant health literacy is in diabetes care and education. The SDOH screener is intended to be administered universally to minimize potential for bias and should be completed by pediatric patients' parent/caregiver or patients

18 years and older. In pediatric T1D settings, the first question should ask for the responder to indicate their relationship to the patient.

Social Determinants of Health Screening Implementation Strategy

Clinical centers diagnosing, treating, and managing patients with diabetes should choose an SDOH screening tool that is most readily available in their electronic health record and most amenable to clinical processes. If no screening tool is accessible, electronic versions can be adapted to paper or self-administration or via an in-person interview during routine check in. Several validated SDOH screening tools exist, which can be used on their own or customized for the organization.

Social Determinants of Health Interventions

No health care organization need reinvent interventions for positive screens. Determine resources available in the office, hospital, and within the community. Facilitate referral to community resources based on patient needs and, if available, optimize care management or care coordination between patient encounters. For smaller centers with little resources, reallocate existing workforces to (1) choose an SDOH screen, (2) implement said screen into existing workflows, (3) address as many screens as feasible for the practice, and (4) render available facility and community resources. Many state Medicaid programs provide an array of services to address SDOH. In fact, in January 2021, the Centers for Medicare & Medicaid Services, released guidelines for states to use detailing opportunities in Medicaid and Children's Health Insurance Plan to address SDOH.[42] Private health insurers are also investing in social programs that better address root causes. It has been purported that private payors have spent close to $2B on housing, food security, employment, education, social and community context, transportation, and general SDOH. Screener completion should be acknowledged, even if no needs were identified. Acknowledgment builds trust with patients and families.

Of note, it is clearly recognized to truly eliminate SDOH disparities in health care requires systemic change, policy initiatives, and governance[17]; however, such change is macroeconomic and beyond scope here.

Proposed scripting

Below is a recommended scripting for discussion of SDOH screener results.

If no social needs are identified through SDOH screener:

I really appreciate you filling out the screener that helps us understand more about your current circumstances. If anything changes, please know we are here to listen, help, and connect you and your family to resources and support.

**Important reminder: Many families have social needs and screen negatively. It is recommended to still ask about concerns and normalize social supports.

If social needs are identified through social determinants of health screener

I noticed you checked some of the items that tell us you may need some support and resources. Thank you for sharing this with me today and I would love to help in any way I can. I would like to ask you some more questions.

In addition to the scripting presented above, some best practices for discussion of social needs include.

- Use normalizing statements.
- Frame questions so caregivers can respond in the positive.
- Determine interventions which have already been implemented.

Clinicians can use framing statements and/or next best questions to facilitate social needs discussions. Examples include.

- Framing statement: Many of my patients are experiencing [insert need].
- Next best question: What supports are you using, or have you used in the past to help you with this?

Screening Frequency

There are no industry standards on screening frequency, and thus, the following recommendations are expert opinion (**Fig. 1**).

Standard minimum screening frequency recommendations include recognizing some primary care practice care for patients living with T1D.

- At all* well visits in primary settings (*not to be administered more frequently than every 55 days)
- Every 6 months regardless of visit type in primary care settings
- Every 6 months in ambulatory specialty settings
- On every admission to the hospital
- At the first ambulatory encounter after admission to the hospital

Introduction of Screener

It is important that patients and families feel safe, empowered, and supported through the screening process. Patients and families must know that they have a right not to complete the SDOH screener.

The following verbiage is recommended as part of the SDOH screener:

We care about our patients. We want to be sure that we support all parts of our patients' lives. This tool helps us address both medical and nonmedical needs of your family. If you would like help with any of these topics, we can talk about resources available. Please answer these questions. It is your choice if you answer them. Filling out this form is not needed to continue your visit.

This verbiage is also recommended for staff when introducing the SDOH screener to patients and families. A warm introduction of the screener is important for patients and families to feel safe, empowered, and supported.

Administration Methods

It is recommended that the SDOH screener is administered automatically via tablet technology.[41] Tablet administration promotes reliability of screening, whereas balancing evidence-based recommendations that SDOH screeners should be administered and completed privately (vs verbal administration).

If administration via tablet is not feasible, administration of the SDOH screener via paper is a recommended alternative. The paper screener should be translated into different languages when possible. Results from the completed paper screener should be transcribed into the medical record, and the paper screener should be submitted to be scanned in the medical record or sent to facilities' comparable health information systems.

For instances in which the parent/caregiver or adult patient would prefer verbal administration, the screener can be verbally administered with results transcribed into the patient's medical record by a clinical staff member. This should be rare.

Recommended Administration Workflow

Below are recommended workflows for screener administration. These are high-level recommendations that can and should be adapted to an individual's organization (**Fig. 2**).

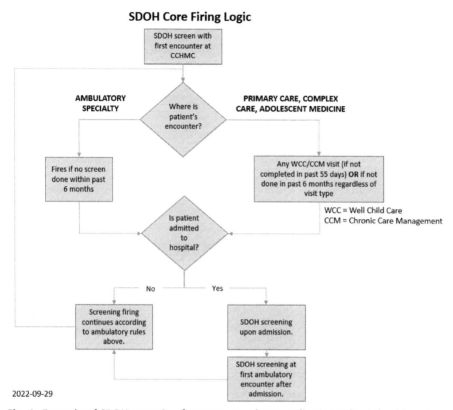

Fig. 1. Example of SDOH screening frequency at a large pediatric academic health system. CCM, chronic care management; WCC, well-child care.

READINESS TOOL KIT

The readiness tool kit is a high-level instrument used to support the development of processes at health care institutions seeking to address SDOH in patients with T1D. To help ensure that all staff members involved in the screening are prepared for

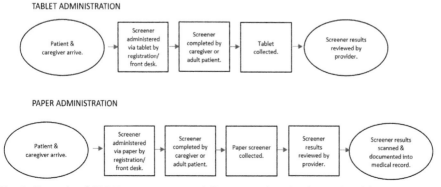

Fig. 2. Example of SDOH process map to deliver screening via electronic tablet or paper.

		Planning
☐	Establish your improvement team.	Possible participants of your improvement team may include physician/provider, nursing/patient services, registration, social work, additional roles included in workflow, QI
☐	Identify unit champions.	Identify unit champions to facilitate testing, implementation, and education.
☐	Obtain tablets & associated equipment.	Ensure you have a sufficient amount of tablets & associated supplies for screening demand. Consider storage and maintenance logistics.
☐	Evaluate screeners currently in use.	Evaluate which screeners are currently in use in your care area. Identify & remove areas of duplication.
☐	Establish measures.	Build process measures (completion & positivity rates). Determine outcome measures that are relevant to your team/care area.
		Screener Administration & Completion Workflow
☐	Identify intended population.	Determine the intended population of screeners in your care setting.
☐	Review SDOH Core Screener firing frequency.	Review screener firing logic. Consider interactions/parameters for other screeners if there are multiple due in the same visit (i.e., max # screeners per visit, prioritization of screeners, etc.)
☐	Establish process for administering screener.	Map out screener administration process. Identify who will administer the screener. When in the workflow is it best to administer screener?
☐	Identify scripting for introduction of screener.	Establish scripting for how screener will be introduced to respondent.
☐	Additional process considerations	Establish back-up processes for when tablet administration is not appropriate. I.e., English is not preferred language
		Screener Response Workflow
☐	Establish process for review of screener.	Determine who will review the screener & who will discuss positive AND negative screener results with respondent.
☐	Identify scripting for screener discussion w/ respondent.	Establish scripting for positive AND negative social risk screens.
☐	Review & complete response tool with team.	Determine how your team will respond to positive screens. Identify on-site responses for judicious utilization of social work team.
☐	Establish process for response.	Determine who will carry out response interventions. i.e., Who will facilitate referrals? Who will provide information and/or carry out onsite responses?
☐	Ensure the team has all necessary resources for onsite responses.	Determine if additional materials or resources are needed for improved onsite response. i.e., up-to-date resource lists, transportation resources, etc.
☐	Established standard documentation practices.	Determine how screener results, response discussion, interventions, and referrals will be documented in medical record. Who will document?
		Training
☐	Identify audience for education.	Review roles affected by screening to ensure all are included in education.
☐	Educate identified roles.	Ensure all necessary roles are educated on why SDOH screening is important and the processes for screening & response, prior to implementation of screening.
☐	Utilize unit champions for just-in-time training.	Utilize unit champions as frontline experts on the process. Can be used to role model screener discussions & responses, answer questions, & promote successful implementation.
		Testing & Learning
☐	Review data	Review data (process & outcome measures) at regular cadence to learn & make adjustments.
☐	Observe screening & collect feedback from staff & patients/families.	Observe screening process & collect feedback to learn. What is going well? What needs improvement?
☐	Run multiple PDSA cycles.	Make adaptations based on learnings through multiple PDSA cycles.

Fig. 3. Readiness tool kit checklist to be used by personnel to implement SDOH screening.

success, the following checklist (**Fig. 3**) helps teams review their current workflows and initiate thought processes helpful in determining screening, response, training, and testing procedures.

SUMMARY

Screening for SDOH in health care settings is crucial for several reasons, including identification of underlying health risks, instituting preventive care and early intervention, tailoring treatment plans to improve outcomes, and most importantly reducing health disparities. Institutions who care for persons living with T1D cannot improve the lives of their patients without first identifying those health risks, which most impact health outcomes and behaviors. Not addressing the social influences of health likely correlates with an inability to reach glycemic targets. Standard practices to implement SDOH screening in any health care organization are now considered standard of care. All institutions should screen and intervene appropriately.

CLINICS CARE POINTS

Implementing SDOH screening in pediatric diabetes clinics is an important step to ensure comprehensive care for young patients. Here is a list of clinic care points to consider when implementing SDOH screening in such clinics:

- Screening Tools Selection: Choose validated SDOH screening tools suitable for pediatric patients.

- Patient Privacy and Comfort: Ensure a private and comfortable setting for screening to encourage open and honest responses from patients and caregivers.

- Training Staff: Train clinic staff on the importance of SDOH screening, how to administer the screening tools, and how to interpret the results.

- Routine Screening: Incorporate SDOH screening into the routine clinic visits for pediatric patients, such as during annual check-ups or follow-up appointments in specialty clinics such as diabetes clinics.

- Culturally Competent Approach: Be sensitive to the cultural and linguistic backgrounds of patients and their families. Offer screening materials in multiple languages and ensure staff are culturally competent.

- Assessment of Basic Needs: Screen for essential needs like food security, housing stability, and access to utilities. Address any immediate needs through referrals to community resources or social services.

- Education and Resources: Provide families with information about available community resources and support services, such as food banks, housing assistance, and transportation assistance.

- Mental Health Screening: Include questions related to emotional and mental well-being, as mental health can significantly impact diabetes management. Provide referrals to mental health services when needed.

- Education on SDOH Impact: Educate patients and families on how SDOH can affect diabetes management and overall health, emphasizing the importance of addressing these factors.

- Care Coordination: Establish clear protocols for sharing SDOH screening results with the diabetes care team. Encourage collaboration between healthcare providers and social workers or case managers.

- Follow-Up and Tracking: Schedule follow-up appointments to monitor changes in SDOH needs and provide ongoing support. Use electronic health records (EHRs) or tracking systems to document and monitor SDOH data.

- Community Partnerships: Collaborate with local community organizations, schools, and social service agencies to strengthen the network of support available to pediatric diabetes patients.

- Quality Improvement: Continuously assess and improve your SDOH screening processes based on feedback from patients, families, and clinic staff.

- Advocacy: Advocate for policies and programs that address SDOH on a broader scale, as this can have a positive impact on the well-being of your patients.

- Research and Evaluation: Consider conducting research or evaluations to measure the effectiveness of your SDOH screening program in improving diabetes management and overall health outcomes.

CONFLICT OF INTEREST

None.

REFERENCES

1. Hill-Briggs F, Adler NE, Berkowitz SA, et al. Social Determinants of Health and Diabetes: A Scientific Review. Diabetes Care 2021;44(1):258–79.
2. Saydah S, Lochner K. Socioeconomic Status and Risk of Diabetes-Related Mortality in the U.S. Public Health Rep 2010;125(3):377–88.
3. Magge SN, Wolf RM, Pyle L, et al. The Coronavirus Disease 2019 Pandemic Is Associated with a Substantial Rise in Frequency and Severity of Presentation of Youth-Onset Type 2 Diabetes. J Pediatr 2022;251:51–9.e2.
4. Wagenknecht LE, Lawrence JM, Isom S, et al. Trends in Incidence of Youth-Onset Type 1 and Type 2 Diabetes in the USA, 2002-18: Results from the Population-Based Search for Diabetes in Youth Study. Lancet Diabetes Endocrinol 2023; 11(4):242–50.
5. WHO, W.H.O. Social Determinants of Health: Evidence on Social Determinants of Health. 2020; Available at: https://www.who.int/health-topics/social-determinants-of-health#tab=tab_1. Accessed 25 October 2020.
6. Fanta M, Ladzekpo D, Unaka N. Racism and Pediatric Health Outcomes. Curr Probl Pediatr Adolesc Health Care 2021;51(10):101087.
7. Karbeah J, Bensignor MO, Vajravelu ME. Multidimensional Approaches to Understanding Structural Racism's Impact on Type 1 Diabetes. Pediatrics 2023;151(5).
8. Maina IW, Belton TD, Ginzberg S, et al. A Decade of Studying Implicit Racial/Ethnic Bias in Healthcare Providers Using the Implicit Association Test. Soc Sci Med 2018;199:219–29.
9. Willis HA, Sosoo EE, Bernard DL, et al. The Associations between Internalized Racism, Racial Identity, and Psychological Distress. Emerg Adulthood 2021; 9(4):384–400.
10. Presumey-Leblanc G, Sandel M. The legacy of slavery and the socialization of black female health and human services workforce members in addressing social determinants of health. J Racial Ethn Health Disparities 2023.
11. Wood PH. Strange new land: Africans in colonial America. New York: Oxford University Press; 2003.
12. Foster NC, Beck RW, Miller KM, et al. State of type 1 diabetes management and outcomes from the T1d Exchange in 2016-2018. Diabetes Technol Ther 2019; 21(2):66–72.
13. Harvey D. Social justice and the city. Rev. Ed. Geographies of justice and social transformation. Athens: University of Georgia Press; 2009. p. 354.
14. Spanakis EK, Golden SH. Race/ethnic difference in diabetes and diabetic complications. Curr Diab Rep 2013;13(6):814–23.
15. Lavik AR, Ebekozien O, Noor N, et al. Trends in type 1 diabetic ketoacidosis during covid-19 surges at 7 us centers: highest burden on non-Hispanic black patients. J Clin Endocrinol Metab 2022;107(7):1948–55.
16. Willi SM, Miller KM, DiMeglio LA, et al. Racial-ethnic disparities in management and outcomes among children with type 1 diabetes. Pediatrics 2015;135(3):424–34.

17. Adler NE, Newman K. Socioeconomic disparities in health: pathways and policies. Health Aff 2002;21(2):60–76.
18. Swope CB, Hernández D, Cushing LJ. The relationship of historical redlining with present-day neighborhood environmental and health outcomes: a scoping review and conceptual model. J Urban Health 2022;99(6):959–83.
19. Berkowitz SA, Orr CJ. Three Lessons About Diabetes and the Social Determinants of Health. Diabetes Care 2023;46(9):1587–9.
20. Apperley LJ, Ng SM. Socioeconomic deprivation, household education, and employment are associated with increased hospital admissions and poor glycemic control in children with type 1 diabetes mellitus. Rev Diabet Stud 2017;14(2–3): 295–300.
21. Link CL, McKinlay JB. Disparities in the prevalence of diabetes: is it race/ethnicity or socioeconomic status? results from the Boston area community health (BACH) survey. Ethn Dis 2009;19(3):288–92.
22. Galvani AP, Parpia AS, Foster EM, et al. Improving the prognosis of health care in the USA. Lancet 2020;395(10223):524–33.
23. Hemmingsen B, Gimenez-Perez G, Mauricio D, et al. Diet, physical activity or both for prevention or delay of type 2 diabetes mellitus and its associated complications in people at increased risk of developing type 2 diabetes mellitus. Cochrane Database Syst Rev 2017;12(12):Cd003054.
24. Maxwell AR, Jones NHY, Taylor S, et al. Socioeconomic and racial disparities in diabetic ketoacidosis admissions in youth with type 1 diabetes. J Hosp Med 2021.
25. Diabetes Control and Complications Trial (DCCT): Results of Feasibility Study. The Dcct Research Group. Diabetes Care 1987;10(1):1–19.
26. Odugbesan O, Addala A, Nelson G, et al. Implicit racial-ethnic and insurance-mediated bias to recommending diabetes technology: insights from t1d exchange multicenter pediatric and adult diabetes provider cohort. Diabetes Technol Ther 2022;24(9):619–27.
27. Alassaf A, Gharaibeh L, Odeh R, et al. Predictors of Glycemic Control in Children and Adolescents with Type 1 Diabetes at 12 Months after Diagnosis. Pediatr Diabetes 2022;23(6):729–35.
28. Bijlsma-Rutte A, Rutters F, Elders PJM, et al. Socio-Economic Status and Hba(1c) in Type 2 Diabetes: A Systematic Review and Meta-Analysis. Diabetes Metab Res Rev 2018;34(6):e3008.
29. Khaw KT, Wareham N, Luben R, et al. Glycated haemoglobin, diabetes, and mortality in men in Norfolk cohort of European prospective investigation of cancer and nutrition (Epic-Norfolk). BMJ 2001;322(7277):15–8.
30. Osborn CY, de Groot M, Wagner JA. Racial and Ethnic Disparities in Diabetes Complications in the Northeastern United States: The Role of Socioeconomic Status. J Natl Med Assoc 2013;105(1):51–8.
31. Suwannaphant K, Laohasiriwong W, Puttanapong N, et al. Association between Socioeconomic Status and Diabetes Mellitus: The National Socioeconomics Survey, 2010 and 2012. J Clin Diagn Res 2017;11(7):LC18–22.
32. Pickett KE, Wilkinson RG. Income Inequality and Health: A Causal Review. Soc Sci Med 2015;128:316–26.
33. Sutherland MW, Ma X, Reboussin BA, et al. Socioeconomic Position Is Associated with Glycemic Control in Youth and Young Adults with Type 1 Diabetes. Pediatr Diabetes 2020;21(8):1412–20.
34. FitzGerald C, Hurst S. Implicit Bias in Healthcare Professionals: A Systematic Review. BMC Med Ethics 2017;18(1):19.

35. Chan AJ, Halperin IJ. Beyond glycated hemoglobin: harnessing data from sensor-based technology to improve glucose variability, time in range and hypoglycemia in adult patients with type 1 diabetes. Can J Diabetes 2021;45(3):269–72.e3.
36. Tanenbaum ML, Adams RN, Lanning MS, et al. Using cluster analysis to understand clinician readiness to promote continuous glucose monitoring adoption. J Diabetes Sci Technol 2018;12(6):1108–15.
37. American Diabetes A. Economic costs of diabetes in the U.S. In 2017. Diabetes Care 2018;41(5):917–28.
38. Velasquez DE, Srinivasan S, Figueroa JF. Trends in social spending by private health insurers. J Gen Intern Med 2023;38(4):1081–3.
39. Wagner EH. Chronic disease management: what will it take to improve care for chronic illness? Eff Clin Pract 1998;1(1):2–4.
40. Langley GJ. The improvement guide : a practical approach to enhancing organizational performance. 2nd edition. San Francisco: Jossey-Bass. xxi; 2009. p. 490.
41. Moen M, Storr C, German D, et al. A review of tools to screen for social determinants of health in the united states: a practice brief. Popul Health Manag 2020; 23(6):422–9.
42. Services CfMM. Opportunities in Medicaid and chip to address social determinants of health (SDOH). Center for Medicaid and Medicare Services: department of health & human services; 2021.

Psychosocial Care for Youth with Type 1 Diabetes
Summary of Reviews to Inform Clinical Practice

Jenna B. Shapiro, PhD[a,b,*], Kimberly P. Garza, PhD, MPH[c],
Marissa A. Feldman, PhD[d], Madeleine C. Suhs, BS[a], Julia Ellis, BS[a],
Amanda Terry, PhD[a,b], Kelsey R. Howard, PhD[a,b],
Jill Weissberg-Benchell, PhD, CDCES[a,b]

KEYWORDS

- Type 1 diabetes • Children • Adolescents • Psychosocial • Intervention

KEY POINTS

- Psychosocial interventions in pediatric type 1 diabetes address barriers to diabetes care and enhance strengths to optimize self-management behaviors and improve emotional well-being.
- Family-based interventions demonstrate the most robust impact across glycemic and psychosocial outcomes. Youth-focused cognitive behavioral theory and motivational interviewing approaches also demonstrate positive effects.
- The most common intervention components include a formal approach to problem-solving and communication skills for healthy discussion and reduced family conflict.
- Interventions to improve health equity, caregiver well-being, and barriers to diabetes technology use show promising preliminary outcomes.

INTRODUCTION

The American Diabetes Association (ADA)[1,2] and the International Society for Pediatric and Adolescent Diabetes (ISPAD)[3] provide psychosocial care recommendations for youth with type 1 diabetes (T1D). Standards of care recognize that the daily demands of diabetes can negatively affect mental health. In addition, mental health, family dynamics, and the broader context in which a family lives impact self-management

[a] Ann & Robert H. Lurie Children's Hospital of Chicago, Pritzker Department of Psychiatry and Behavioral Health, 225 East Chicago Avenue, Box 10, Chicago, IL 60611, USA; [b] Northwestern University Feinberg School of Medicine, Department of Psychiatry & Behavioral Sciences, 446 E Ontario Street, Chicago, IL, USA; [c] Roanoke College, 221 College Lane, Salem, VA 24153, USA; [d] Johns Hopkins All Children's Hospital, Child Development and Rehabilitation Center, 880 Sixth Street South #170, Saint Petersburg, FL 33701, USA
* Corresponding author.
E-mail address: jeshapiro@luriechildrens.org

Endocrinol Metab Clin N Am 53 (2024) 107–122
https://doi.org/10.1016/j.ecl.2023.10.002
0889-8529/24/© 2023 Elsevier Inc. All rights reserved.

behaviors and glycemic outcomes.[1] Guidelines support creating a psychosocially-minded multidisciplinary team that offers routine psychological assessment and ongoing support beyond merely offering services when problems are identified.[1,3]

ADA and ISPAD both recommend administration of age-appropriate psychosocial screening tools (patient-reported outcomes) at diagnosis, in periodic intervals (eg, annually), when there are diabetes difficulties, and during life transitions.[1–4] Although generic measures of mental health are important to evaluate (eg, depression, anxiety, psychiatric history), diabetes-specific factors that affect self-management should also be assessed for youth and their caregivers.[1,3] Diabetes-related screening may include attitudes related to diabetes, expectations about and barriers to diabetes management, the emotional impact of diabetes (eg, diabetes distress, fear of hypoglycemia [FOH], health-related quality of life [HRQOL]), and family dynamics (eg, family communication and conflict, family involvement in diabetes tasks).[1–4] Screeners also assess for disordered eating behaviors and intentional insulin omission for weight loss, diabetes-related strengths, cognitive assessment and school functioning, sleep problems, health literacy, and access to resources.[1–4] Validated measures are often available for self-report by youth starting around age 8 years and for caregiver report.[3] Parent-proxy report is also available for screening emotional and behavioral challenges in younger children.[3]

When indicated, evidence-based behavioral health interventions address barriers to optimal self-care behaviors and build skills for enhanced diabetes and psychological outcomes.[1,3–5] ISPAD also encourages proactive interventions to prevent distress and optimize diabetes management.[3] The current review summarizes findings from select systematic reviews and meta-analyses on psychosocial interventions in pediatric diabetes to inform recommendations for care (**Table 1**, for a list of included reviews). Evidence-based interventions are organized around key behavioral health targets, including (1) emotional impact of diabetes and coping skills for youth with T1D, (2) family dynamics and caregiver mental health, (3) systemic factors contributing to health disparities, and (4) psychosocial factors affecting diabetes technology uptake and use.

YOUTH-FOCUSED BEHAVIORAL HEALTH INTERVENTIONS
Psychosocial Factors Impacting Youth Diabetes Outcomes

The time-intensive, complex, and relentless nature of diabetes self-management can impact youth mental health. Diabetes-specific distress refers to the negative emotions people experience (eg, worry, guilt, anger) when living with diabetes and the burden of daily self-management.[6] Diabetes-specific distress is recommended to be routinely monitored in youth ages 7 or 8 years and up and caregivers due to its high prevalence and negative impact on self-management and glycemic outcomes.[1,2] FOH can lead to purposefully maintaining suboptimally higher glucose levels to prevent hypoglycemia.[7] HRQOL, and diabetes HRQOL specifically, refers to an individual's subjective experience of the impact that diabetes and its management have on daily functioning.[8]

The diabetes resilience model[9] recognizes the challenges of managing diabetes and posits that protective processes are used to achieve optimal health and emotional outcomes. Protective processes include goal setting, problem-solving, stress management, and the ability to make meaning out of adverse experiences.[9] Diabetes strengths refer to adaptive skills including the perceived ability to manage the demands of diabetes and rely on others for help when needed.[10]

Although diabetes-specific distress and FOH are associated with suboptimal self-care behaviors and glycemic outcomes,[6,7] higher levels of diabetes-specific HRQOL

Table 1
Summary of select reviews on psychosocial interventions in pediatric diabetes

Reference, Date	Summary of Focus Area
Barry-Menkhaus et al,[24] 2020	Review of brief strategies for distress and self-management that can be delivered alongside usual medical care
Bergmame & Shaw,[11] 2021	Systematic and scoping review of psychosocial interventions to improve diabetes management
Boland et al,[37] 2019	Systematic review of barriers and facilitators to shared decision-making in pediatric health care settings
Butler et al,[57] 2022	Review of health disparities and promising approaches to improve health equity
Ellis & Naar,[25] 2023	Review of interventions to improve health disparities for racial and ethnic minoritized youth
Feldman et al,[32] 2018	Systematic review of family-based interventions
Fitzpatrick et al,[12] 2013	Systematic review of problem-solving interventions for diabetes self-management and glycemic outcomes
Gayes & Steele,[23] 2014	Meta-analysis of motivational interviewing for pediatric health behavior change
Hilliard et al,[13] 2016	Review of behavioral interventions to promote diabetes management
Hood et al,[14] 2010	Systematic review and meta-analysis of interventions with adherence-promoting components on glycemic control
Ispriantari et al,[34] 2023	Systematic review of family-based interventions on health outcomes
Lohan et al,[43] 2015	Systematic review of parenting interventions
McBroom & Enriquez,[33] 2009	Systematic review of family-based interventions on health outcomes and family dynamics
Savage et al,[18] 2010	Systematic review of psychosocial interventions on health outcomes
Tully et al,[44] 2017	Review of peer coaching interventions for caregivers
Wagner et al,[61] 2019	Review of interventions addressing diabetes-related challenges organized by social ecological systems
Winkley et al,[17] 2006	Systematic review and meta-analysis of psychological interventions on glycemic outcomes for children and adults
Winkley et al,[15] 2020	Systematic review and meta-analysis of psychological interventions on glycemic outcomes for children and adults
Wu et al,[16] 2023	Systematic review and meta-analysis of resilience-promoting interventions in adolescents
Zhao et al,[45] 2019	Meta-analysis of parenting interventions on psychosocial adjustment in caregivers of youth

and diabetes strengths are associated with more optimal self-care behaviors and glycemic outcomes.[8,10] By identifying an individual's strengths and struggles related to diabetes, effective behavioral health programs can be provided that build skills and target areas of concern. Diabetes-specific interventions differ from general approaches for mental health difficulties that do not address challenges directly related to diabetes.

Interventions for Children and Adolescents

Several published reviews evaluate the impact of youth-focused psychosocial interventions for diabetes-specific challenges.[11-16] Some reviews and meta-analyses combine different youth-focused and family-based interventions and have mixed findings. Some show small effects on glycemic outcomes,[14,17] others show no treatment effect,[15] and some show mixed effects for glycemic, self-management, and psychosocial outcomes.[11,12,16] Results suggest that theory-based interventions contribute to more positive health outcomes than a-theoretical interventions.[18]

Of the promising youth-focused behavioral health interventions, many are based on social cognitive theory (SCT), cognitive behavioral theory (CBT), or motivational interviewing (MI).[11,13] SCT suggests that an individual's belief in their ability to engage in diabetes self-care behaviors and the anticipated positive or negative consequences of each behavior influence the likelihood of completing self-management behaviors.[19] CBT recognizes interrelationships between thoughts, emotions, and behaviors. Negative thoughts are modified about diabetes and other situations, and adaptive coping behaviors are increased (eg, problem-solving, relaxation, assertive communication, organizational skills) to improve self-management behaviors and emotional well-being. MI recognizes that individuals vary in their readiness and willingness to change and that the likelihood of change, such as engaging in new or more frequent diabetes self-management behaviors, is enhanced when individuals articulate their own self-motivating change-focused statements.[20]

Resilience promotion interventions, or positive psychology interventions, use CBT and SCT to promote positive health and psychosocial outcomes.[13,16] Although resilience promotion interventions often teach more than one skill, the common thread is problem-solving, including identifying the problem, evaluating possible solutions, selecting the best option, and assessing impact.[12,16] Coping skills training is one group-based resilience promotion intervention that teaches problem-solving, stress management, assertive communication skills, positive self-talk, and conflict resolution and is associated with improved glycemic outcomes and HRQOL for teenagers 1-year post-intervention.[21] Supporting Teen Problem-Solving (STePS) is another teen-focused group-based intervention that builds diabetes strengths by improving emotion regulation, perspective-taking, problem-solving, and communication.[22] STePS reduces diabetes distress and depressive symptoms with effects increasing over 3 years.[22]

MI is a patient-centered empathy-led communication approach that increases the likelihood of behavior change by understanding the barriers to change and enhancing a youth's intrinsic motivation.[20] MI involves building awareness of discrepancies between current and desired behaviors, selectively reflecting youths' statements about reasons and ability to change, and setting and achieving attainable goals. MI is associated with improvements in hemoglobin A1c (HbA1c) and diabetes self-management behaviors for adolescents in the short and long term.[23]

Some reviews highlight the importance of mobile health approaches for teenagers given their relevance and potential for dissemination.[13] Technology-based interventions include reminders or positive affirmations via text message, apps for self-management monitoring, and reward-based gamified programs for self-management behaviors.[13] Although electronic interventions show some promise for self-efficacy and self-management behaviors, findings are mixed and youth-focused interventions do not appear to improve glycemic outcomes.[13,24,25]

Another review described brief interventions, referring to single session or low time commitment approaches that are potentially scalable in clinic settings and for families with low resources who may have limited availability to attend multiple sessions.[24] Examples include a resilience-based intervention, as part of the Diabetes Strengths Study that trained providers to emphasize what the youth is doing well and praise self-care behaviors, finding a positive impact on diabetes strengths, self-management behaviors, and diabetes distress.[26] In addition, MI can be delivered by any provider in a clinic setting by understanding what is important to a youth, focusing on the benefit of engaging in specific self-management behaviors to improve personal priority areas in the short term, and encouraging self-articulated reasons for change, though mental health professionals may be able to garner more robust effects. Other brief strategies include recommendations to pair diabetes tasks with other specific routine activities and teaching components of interventions that would typically be delivered over multiple sessions (eg, role playing to practice telling peers about diabetes; problem-solving to address a diabetes-related stressor; encouraging youth "delegation" of tasks to others increase tangible support).[24]

FAMILY-BASED BEHAVIORAL HEALTH INTERVENTIONS
Role of Parenting and Family Factors on Diabetes Outcomes

T1D impacts the entire family. When children are young, caregivers are directly responsible for diabetes management.[27] Young children may have difficulty communicating symptoms, engage in inconsistent food intake and physical activity, and may have difficulty tolerating finger sticks, insulin injections, or technology insertion.[27] Parenting behaviors around diabetes tasks and mealtime, and caregiver coping and psychological adjustment, affect diabetes management.[27] Diabetes distress and FOH are common for caregivers and affect glycemic outcomes, the latter increasing risk for intentionally maintaining higher glucose levels.[27]

Family involvement ideally becomes more collaborative in nature with as youth age. Open communication, shared responsibility for diabetes tasks, and emotional support from caregivers can enable self-efficacy (eg, parents' transition from administration of tasks to monitoring).[28] Authoritative parenting, family cohesion, and positive communication are associated with better child adjustment, psychological functioning, and glycemic outcomes.[29,30] Conversely, authoritarian parenting, high levels of diabetes-related family conflict, and diabetes-specific distress in caregivers are related to decreased adherence and worse glycemic outcomes.[31] Premature transition to independence in self-care, especially as competing demands increase during adolescence, can worsen self-management and glycemic control.[29] "Miscarried helping," an overinvolved and intrusive parenting behavior that is negatively perceived by adolescents, can also result in less engagement in self-care tasks, suboptimal glycemia, and negative psychological outcomes.[28]

Family-Focused Interventions

Several reviews evaluate family-based interventions, which broadly improve HbA1c, self-management behaviors, family functioning, and HRQOL.[32–34] Behavioral Family Systems Therapy (BFST) improves maladaptive family interactions and rules, changes negative assumptions about other family members' behaviors, and enhances collaborative problem-solving and communication skills (eg, reducing blame and lecturing through practicing non-accusatory statements, praise, and reflective listening).[35] With positive outcomes on diabetes-related family conflict, self-management behaviors, and parent–child relationships, revisions were made to include content specific to diabetes. The revised intervention, BFST for Diabetes (BFST-D), included behavioral contracting in which attainable goals and the behavioral steps to achieve them were identified along with associated privileges and consequences. Modifications resulted in improved self-management behaviors and HbA1c.[36]

Within the clinic setting, shared decision-making reflects a general approach to collaborating with patients and families in goal setting and other aspects of care by centering youth and caregiver preferences and values.[24,37] Another in-clinic intervention, Family Teamwork, involves four visits during diabetes appointments in which psychoeducation is provided on diabetes in the context of child development (eg, explaining the many factors affecting blood glucose and the need for active parental involvement).[38,39] An individualized responsibility sharing plan delineates caregiver versus youth task responsibilities. Collaborative problem-solving, emotional support, and communication with calm and neutral language are encouraged for out-of-range numbers, meals, and exercise. Family Teamwork improves family conflict, parent involvement, and HbA1c.[38,39]

Multifamily group therapy provides support to youth and their parents in a group setting and incorporates approaches such as behavioral contracting,[40] problem-solving,[40,41] communication skills,[40,41] and parent simulation of living with diabetes.[42] Multifamily groups improve glycemic outcomes under certain circumstances[41,42] and enhance psychosocial outcomes (eg, responsibility sharing, HRQOL).[40]

Caregiver-Only Interventions

Many family-based interventions include the youth with T1D, but some reviews focus on caregiver-only interventions.[43–46] One review evaluated peer coaching in which trained caregivers of youth with T1D provided emotional support and practical guidance on daily tasks.[44] Mothers receiving peer coaching experienced less diabetes distress, fewer management concerns, and more self-confidence.[47] However, follow-up studies resulted in inconsistent findings.[48,49] A stepped care approach, in which peer coaching was augmented by telephone-based CBT skills and then consultation with a diabetes educator and psychologist if needed (First STEPS [Study of Type 1 in Early childhood and Parenting Support]), found significant improvements in parent depressive symptoms over time.[46,50]

A few studies have focused on teaching CBT skills to support caregiver mental health and diabetes management. The Reducing Emotional Distress for Childhood Hypoglycemia in Parents (REDCHiP) intervention taught caregivers to identify worried thoughts related to hypoglycemia, enhance coping strategies (eg, relaxation, positive self-talk) and develop a fear hierarchy to engage in or imagine hypoglycemia-related situations (eg, having another adult treat a low). REDCHiP improved caregiver FOH at post-intervention and 3-month follow-up.[51] A telephone-based parent support program also taught CBT skills including problem-solving, resulting in improved short-term parenting stress.[52]

Parenting training enhances positive parenting strategies to improve behavioral functioning in youth. The standardized Positive Parenting Program (Triple P) was conducted with parents of young children with T1D and teaches parent behavior management skills to increase positive behaviors (eg, praise, quality time, giving instructions) and reduce misbehavior (eg, planned ignoring, setting ground rules, consequences, time out). Triple P improved caregiver depressive symptoms, anxiety, diabetes-related family conflict, and child disruptive behaviors for youth with preexisting challenges in the short term.[53] The DELFIN (Das Elterntraining für Eltern von Kindern mit Diabetes Typ 1 [The parenting program for parents of children with type 1 diabetes]) caregiver group intervention taught communication skills for diabetes-specific conflict situations. Metabolic outcomes remained stable for the intervention group while the control group declined.[54]

HEALTH EQUITY INTERVENTIONS
Health and Mental Health Disparities in Pediatric Type 1 Diabetes

Health equity is a fundamental goal in pediatric diabetes that refers to the absence of unfair differences in health across groups of people.[55] Health disparities occur in the context of systemic unfair distribution of resources and opportunities, historical disinvestment, hierarchical social structures, and discriminatory laws and policies that continue to enact harm on specific communities and result in systematic differences in health. Disparities in diabetes are well-documented; racially and ethnically minoritized youth with T1D experience worse health and psychosocial outcomes, including higher HbA1c levels, diabetes-related complications, less access to diabetes technologies, more difficulty engaging in diabetes care, higher diabetes distress, and lower social support than non-Hispanic White youth.[56,57] Youth and families with lower socioeconomic resources also experience higher HbA1c levels, more hospital admissions, and diabetes distress, and fewer opportunities to meet peers with diabetes.[57–59]

Social determinants of health are the circumstances in which people live, work, and grow and have been identified as important intervention targets to improve disparities in health.[55] Examples include difficulty accessing a treatment provider due to living far away from a medical setting, lack of access to affordable transportation, food and housing instability, financial difficulty, and exposure to chronic stress directly and indirectly impacting glycemic control and psychosocial outcomes.[25,55,57] A recent study found that implicit bias in medical providers reduces diabetes technology access such that families with public insurance are less likely to be offered technology, a practice that disproportionately affects racially and ethnically minoritized youth.[60] Mental health care stigma, low access to diabetes-related psychosocial support, and lack of experienced and diverse mental health providers are barriers to care that also disproportionately affect minoritized populations.[57]

Behavioral Health Interventions to Improve Health Equity

In addition to policy-related advocacy, culturally informed behavioral health interventions and those designed to improve access to equitable health care are critical for improving health and mental health equity.[25,57,61] Culturally sensitive intervention adaptations for racially and ethnically minoritized families include sharing short stories about other families' experiences to destigmatize challenges, using culturally tailored materials, offering culturally relevant faith-based coping strategies, and creating language-congruent clinics for Spanish-speaking families.[25,57,62] One three-session clinic-administered e-health intervention to increase caregiver monitoring for Black teenagers, The 3Ms (standing for *medicine*, *meter*, and *meals*), was developed with community partners, showing positive effects on HbA1c.[63]

To improve social determinants of health, Care Ambassadors increase clinic attendance by focusing on scheduling/rescheduling and confirming appointments.[64] In-person service navigators who provide community referrals to address social needs positively impact child health in other pediatric settings, with research in diabetes underway.[57,65] Providers can also be educated about insurance coverage for technology and risk for implicit bias to reduce gatekeeping devices.[25,60,66]

For families with frequent diabetes care difficulties, Multisystemic Therapy (MST) for diabetes involves intensive, home-based, individualized support to improve factors affecting diabetes in family, peer, school, neighborhood/community, and medical care settings.[67] At the youth and family levels, MST may incorporate CBT, parenting training, problem-solving, and communication skills. Within school, peer, and community settings, diabetes support and monitoring are increased. In the medical setting, clinic attendance barriers are addressed and family medical team communication and collaboration is facilitated. MST reduces diabetes-specific distress, HbA1c, and hospital admissions[67] and has been adapted with preliminary positive findings to be delivered by community health workers.[68]

Novel Interventions in Children's Healthcare (NICH) is a multisystemic intervention focused on improving social determinants of health and diabetes management within the broader environmental context.[69] NICH involves 24/7 care coordination and case management with frequent points of contact to advocate and communicate with the health care team, access basic needs and resources, and organize services and meetings with school and community agencies (eg, mental health care). For some families, NICH has also involved BFST-D[36] to enhance diabetes-related family dynamics.[69] NICH lowers HbA1c, reduces medical costs, and improves emergency department visits and hospital admissions for preventable diabetes concerns.[70]

Diabetes Technology Considerations and Interventions

Diabetes technology provides psychosocial advantages for youth and their families, including decreased distress, improved HRQOL, greater freedom, and greater control over life and diabetes.[66,71] Among the challenges that could contribute to discontinuation are information overload, device or insertion discomfort, size and visibility of devices, alarm intrusiveness, sensor/adhesive failures, or other technical difficulties.[66] In addition, some youth feel that wearing devices is a constant reminder of diabetes.[66]

Many challenges can be addressed by provider education and psychosocial support. One crucial element may be expectation setting when starting a device. Youth and caregivers may expect technologies to be hands-off[66] and disappointment may lead to device discontinuation. Education should include realistic expectations for what a device can do and what the experience of placing, wearing, and using it entails. Anticipatory guidance can be provided around common challenges with technology to proactively identify and problem solve around concerns (eg, guidelines for caregiver–adolescent communication related to remote monitoring; troubleshooting common issues related to adhesive or sensor malfunctions; strategies to optimize alarms and reduce "fatigue").

Although no reviews have been published specifically on interventions for technology uptake and use, one study on a caregiver-focused intervention for CGM use, Strategies to Enhance New CGM Use in Early Childhood (SENCE),[72] was noted in a review of family-based interventions.[46] Caregivers of young children were taught CBT skills for CGM-related situations (eg, identifying caregiver emotions related to out-of-range glucose levels, cognitive restructuring for negative thoughts about alarms, relaxation, problem-solving, communication skills), resulting in improved caregiver diabetes distress and FOH.[72]

DISCUSSION

Psychosocial care involves understanding the factors that affect diabetes outcomes for youth and families and providing evidence-based interventions to address barriers and build strengths to optimize diabetes care, mental health, and daily functioning. Family-focused interventions that improve communication, collaborative problem-solving, and responsibility sharing are the most robust for improving both glycemic and psychosocial outcomes.[32] Youth-focused interventions frequently teach CBT skills or use MI to increase motivation for change, significantly improving diabetes distress,[22] self-management behaviors,[11] and glycemic outcomes.[11,21] **Fig. 1** summarizes the components from the evidence-based interventions that improve psychosocial, behavioral, or glycemic outcomes in youth with T1D.

Problem-solving and communication skills are both components of effective youth-focused and family-based interventions, suggesting that these approaches are particularly impactful. However, one review identified that problem-solving as a stand-alone

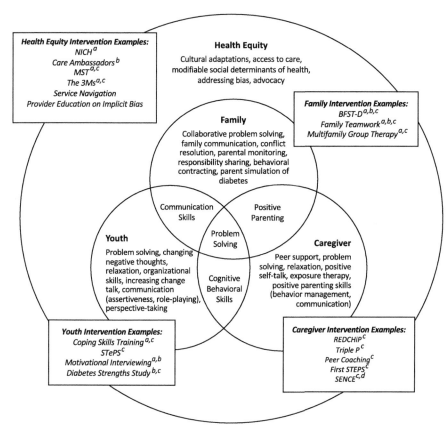

Fig. 1. Intervention components included in evidence-based psychosocial interventions in pediatric diabetes. [a]Improves glycemic outcomes. [b]Improve health behaviors. [c]Improve psychosocial outcomes. [d]Intervention focused on psychosocial aspects of diabetes technology use. NICH, Novel Interventions in Children's Healthcare[69,70]; Care Ambassadors[64]; MST, Multisystemic Therapy[67,68]; The 3Ms[63]; Service Navigation[57,65]; provider education on implicit bias[25,60,66]; BFST-D, Behavioral Family Systems Therapy for Diabetes[35,36]; Family Teamwork[38,39]; multifamily group therapy[40-42]; Coping Skills Training[21]; STePS, Supporting Teen Problem-Solving[22]; motivational interviewing[23]; Diabetes Strengths Study[26]; REDCHiP, Reducing Emotional Distress for Childhood Hypoglycemia in Parents[51]; Triple P, Positive Parenting Program[53]; peer coaching[44,47]; First STEPS, Study of Type 1 in Early Childhood and Parenting Support[46,50]; SENCE, Strategies to Enhance New CGM Use in Early childhood.[72]

approach seems insufficient for improving outcomes, noting that interventions seem most impactful when problem-solving is delivered along with other family-based or youth-focused intervention components over multiple sessions.[12] Further, when problem-solving and communication skills are delivered within a family context, the skills differ from those delivered within a youth-only framework. Specifically, family-based problem-solving refers to a collaborative process involving jointly identifying a problem, setting an attainable goal, listening to feedback from other family members, and selecting a solution that is mutually satisfactory, sometimes requiring negotiation and conflict resolution. In contrast, when conducted individually, youth unilaterally brainstorm, evaluate, select, and implement a chosen solution. Similarly, communication training in the context of youth-focused interventions teaches youth how to assertively ask for what they need or set boundaries. Family-based communication skills involve open and healthy dialogue to reduce blame, conflict, and miscommunication while increasing productive discussion, perspective-taking, and ability to listen. Both formats improve coping, but only family-based interventions improve conflictual interactions and shared responsibility for diabetes management within the family system; a possible reason family-based interventions seem more successful in improving outcomes. To further develop and study these and other diabetes-specific interventions, researchers should evaluate and compare intervention components to identify specific factors driving outcomes.

Interventions to improve caregiver well-being beyond parenting strategies alone are emerging with preliminary positive effects for caregiver FOH[51] and depressive symptoms.[50] Similarly, health equity interventions are being developed and evaluated, including culturally relevant adaptations and approaches to improving modifiable social determinants of health.[29,61] Interventions addressing technology-based psychosocial challenges are emerging.

Although psychosocial interventions are effective for improving glycemic, behavioral, and psychosocial outcomes for youth and caregivers, access remains limited. In recent studies on implementation of psychosocial screening, the most common barriers to screening in pediatric settings include time constraints, limited perceived impact of screening on medical decision-making, and difficulty knowing how to respond to elevations, including challenges identifying referrals.[73,74] The existing shortage of mental health providers,[75] worsened by the spike in mental health needs during the COVID-19 pandemic,[76] has only increased the barriers families face in accessing psychosocial care.

Solutions are needed to improve access to evidence-based psychosocial care for youth with diabetes. Embedding trained mental health providers within multidisciplinary clinics can improve access to evidence-based, diabetes-specific interventions and reduce the burden of finding and following up with external referrals. Training for diabetes care providers to effectively and thoughtfully deliver components of interventions in brief formats (eg, MI, problem-solving, family communication) may address some diabetes-specific challenges for some families. Community resources and programs can also be provided to families, including organizations providing peer connection, resources to help families with high social needs, and referrals to outpatient therapeutic support via the American Diabetes Association's mental health provider directory.[77] Ongoing training for mental health providers in the community about diabetes-specific considerations and interventions[78] will also increase availability of evidence-based psychosocial care.

The current review summarizes findings from other published reviews, and limitations reflect limited diversity (participants predominately identified as non-Hispanic White and were well-resourced) and small sample sizes. Future research is needed with increased demographic diversity in terms of race, ethnicity, socioeconomic status, and family structure.[11,15] This review also may not include more recent studies published after these prior reviews were completed. To date, no interventions included in reviews target child FOH, disordered eating behaviors (or the diabetes-specific behavior of intentional insulin omission for weight loss), sleep difficulty related to diabetes, or cognitive difficulties (eg, executive function challenges), reflecting unique risks in pediatric diabetes that can negatively impact health and psychological well-being.[3] Additional research is needed to examine pathways to improve glycemic outcomes given mixed findings. Research should also investigate which approach to use for specific individuals and families. Finally, a focus on implementation and dissemination is critical to increase access to effective interventions. Assessment of cost-effectiveness and facilitators and barriers to implementation are also needed.

CLINICS CARE POINTS

- Psychosocial assessment and evidence-based interventions are of critical importance when working with youth with type 1 diabetes.
- Diabetes-specific psychosocial interventions address barriers to care and build individual and family-based strengths to optimize self-management behaviors and improve psychological well-being.
- Family-based interventions seem strongest for improving outcomes and teach collaborative problem-solving and family communication to resolve common diabetes challenges.
- Youth- and caregiver-only interventions that provide cognitive behavioral and motivational interviewing strategies can also improve diabetes distress, diabetes strengths, quality of life, and glycemic outcomes.
- Clinicians should recognize barriers contributing to health disparities and provide culturally sensitive recommendations and referrals. There are systems-level interventions that can comprehensively support families with the greatest social needs.
- When starting diabetes technology, set realistic expectations and proactively address common challenges to support continued use.

DISCLOSURE

The authors have no conflicts to report.

REFERENCES

1. ElSayed NA, Aleppo G, Aroda VR, et al. Facilitating positive health behaviors and well-being to improve health outcomes: Standards of care in diabetes-2023. Diabetes Care 2023;46(Suppl 1):S68–96.
2. ElSayed NA, Aleppo G, Aroda VR, et al. 14. Children and adolescents: Standards of care in diabetes-2023. Diabetes Care 2023;46(Suppl 1):S230–53.
3. de Wit M, Gajewska KA, Goethals ER, et al. ISPAD Clinical Practice Consensus Guidelines 2022: Psychological care of children, adolescents and young adults with diabetes. Pediatr Diabetes 2022;23(8):1373–89.
4. Gregory JW, Cameron FJ, Joshi K, et al. ISPAD clinical practice consensus guidelines 2022: diabetes in adolescence. Pediatr Diabetes 2022;23(7):857–71.
5. de Bock M, Codner E, Craig ME, et al. ISPAD clinical practice consensus guidelines 2022: glycemic targets and glucose monitoring for children, adolescents, and young people with diabetes. Pediatr Diabetes 2022;23(8):1270–6.
6. Rechenberg K, Whittemore R, Holland M, et al. General and diabetes-specific stress in adolescents with type 1 diabetes. Diabetes Res Clin Pract 2017;130:1–8.
7. Johnson SR, Cooper MN, Davis EA, et al. Hypoglycaemia, fear of hypoglycaemia and quality of life in children with type 1 diabetes and their parents. Diabet Med 2013;30(9):1126–31.
8. Hilliard ME, Minard CG, Marrero DG, et al. Assessing health-related quality of life in children and adolescents with diabetes: Development and psychometrics of the Type 1 Diabetes and Life (T1DAL) measures. J Pediatr Psychol 2020;45(3):328–39.

9. Hilliard ME, Harris MA, Weissberg-Benchell J. Diabetes resilience: a model of risk and protection in type 1 diabetes. Curr Diab Rep 2012;12(6):739–48.

10. Hilliard ME, Iturralde E, Weissberg-Benchell J, et al. The Diabetes Strengths and Resilience Measure for Adolescents with Type 1 Diabetes (DSTAR-Teen): Validation of a new, brief self-report measure. J Pediatr Psychol 2017;42(9):995–1005.

11. Bergmame L, Shaw S. Clinical utility of psychoeducational interventions for youth with type 1 diabetes: a scoping review. Continuity in Education 2021;2(1):76–108.

12. Fitzpatrick SL, Schumann KP, Hill-Briggs F. Problem solving interventions for diabetes self-management and control: a systematic review of the literature. Diabetes Res Clin Pract 2013;100(2):145–61.

13. Hilliard ME, Powell PW, Anderson BJ. Evidence-based behavioral interventions to promote diabetes management in children, adolescents, and families. Am Psychol 2016;71(7):590–601.

14. Hood KK, Rohan JM, Peterson CM, et al. Interventions with adherence-promoting components in pediatric type 1 diabetes. Diabetes Care 2010;33(7):1658–64.

15. Winkley K, Upsher R, Stahl D, et al. Systematic review and meta-analysis of randomized controlled trials of psychological interventions to improve glycaemic control in children and adults with type 1 diabetes. Diabet Med 2020;37(5): 735–46.

16. Wu Y, Zhang YY, Zhang YT, et al. Effectiveness of resilience-promoting interventions in adolescents with diabetes mellitus: a systematic review and meta-analysis. World J Pediatr 2023;19(4):323–39.

17. Winkley K, Ismail K, Landau S, et al. Psychological interventions to improve glycaemic control in patients with type 1 diabetes: Systematic review and meta-analysis of randomized controlled trials. BMJ 2006;333(7558):65.

18. Savage E, Farrell D, McManus V, et al. The science of intervention development for type 1 diabetes in childhood: Systematic review. J Adv Nurs 2010;66(12): 2604–19.

19. Bandura A. Health promotion from the perspective of social cognitive theory. Psychol Health 1998;13(4):623–49.

20. Miller WR, Rose GS. Toward a theory of motivational interviewing. Am Psychol 2009;64(6):527–37.

21. Grey M, Boland EA, Davidson M, et al. Coping skills training for youth with diabetes mellitus has long-lasting effects on metabolic control and quality of life. J Pediatr 2000;137(1):107–13.

22. Weissberg-Benchell J, Shapiro JB, Bryant FB, et al. Supporting Teen Problem-Solving (STePS) 3 year outcomes: Preventing diabetes-specific emotional distress and depressive symptoms in adolescents with type 1 diabetes. J Consult Clin Psychol 2020;88(11):1019–31.

23. Gayes LA, Steele RG. A meta-analysis of motivational interviewing interventions for pediatric health behavior change. J Consult Clin Psychol 2014;82(3):521–35.

24. Barry-Menkhaus SA, Wagner DV, Riley AR. Small interventions for big change: Brief strategies for distress and self-management amongst youth with type 1 diabetes. Curr Diab Rep 2020;20(1):3.

25. Ellis D.A. and Naar S., Interventions across the translational research spectrum: Addressing disparities among racial and ethnic minoritized youth with type 1 diabetes, Endocrinol Metab Clin North Am, 52 (4), 2023, 585-602.

26. Hilliard ME, Eshtehardi SS, Minard CG, et al. Featured article: Strengths-based, clinic-integrated nonrandomized pilot intervention to promote type 1 diabetes adherence and well-being. J Pediatr Psychol 2019;44(1):5–15.

27. Pierce JS, Kozikowski C, Lee JM, et al. Type 1 diabetes in very young children: a model of parent and child influences on management and outcomes. Pediatr Diabetes 2017;18(1):17–25.

28. Gruhn MA, Lord JH, Jaser SS. Collaborative and overinvolved parenting differentially predict outcomes in adolescents with type 1 diabetes. Health Psychol 2016; 35(7):652–60.

29. Butler A, Georges T, Anderson B. Family Influences. In: Delamater A, Marrero D, editors. *Behavioral diabetes*. Cham, Switzerland: Springer; 2020. p. 105–20.

30. Monaghan M, Horn IB, Alvarez V, et al. Authoritative parenting, parenting stress, and self-care in pre-adolescents with type 1 diabetes. J Clin Psychol Med Settings 2012;19(3):255–61.

31. Tsiouli E, Alexopoulos EC, Stefanaki C, et al. Effects of diabetes-related family stress on glycemic control in young patients with type 1 diabetes: Systematic review. Can Fam Physician 2013;59(2):143–9.

32. Feldman MA, Anderson LM, Shapiro JB, et al. Family-based interventions targeting improvements in health and family outcomes of children and adolescents with type 1 diabetes: a systematic review. Curr Diab Rep 2018;18(3):15.

33. McBroom LA, Enriquez M. Review of family-centered interventions to enhance the health outcomes of children with type 1 diabetes. Diabetes Educ 2009;35(3): 428–38.

34. Ispriantari A, Agustina R, Konlan KD, et al. Family-centered interventions for children and adolescents with type 1 diabetes mellitus: an integrative review. Child Health Nurs Res 2023;29(1):7–23.

35. Wysocki T, Greco P, Harris MA, et al. Behavior therapy for families and adolescents with diabetes: Maintenance of treatment effects. Diabetes Care 2001; 24(3):441–6.

36. Wysocki T, Harris MA, Buckloh LM, et al. Randomized trial of behavioral family systems therapy for diabetes: maintenance of effects on diabetes outcomes in adolescents. Diabetes Care 2007 Mar;30(3):555–60.

37. Boland L, Graham ID, Légaré F, et al. Barriers and facilitators of pediatric shared decision-making: a systematic review. Implement Sci 2019;14(1):7.

38. Anderson BJ, Brackett J, Ho J, et al. An office-based intervention to maintain parent-adolescent teamwork in diabetes management. Impact on parent involvement, family conflict, and subsequent glycemic control. Diabetes Care 1999; 22(5):713–21.

39. Laffel LMB, Vangsness L, Connell A, et al. Impact of ambulatory, family-focused teamwork intervention on glycemic control in youth with type 1 diabetes. J Pediatr 2003;142(4):409–16.

40. Kichler JC, Kaugars AS, Marik P, et al. Effectiveness of groups for adolescents with type 1 diabetes mellitus and their parents. Fam Syst Health 2013;31(3): 280–93.

41. Carpenter JL, Price JEW, Cohen MJ, et al. Multifamily group problem-solving intervention for adherence challenges in pediatric insulin-dependent diabetes. Clin Pract Pediatr Psychol 2014;2(2):101–15.

42. Satin W, La Greca AM, Zigo MA, et al. Diabetes in adolescence: Effects of multifamily group intervention and parent simulation of diabetes. J Pediatr Psychol 1989;14(2):259–75.

43. Lohan A, Morawska A, Mitchell A. A systematic review of parenting interventions for parents of children with type 1 diabetes. Child Care Health Dev 2015;41(6): 803–17.

44. Tully C, Shneider C, Monaghan M, et al. Peer coaching interventions for parents of children with type 1 diabetes. Curr Diab Rep 2017;17(6):39.

45. Zhao X, Ai Z, Chen Y, et al. The effectiveness of parenting interventions on psychosocial adjustment in parents of children and adolescents with type 1 diabetes: a meta-analysis. Worldviews Evid Based Nurs 2019;16(6):462–9.

46. Monaghan M, Bryant BL, Inverso H, et al. Young children with type 1 diabetes: Recent advances in behavioral research. Curr Diab Rep 2022;22(6):247–56.

47. Sullivan-Bolyai S, Grey M, Deatrick J, et al. Helping other mothers effectively work at raising young children with type 1 diabetes. Diabetes Educ 2004;30(3): 476–84.

48. Mackey ER, Herbert L, Monaghan M, et al. The feasibility of a pilot intervention for parents of young children newly diagnosed with type 1 diabetes. Clin Pract Pediatr Psychol 2016;4(1):35–50.

49. Sullivan-Bolyai S, Bova C, Leung K, et al. Social Support to Empower Parents (STEP): an intervention for parents of young children newly diagnosed with type 1 diabetes. Diabetes Educ 2010;36(1):88–97.

50. Hilliard ME, Tully C, Monaghan M, et al. First STEPS: Primary outcomes of a randomized, stepped-care behavioral clinical trial for parents of young children with new-onset type 1 diabetes. Diabetes Care 2022;45(10):2238–46.

51. Patton SR, Clements MA, Marker AM, et al. Intervention to reduce hypoglycemia fear in parents of young kids using video-based telehealth (REDCHiP). Pediatr Diabetes 2020;21(1):112–9.

52. Monaghan M, Hilliard ME, Cogen FR, et al. Supporting parents of very young children with type 1 diabetes: Results from a pilot study. Patient Educ Couns 2011; 82(2):271–4.

53. Westrupp EM, Northam E, Lee KJ, et al. Reducing and preventing internalizing and externalizing behavior problems in children with type 1 diabetes: a randomized controlled trial of the Triple P-Positive Parenting Program. Pediatr Diabetes 2015;16(7):554–63.

54. Saßmann H, de Hair M, Danne T, et al. Reducing stress and supporting positive relations in families of young children with type 1 diabetes: a randomized controlled study for evaluating the effects of the DELFIN parenting program. BMC Pediatr 2012;12:152.

55. Hill-Briggs F, Adler NE, Berkowitz SA, et al. Social determinants of health and diabetes: a scientific review. Diabetes Care 2021;44(1):258–79.

56. Borschuk AP, Everhart RS. Health disparities among youth with type 1 diabetes: a systematic review of the current literature. Fam Syst Health 2015;33(3):297–313.

57. Butler AM, Brown SD, Carreon SA, et al. Equity in psychosocial outcomes and care for racial and ethnic minorities and socioeconomically disadvantaged people with diabetes. Diabetes Spectr 2022;35(3):276–83.

58. Hagger V, Hendrieckx C, Sturt J, et al. Diabetes distress among adolescents with type 1 diabetes: a systematic review. Curr Diab Rep 2016;16(1):9.

59. Walker AF, Schatz DA, Johnson C, et al. Disparities in social support systems for youth with type 1 diabetes. Clin Diabetes 2015;33(2):62–9.

60. Addala A, Hanes S, Naranjo D, et al. Provider implicit bias impacts pediatric type 1 diabetes technology recommendations in the United States: Findings from The Gatekeeper Study. J Diabetes Sci Technol 2021;15(5):1027–33.

61. Wagner DV, Koskela-Staples N, Harris MA, et al. All systems go: an ecological perspective of behavioral health for youth with type 1 diabetes. Fam Syst Health 2019;37:10–29.

62. Akindana A, Owens-Gary M, Williams A. When it all gets to be too much: Addressing diabetes distress in African Americans. AADE Pract 2016;4(4):44–9.
63. Ellis DA, Idalski Carcone A, Ondersma SJ, et al. Brief computer-delivered intervention to increase parental monitoring in families of African American adolescents with type 1 diabetes: A randomized controlled trial. Telemed J e Health 2017; 23(6):493–502.
64. Svoren BM, Butler D, Levine BS, et al. Reducing acute adverse outcomes in youths with type 1 diabetes: a randomized, controlled trial. Pediatrics 2003; 112(4):914–22.
65. Gottlieb LM, Hessler D, Long D, et al. Effects of social needs screening and in-person service navigation on child health: a randomized clinical trial. JAMA Pediatr 2016;170(11):e162521.
66. Brew-Sam N, Chhabra M, Parkinson A, et al. Experiences of young people and their caregivers of using technology to manage type 1 diabetes mellitus: Systematic literature review and narrative synthesis. JMIR Diabetes 2021;6(1):e20973.
67. Ellis DA, Frey MA, Naar-King S, et al. The effects of multisystemic therapy on diabetes stress among adolescents with chronically poorly controlled type 1 diabetes: Findings from a randomized, controlled trial. Pediatrics 2005;116(6): e826–32.
68. Ellis DA, Carcone AI, Naar-King S, et al. Adaptation of an evidence-based diabetes management intervention for delivery in community settings: Findings from a pilot randomized effectiveness trial. J Pediatr Psychol 2019;44(1): 110–25.
69. Harris MA, Wagner DV, Heywood M, et al. Youth repeatedly hospitalized for DKA: proof of concept for novel interventions in children's healthcare (NICH). Diabetes Care 2014;37(6):e125–6.
70. Wagner DV, Barry SA, Stoeckel M, et al. NICH at its best for diabetes at its worst: Texting teens and their caregivers for better outcomes. J Diabetes Sci Technol 2017;11(3):468–75.
71. Papadakis JL, Anderson LM, Garza K, et al. Psychosocial aspects of diabetes technology use. Endocrinol Metab Clin North Am 2020;49(1):127–41.
72. Strategies to Enhance New CGM Use in Early Childhood SENCE Study Group. A randomized clinical trial assessing continuous glucose monitoring (CGM) use with standardized education with or without a family behavioral intervention compared with fingerstick blood glucose monitoring in very young children with type 1 diabetes. Diabetes Care 2021;44(2):464–72.
73. Anderson LM, Papadakis JL, Vesco AT, et al. Patient-reported and parent proxy-reported outcomes in pediatric medical specialty clinical settings: A systematic review of implementation. J Pediatr Psychol 2020;45(3):247–65.
74. Corathers S, Williford DN, Kichler J, et al. Implementation of psychosocial screening into diabetes clinics: Experience from the type 1 diabetes exchange quality improvement network. Curr Diab Rep 2023;23(2):29.
75. Butryn T, Bryant L, Marchionni C, et al. The shortage of psychiatrists and other mental health providers: Causes, current state, and potential solutions. Int J Acad Med 2017;3:5–9.
76. Radhakrishnan L, Leeb RT, Bitsko RH, et al. Pediatric emergency department visits associated with mental health conditions before and during the COVID-19 pandemic - United States, January 2019-January 2022. MMWR Morb Mortal Wkly Rep 2022;71(8):319–24.

77. Mental health directory. In: American Diabetes Association: DiabetesPro. 1995–2022. Available at: https://my.diabetes.org/health-directory. Accessed August 1, 2023.

78. Behavioral health resources. In: American Diabetes Association: DiabetesPro. 1995-2022. Available at: https://professional.diabetes.org/meeting/other/behavioral-health-resources. Accessed August 1, 2023.

Acute and Chronic Adverse Outcomes of Type 1 Diabetes

Rachel Longendyke, MD*, Jody B. Grundman, MD, MPH,
Shideh Majidi, MD, MSCS

KEYWORDS

- Type 1 diabetes • Complications • Diabetic ketoacidosis • Severe hypoglycemia
- Macrovascular • Microvascular

KEY POINTS

- The Diabetes Control and Complications Trial (DCCT) and the follow-up Epidemiology of Diabetes Interventions and Complications (EDIC) study showed that improving glycemic management is associated with lower rates of complications.
- Acute complications can occur in youth and adolescents, and chronic complications can occur as early as the adolescent period.
- Guidelines exist for screening and management of complications.
- New technologies, including continuous glucose monitors and insulin pumps, have the potential to better understand/address glycemic patterns and decrease rates of both acute and chronic complications.

INTRODUCTION

Despite significant advances in diabetes treatment and technology in recent history, type 1 diabetes (T1D) continues to be associated with significant complications, both acute and chronic. In the acute setting, complications associated with T1D include hypoglycemia and diabetic ketoacidosis (DKA). Chronic complications can be categorized as either microvascular or macrovascular. Microvascular complications of T1D most commonly manifest as retinopathy, neuropathy, and nephropathy,[1] while macrovascular complications include various types of cardiovascular disease such as coronary artery disease, cerebrovascular disease, and peripheral vascular disease.[2]

The Diabetes Control and Complications Trial (DCCT) and the follow-up Epidemiology of Diabetes Interventions and Complications (EDIC) study showed that interventions aimed at maintaining glucose levels as close to the non-diabetic range as safely possible were associated with lower rates of both microvascular and macrovascular

Children's National Hospital, 111 Michigan Avenue Northwest, Washington, DC 20010, USA
* Corresponding author.
E-mail address: RLongendyke@childrensnational.org

Endocrinol Metab Clin N Am 53 (2024) 123–133
https://doi.org/10.1016/j.ecl.2023.09.004
0889-8529/24/© 2023 Elsevier Inc. All rights reserved.

complications.[3] However, achieving target hemoglobin (Hb)A1c levels remains a difficult challenge at any age, especially during youth and young adulthood.[4] As the prevalence of T1D continues to increase, concern for complications also rises.[2] Despite recent improvements in diabetes care, T1D continues to be associated with risk for substantial medical burden.[1] This article reviews the acute and chronic complications that are seen in youth and adults with T1D.

ACUTE COMPLICATIONS
Diabetic Ketoacidosis (DKA)

Diabetic ketoacidosis (DKA) is one of the most serious acute complications of T1D and is classically characterized by the triad of hyperglycemia, metabolic acidosis, and hyperketonemia.[5] Typical diagnostic criteria include elevated glucose of greater than 250 mg/dL, ketones detected in serum or urine, and metabolic acidosis (serum bicarbonate <18mEq/L and/or pH < 7.30).[6] DKA can be further classified as mild, moderate, or severe based on the severity of a patient's metabolic acidosis and the presence of altered mental status.[7] DKA typically presents with symptoms of nausea, vomiting, abdominal pain, declining mental status, and altered breathing patterns.[8] Patients may also report a history of polyuria, polydipsia, polyphagia, weakness, malaise, or lethargy.[8]

Approximately 30% of people with new-onset T1D present with DKA, with higher rates in children compared to adults.[5] In adults with known T1D, the incidence of DKA ranged from 0 to 263 per 1000 person-years (PYs) and prevalence ranged from 0 to 128 per 1000 people.[6] In children with established T1D, data published in 2015 from a German database of 31,330 individuals showed that in those aged 0.5 to 20 years the rate of ketoacidosis is 4.82 per 100 PYs.[9]

There are several established risk factors for DKA in people with previously diagnosed T1D. Non-modifiable risk factors include age, socioeconomic status, sex, and ethnicity.[9] Risk of DKA increases after early childhood (>5 year old) and then plateaus between 13 and 25 year old. After 25 years, the risk of DKA decreases as age increases.[9] People with socioeconomic disadvantages and females have also been shown to be at higher risk for DKA.[9] Modifiable risk factors for DKA include prior DKA admissions, elevated HbA1c, co-morbid psychiatric disorders, and acute infections.[9] The practice setting where people with T1D receive care may also be associated with risk of DKA. Individuals who are cared for in settings with less experience treating T1D had higher rates of DKA. Additionally, regular contact with an endocrinologist may protect against DKA, as people with poor clinic attendance and less contact with their diabetes health care team were more likely to have recurrent DKA.[9] The advancement of diabetes technology has associated with a decrease in DKA, with data from the type 1 diabetes exchange registry showed that individuals using a pump were less likely to report an episode of DKA compared to those using injection therapy (2% vs 4%; $P = .002$).[10]

DKA can be associated with significant morbidity and mortality, underscoring the importance of prompt treatment. The most common cause of death in DKA is cerebral edema.[11] Cerebral edema occurs in 0.7% to 1% of children with DKA, particularly in those with new-onset diabetes and presents with headache followed by altered mental status and lethargy.[7] Continued deterioration may lead to seizures, incontinence, pupillary changes, bradycardia, and respiratory arrest.[7] Mannitol is used in the treatment of cerebral edema.[7] Other complications of DKA are numerous and include electrolyte derangements (such as hypokalemia and hyperkalemia), thrombosis, stroke, and sepsis.[11]

Treatment of DKA is typically by protocol and specific to each institution. Nevertheless, the goals of treatment are the same, which include resolution of dehydration and correction of hyperglycemia, ketosis, and acidosis.[8] The 3 main components of treatment are intravenous hydration, insulin, and electrolyte management.

Of note, in pediatrics, the fluid resuscitation regimen is controversial, due at least in part to the lack of consensus regarding the cause of cerebral edema, which is a more common complication in the pediatric population.[8] Due to the proposed association between cerebral edema and the osmotic shifts from the rate of fluid or electrolyte replacement, the Pediatric Emergency Care Applied Research Network FLUID study compared the acute and long-term neurologic outcomes with subsequent rapid or slow fluid replacement of either 0.45% or 0.9% saline.[12] Ultimately, it did not show a significant difference between the various fluid administration protocols and neurologic outcomes.[12]

Severe Hypoglycemia

Hypoglycemia is the most common life-threatening acute complication of T1D treatment.[11] It is associated with significant morbidity and mortality with outcomes ranging from mild cognitive impairment to coma, seizure, and sudden death.[11] Also of importance, hypoglycemia can be a limiting factor in people with T1D obtaining tight glycemic control.[13]

Symptoms of hypoglycemia in general include tremor, palpitations, anxiety, sweating, hunger, and paresthesias.[13] The American Diabetes Association (ADA) defines level 3 hypoglycemia as a severe event that involves altered mental and/or physical function during which an individual requires assistance to recover.[14] Level 3 hypoglycemia may progress to unseriousness, seizure, coma, or death.[14]

Counterregulatory responses to hypoglycemia are impaired in people with T1D.[11] The first 2 physiologic protections against hypoglycemia (decrease in insulin secretion and increase in glucagon secretion) are lost and the third physiologic defense, release of epinephrine, is often attenuated.[13] The attenuated epinephrine response to declining glucose levels is responsible for defective glucose counterregulation. While the mechanism behind the attenuated sympathoadrenal response to hypoglycemia in those with T1D is not known, the loss of its sympathetic neural component causes hypoglycemia unawareness.[13] Hypoglycemia-associated autonomic failure is the concept that recent episodes of hypoglycemia or prior exercise or sleep causes defective glucose counterregulation as well as hypoglycemia unawareness, leading to recurrent hypoglycemia.[13]

Causes of hypoglycemia include missed meals, insulin dosing errors, and rapid insulin absorption due to intramuscular injection or taking a hot shower or bath soon after injection.[11] In addition, patients may overdose on insulin intentionally for secondary gain or suicide attempt.[11] In these situations, insulin overdose causes decreased hepatic glucose output.[11] Physical activity can also lead to hypoglycemia due to increased glucose utilization.[11]

Alcohol consumption suppresses gluconeogenesis and glycogenolysis and improves insulin sensitivity, therefore alcohol consumption is another risk factor for hypoglycemia.[11] Frequent hypoglycemia can lead to hypoglycemia unawareness, which can increase the risk for even lower blood sugars without detection and severe hypoglycemia.[11]

Since the DCCT, there have been several studies investigating the incidence rates of severe hypoglycemia in youth with T1D. In 1 study of children aged 0 to 19 years, where severe hypoglycemia was defined as a hypoglycemic episode causing loss of consciousness or seizure or resulting in an emergency department (ED) visit or admission, an incidence rate of 19 per 100 patient-years was reported.[15]

Exercise, which lowers blood glucose levels via skeletal muscle uptake, can also result in hypoglycemia.[11] Numerous studies in both adults and children have shown severe hypoglycemia events are more common at night, particularly following days with increased physical activity.[16] One study on adolescents with T1D participating in moderate-intensity exercise in the afternoon showed that glucose requirements to maintain euglycemia increased in a biphasic manner, with increased requirements during and shortly after exercise as well as between 24:00 and 04:00 hours.[17]

The use of insulin pumps has the benefit of lowering HbA1c levels without increasing the risk of hypoglycemia in pediatric patients. Adding continuous glucose monitors (CGM) to insulin pump therapy further decreases the rates of hypoglycemia.[11] Results of a systematic review of commercial hybrid closed-loop (HCL) automated insulin delivery (AID) systems showed that these technologies improve glycemic control without increasing the incidence of severe hypoglycemia.[18] In adults, use of CGM has also been shown to decrease time with glucose less than 70 mg/dL.[19] HCL systems also decrease hypoglycemia in this population.[20]

Most episodes of asymptomatic or symptomatic hypoglycemia can be effectively treated with glucose tablets or carbohydrate-containing food or drink.[13] Glucose gel is another option, particularly when a person is conscious but not oriented.[21] Glucagon injections have been used for decades to manage severe hypoglycemia.[11] More recently, glucagon nasal powder has been approved for management of severe hypoglycemia.[22] In the hospital setting, dextrose infusion is another option for treatment.[11]

CHRONIC COMPLICATIONS
Microvascular Complications

Diabetic retinopathy
Diabetic retinopathy (DR) is a microvascular complication that causes progressive vision loss in people with T1D. Its prevalence is highly correlated with the individual's duration of diabetes, and it is the most frequent cause of new cases of blindness in adults aged 20 to 74 years.[2] DR is characterized by abnormalities of the retina and is divided into 2 main categories: non-proliferative diabetic retinopathy (NPDR) and proliferative diabetic retinopathy (PDR).[23] The global prevalence for any DR is 27%. There is a 25% prevalence of NPDR, 1.4% PDR, and 4.6% diabetic macular edema.[24]

In addition to duration of diabetes, chronic hyperglycemia is a major risk factor for the development of DR.[2] The development of DR is also strongly correlated with hypertension.[25] Higher Hb A1C levels are associated with the progression of DR, while intensive glycemic control decreases the incidence and deterioration of retinopathy.[25] Other risk factors include nephropathy, dyslipidemia, smoking, and higher body mass axis (BMI).[25] Interestingly, worsening of DR is also associated with initiation of effective treatment and large and rapid reductions in blood glucose levels.[26]

The ADA currently recommends that adults with T1D have an initial dilated and comprehensive eye examination within 5 years after onset of diabetes.[27] Following initial examination, if there is no retinopathy for 1 or more annual examinations and glycemia is well controlled, screening every 1 to 2 years can be considered.[27] However, if retinopathy is present, eye examinations should be repeated at least annually, and if progressing or sight-threatening, eye examinations will need to be more frequent.[27] For children and adolescents, the first dilated and comprehensive eye examination is recommended 3 to 5 years after diagnosis, provided the child is $\geq$ 11 year old or puberty has started, whichever is earlier.[28] Following the initial examination, repeated dilated and comprehensive eye examinations should occur every 2 years; however, less frequent examinations may be appropriate based on risk factor assessment.[28]

Treating diabetic retinopathy depends on treating both the underlying metabolic conditions that lead to the development of retinopathy as well as treating the particular abnormalities identified.[2] Therefore, intensive diabetes management aimed at achieving near normoglycemia is 1 goal of treatment. Improved glycemic control has been shown to prevent DR as well as delay its progression.[2] In addition to optimizing blood glucose management, high blood pressure and dyslipidemia should also be addressed to avoid progression of retinopathy.[2,25]

In addition to the medical management discussed previously, there are several intraocular therapies for DR.[25] For those with diabetic macular edema, anti-vascular endothelial growth factor (VEGF) therapy (such as ranibizumab, bevacizumab, and aflibercept) has been shown to reduce diabetic macular edema and improve vision.[25] Laser photocoagulation is another well-established treatment for those with diabetic retinopathy.[2] Panretinal laser photocoagulation is the preferred treatment for all patients with PDR as well as those with severe NPDR.[25] In addition, recent studies have shown that intravitreous injection of anti-VEGF may be an alternative treatment to panretinal laser photocoagulation for those with PDR.[25]

Nephropathy

Diabetic nephropathy (DN) is one of the most frequent and severe complications of diabetes.[29] DN most commonly presents 5 to 15 years after diagnosis of T1D.[30] DN is estimated to occur in 20% to 40% of people with diabetes, is the most common cause of end-stage renal disease (ESRD), and is associated with an increased risk of death, primarily from cardiovascular causes.[2]

Albuminuria is a marker of many of the pathologic findings associated with DN, including elevated glomerular pressure, glomerular basement membrane abnormalities, and injury to endothelial cells and kidney tubules.[31] The earliest stage of DN is microalbuminuria, which is defined as albumin excretion of 30 to 299 mg/24 hours.[2] Macroalbuminuria, a more advanced stage of DN, represents albuminuria $\geq$ 300 mg/24 hours.[2] People with T1D who progress from microalbuminuria to macroalbuminuria are likely to develop ESRD.[32] While, classically, DN has been characterized by persistent albuminuria followed by a decline in glomerular filtration rate (GFR), there are several alternative phenotypes including albuminuria regression, rapid decline in GFR, and non-proteinuric or non-albuminuric DKA, which are characterized by a decreased GFR without proteinuria.[33]

A longer duration of diabetes has been found to be associated with a higher prevalence of DN.[31] Persistent hyperglycemia is also directly associated with DN.[31] It is well established that the main risk factors for DN are hyperglycemia, hypertension, and genetic predisposition.[2] Other risk factors include elevated serum lipids, obesity, smoking, and a family history of DN.[31]

Screening for DN is important as people with T1D are often asymptomatic until their GFR has significantly declined.[31] The main method of screening for DN is by urine albumin excretion, measured by an albumin-to- creatinine ratio in random spot urine.[2] For those with T1D, the ADA recommends considering annual screening for albuminuria with annual urine albumin at puberty or age greater than 10 year old or puberty (whichever is earlier) and have had diabetes for $\geq$5 years.[28] The ADA currently recommends that all adults with T1D for $\geq$5 years also obtain an annual estimated GFR.[30] In patients who have a diagnosis of DN, urinary albumin should be assessed more frequently, anywhere from 1 to 4 times per year depending on the stage of the disease.[30]

Prevention of DN involves effective treatment for the known risk factors, including hypertension, hyperglycemia, smoking, and dyslipidemia.[2] In individuals who have evidence of nephropathy, the goal of treatment is to prevent the progression from microalbuminuria to macroalbuminuria which helps to prevent decline in renal function and reduces the risk of cardiovascular events.[2] Intensive diabetes management, specifically targeting an HbA1c $\leq$ 7%, has been shown to prevent progression from microalbuminuria to macroalbuminuria.[31] In people with T1D who have hypertension, angiotensin converting enzyme (ACE) inhibitors and/or angiotensin-receptor blockers (ARBs) are the first-line treatment.[31] These agents have been shown to prevent or forestall progression to albuminuria and decreased renal function in people with T1D and hypertension.[31]

Neuropathy

Microvascular complications of the nervous system also occur in those with T1D. The diabetic neuropathies represent a heterogenous group of different disorders that can present with diverse clinical symptoms and may be focal or diffuse in presentation.[2] Distal symmetric polyneuropathy, also referred to as peripheral neuropathy, is the most common neuropathy in people with diabetes.[31] Diabetic peripheral neuropathy (DPN) occurs in a "stocking and glove" distribution, affecting the hands and lower limbs.[34] Diabetic autonomic neuropathies (DAN) are also common in those with T1D.[2] Various types of autonomic neuropathies can occur, including cardiac autonomic neuropathy, gastrointestinal dysmotility, diabetic cytopathy, and erectile dysfunction.[34]

It is estimated that at least 20% of adults with diabetes have at least 1 manifestation of DPN.[2] In youth with T1D, the prevalence of peripheral neuropathy has been estimated to be anywhere from 7% to 90%, the large range likely reflecting both symptomatic and asymptomatic patients as well as various measures used in different studies.[31] The prevalence of DAN is reported to range from 1.6% to 90%, depending on the test used for assessment.[2] When looking specifically at cardiac autonomic neuropathy (CAN) in young people with T1D, the prevalence was found to be 12%.[34]

Poor glycemic control is the main risk factor in the development and progression of DPN in both youth and adults with diabetes.[31] Near-normal glycemic control has been shown to delay or prevent the development of DPN and CAN in those with T1D.[27] DPN has also been associated with other risk factors, including lipid and blood pressure indexes and duration of diabetes.[35] Risk factors for DAN include diabetes duration, age, poor glycemic control, hypertension, and dyslipidemia.[2]

Up to half of people with DPN may be asymptomatic and therefore at high risk of injury, emphasizing the importance of screening for peripheral neuropathy to prevent further loss of sensory function and improve quality of life.[2] Clinical screening for peripheral neuropathy by physical examination can be via pinprick of the foot, ankle reflexes, vibratory sensation via tuning fork, and examination of proprioception.[31] Screening for autonomic neuropathy can include asking patients about symptoms of orthostatic dizziness, syncope, or dry, cracked skin in the extremities.[27] In adults, screening for DPN and DAN should begin 5 years after diagnosis of T1D and should occur annually thereafter.[27] For children and adolescents, the ADA recommends screening for DPN with a yearly comprehensive foot examination beginning at the start of puberty or at age $\geq$10 years, whichever is earlier once the patient has had a diabetes duration of 5 years.[28]

It is recommended that control of glucose, blood pressure, and serum lipids be optimized to prevent or delay the development of neuropathy.[27] Furthermore, while treatments aimed at reversing underlying nerve damage in diabetic neuropathy are currently not available, both pharmacologic and non-pharmacologic strategies for pain relief in DPN and for relief of symptoms in DAN are available.[27] For neuropathic pain in diabetes, pregabalin or duloxetine are the recommended initial treatments.[36] Treatments for autonomic neuropathy are aimed at the specific organ affected.[2] In CAN, treatment is aimed at alleviating symptoms specific to the patient's clinical manifestation.[36] For example, postural hypotension and dizziness may be treated with mechanical measures or pharmacologic agents.[2] Gastroparesis may be treated by eating small frequent meals.[2] Metoclopramide, a prokinetic agent, is the only FDA- approved treatment for gastroparesis at the present time.[27] Lastly, potential treatments for erectile dysfunction include phosphodiesterase type 5 inhibitors.[2] Other treatment options include intracorporeal or intraurethral prostaglandins, vacuum devices, or penile prostheses.[27] The ADA does not currently have recommendations for treatment of neuropathy in children or adolescents.[28]

As a result of multiple factors, including peripheral neuropathy, foot ulcerations and amputations are associated with diabetes.[27] Therefore, the ADA recommends a comprehensive foot examination for adults at least annually to identify those at risk for ulceration and amputation.[27] Those with evidence of sensory loss or a history of ulceration or amputation should have foot inspections more frequently.[27]

Macrovascular Complications

Cardiovascular disease (CVD) is a broad term that encompasses numerous conditions that affect the heart and the major blood vessels, including coronary artery disease (CAD), cerebrovascular disease, and peripheral vascular disease (PVD).[37] There is significant overlap in the disease processes involved in all 3 subtypes of cardiovascular disease.[37] Prior studies have revealed that patients with T1D have an increased incidence of cardiovascular events as well as increased cardiovascular disease mortality.[38]

CVD is characterized by vascular dysfunction and in diabetes this is a result of endothelial dysfunction and chronic vascular inflammation which cause atherosclerosis and vascular obstruction.[37] In the macrovasculature, these pathologic changes lead to CAD, PVD, and cerebrovascular disease.[37] It is theorized that hyperglycemia itself may cause both endothelial dysfunction and vascular inflammation through numerous metabolic processes that involve oxidative stress.[37]

The long-term cumulative incidence of CVD in those with T1D from the DCCT/EDIC study was 14% after 30 years of diabetes duration.[39] The risk of mortality from CVD in those with T1D is 3 to 10 fold higher than those without T1D.[40] In youth with T1D, subclinical signs of CVD are evident based on assessment of carotid intima-media thickness and arterial stiffness.[41,42] Youth with T1D also have higher rates of CVD risk factors with anywhere from 14% to 45% having 2 or more risk factors.[43,44]

The increased cardiovascular risk in patients with T1D is multifactorial with risk factors of chronic hyperglycemia, diabetic nephropathy, and cardiac autonomic neuropathy, as well as the usual cardiovascular risk factors of tobacco smoking, elevated LDL cholesterol, and hypertension.[38] Several other factors are also suspected to play a role in the increased cardiovascular risk in T1D, including hypoglycemia, increased glycemic variability, insulin resistance in overweight/obese patients, other lipid disorders, and potentially a dysfunctional immune system response.[38]

The ADA provides recommendations for the screening of cardiovascular risk factors in people with T1D. For both children and adults with T1D, blood pressure should be monitored at every visit.[28,45] In children (age $\geq$2 years) and adolescents, dyslipidemia should be screened with an initial lipid profile soon after diagnosis, once glycemia has improved .[28] If initial LDL is $\leq$ 100 mg/dL, testing should be repeated at 9 to 11 years of age.[28] If repeated LDL is <100 mg/dL, then lipid panel should be repeated every

3 years.[28] For adults not taking statins or other lipid-lowering therapy, the ADA recommends obtaining a lipid profile at the time of diabetes diagnosis and at least every 5 years thereafter if under the age of 40 years.[45] Screening for signs and symptoms of CV autonomic neuropathy should begin 5 years after diagnosis of T1D.[46] Currently, in asymptomatic adults with T1D, the ADA does not recommend routine screening for CAD, as it does not improve outcomes as long as atherosclerotic cardiovascular disease risk factors are treated.[45]

Treatment for CVD depends on the specific condition and can include lifestyle modifications, lipid-lowering medications, and anti-hypertensives. Recent studies have also suggested the potential of metformin to improve cardiovascular and cerebrovascular risk factors.[47]

SUMMARY

T1D is associated with acute and chronic complications in youth and adults. Chronically elevated HbA1c levels are the most common risk factor associated with complications. Following the DCCT, HbA1c became the gold standard for the assessment of glycemic control.[48] While there is a substantial body of data that links increasingly high HbA1c levels to increased rate of complications, people with the same HbA1c sometimes have significantly different rates of complications.[48] HbA1c does not capture fluctuations in glucose levels between different days or throughout any given day and is affected by non–diabetes-related conditions, including hemoglobinopathies, liver disease, pregnancy, and chronic kidney disease.[49] Limitations in the utility of HbA1c measurements have led to a desire to find other methods of assessment of glycemic control.

Usage of continuous glucose monitors (CGMs) has become more widespread in recent years, providing data that can complement monitoring of HbA1c in the clinical setting.[48] The ADA recommends that a CGM should be offered to adults and children using multiple daily injections or continuous subcutaneous insulin.[50] CGM has resulted in the development of core metrics for comprehensive understanding of glycemic status, including time in range (TIR), which is defined as 70 to 180 mg/dL.[49] A TIR of 70% correlated with an HbA1c of 7.0%, while a TIR of 80% approximates a HbA1c of 6.5%.[49] As TIR becomes a more prominent method for assessing glycemic control, numerous studies have evaluated the impact of TIR on diabetes complications.[49] Various studies have associated TIR with DR, albuminuria, and diabetic polyneuropathy.[49] Recent evidence has shown that AID systems increase TIR and improve A1C in those with diabetes.[50]

Improvements have been made to decrease the risk of complications, including the expansion of types of insulin available and advancement of technologies. Early identification of autoantibodies before diabetes diagnosis may help decrease the high rates of DKA at T1D diagnosis. However, despite recent advancements, there is still a significant burden from complications. Continued efforts and interventions are needed to decrease complication rates further, including earlier identification of diabetes and interventions to improve diabetes management as early as possible.

CLINICS CARE POINTS

- DKA is still prevalent at diagnosis in youth, occurring with ~30% of new-onset diagnoses in children. The risk of cerebral edema, and its associated morbidity and mortality, remains a severe potential consequence of DKA.

- Elevated HbA1c levels are associated with the development of acute and chronic complications. Greater percent TIR has been associated with less DR, albuminuria, and polyneuropathy.

- Use of insulin pumps has the benefit of lowering HbA1c levels without increasing the risk of hypoglycemia in pediatric patients. Adding CGM to insulin pump therapy further decreases the rates of hypoglycemia.

- Use of CGM in adults using both multiple daily insulin injections and insulin pump therapy not only lowers HbA1c but also increases TIR and reduces hypoglycemia.

- HCL AID systems further improve glycemic control in both children and adults.

- Attention to improving glycemic, blood pressure, and lipid control can reduce chronic diabetes complications. A rapid decrease in HbA1c has been associated with transient worsening of DR.

DISCLOSURE

The authors have no conflicts of interest to disclose.

REFERENCES

1. DiMeglio LA, Evans-Molina C, Oram RA. Type 1 diabetes. Lancet 2018;391: 2449–62.
2. Melendez-Ramirez LY, Richards RJ, Cefalu WT, et al. Complications of type 1 diabetes. Endocrinol Metab Clin North Am 2010;39(3):625–40.
3. Nathan DM. The diabetes control and complications trial/epidemiology of diabetes interventions and complications study at 30 years: overview. Diabetes Care 2014;37:9–16.
4. Miller KM, Beck RW, Foster NC, et al. HbA1c Levels in Type 1 Diabetes from Early Childhood to Older Adults: A Deeper Dive into the Influence of Technology and Socioeconomic Status on HbA1c in the T1D Exchange Clinic Registry Findings. Diabetes Technol Ther 2020;22(9):645–50.
5. Ehrmann D, Kulzer B, Roos T, et al. Risk factors and prevention strategies for diabetic ketoacidosis in people with established type 1 diabetes. Lancet Diabetes Endocrinol 2020;8(5):436–46.
6. Fazeli Farsani S, Brodovicz K, Soleymanlou N, et al. Incidence and prevalence of diabetic ketoacidosis (DKA) among adults with type 1 diabetes mellitus (T1D): a systematic literature review. BMJ Open 2017;7(7):e016587.
7. Gosmanov AR, Gosmanova EO, Kitabchi AE. Hyperglycemic crises: diabetic ketoacidosis and hyperglycemic hyperosmolar state. South; Dartmouth (MA): MDText.com; 2000. https://www.endotext.org/section/diabetes/.
8. Calimag APP, Chlebek S, Lerma EV, et al. Diabetic ketoacidosis. Dis Mon 2023; 69(3):101418.
9. Karges B, Rosenbauer J, Holterhus PM, et al. Hospital admission for diabetic ketoacidosis or severe hypoglycemia in 31,330 young patients with type 1 diabetes. Eur J Endocrinol 2015;173(3):341–50.
10. Foster NC, Beck RW, Miller KM, et al. State of Type 1 Diabetes Management and Outcomes from the T1D Exchange in 2016-2018. Diabetes Technol Ther 2019; 21(2):66–72.
11. Rewers A. Acute Metabolic Complications in Diabetes. In: Cowie CC, Casagrande SS, Menke A, et al, editors. Diabetes in America. 3rd edition. Bethesda (MD): National Institute of Diabetes and Digestive and Kidney Diseases (US); 2018. CHAPTER 17.

12. Kuppermann N, Ghetti S, Schunk JE, et al. PECARN DKA FLUID Study Group. Clinical Trial of Fluid Infusion Rates for Pediatric Diabetic Ketoacidosis. N Engl J Med 2018;378(24):2275–87.

13. Cryer PE. Hypoglycemia in type 1 diabetes mellitus. Endocrinol Metab Clin North Am 2010;39(3):641–54.

14. ElSayed NA, Aleppo G, Aroda VA, et al. 6. Glycemic Targets: Standards of Care in Diabetes—2023. Diabetes Care 2023;46(Supplement_1):S97–110.

15. Rewers A, Chase HP, Mackenzie T, et al. Predictors of Acute Complications in Children With Type 1 Diabetes. JAMA 2002;287(19):2511–8.

16. Tsalikian E, Mauras N, Beck RW, et al. Impact of exercise on overnight glycemic control in children with type 1 diabetes mellitus. J Pediatr 2005;147(4):528–34.

17. McMahon SK, Ferreira LD, Ratnam N, et al. Glucose requirements to maintain euglycemia after moderate-intensity afternoon exercise in adolescents with type 1 diabetes are increased in a biphasic manner. J Clin Endocrinol Metab 2007;92(3):963–8.

18. Peacock S, Frizelle I, Hussain S. A Systematic Review of Commercial Hybrid Closed-Loop Automated Insulin Delivery Systems. Diabetes Ther 2023;14(5):839–55.

19. Beck RW, Riddlesworth T, Ruedy K, et al. Effect of Continuous Glucose Monitoring on Glycemic Control in Adults With Type 1 Diabetes Using Insulin Injections: The DIAMOND Randomized Clinical Trial. JAMA 2017;317(4):371–8.

20. Garg SK, Weinzimer SA, Tamborlane WV, et al. Glucose Outcomes with the In-Home Use of a Hybrid Closed-Loop Insulin Delivery System in Adolescents and Adults with Type 1 Diabetes. Diabetes Technol Ther 2017;19(3):155–63.

21. Iqbal A, Heller S. Managing hypoglycaemia. Best Pract Res Clin Endocrinol Metab 2016;30(3):413–30.

22. Sherr JL, Ruedy KJ, Foster NC, et al. Glucagon Nasal Powder: A Promising Alternative to Intramuscular Glucagon in Youth With Type 1 Diabetes. Diabetes Care 2016;39(4):555–62.

23. Wang W, Lo ACY. Diabetic Retinopathy: Pathophysiology and Treatments. Int Journal Mol Sci 2018;19(6):1816–30.

24. Thomas RL, Halim S, Gurudas S, et al. IDF Diabetes Atlas: A review of studies utilising retinal photography on the global prevalence of diabetes related retinopathy between 2015 and 2018. Diabetes Res Clin Pract 2019;157:107840.

25. Lin KY, Hsih WH, Lin YB, et al. Update in the epidemiology, risk factors, screening, and treatment of diabetic retinopathy. J Diabetes Investig 2021;12(8):1322–5.

26. Bain SC, Klufas MA, Ho A, et al. Worsening of diabetic retinopathy with rapid improvement in systemic glucose control: A review. Diabetes Obes Metab 2019;21(3):454–66.

27. ElSayed NA, Aleppo G, Aroda VA, et al. 12. Retinopathy, Neuropathy, and Foot Care: Standards of Care in Diabetes—2023. Diabetes Care 2023;46(Supplement_1):S203–15.

28. ElSayed NA, Aleppo G, Aroda VA, et al. 14. Children and Adolescents: Standards of Care in Diabetes— 2023. Diabetes Care 2023;46(Supplement_1):S230–53.

29. Samsu N. Diabetic Nephropathy: Challenges in Pathogenesis, Diagnosis, and Treatment. BioMed Res Int 2021;2021:1497449.

30. ElSayed NA, Aleppo G, Aroda VA, et al. 11. Chronic Kidney Disease and Risk Management: Standards of Care in Diabetes—2023. Diabetes Care 2023;46(Supplement 1):S191–202.

31. Tommerdahl KL, Shapiro ALB, Nehus EJ, et al. Early microvascular complications in type 1 and type 2 diabetes: recent developments and updates. Pediatr Nephrol 2022;37(1):79–93.
32. American Diabetes Association. Standards of Medical Care in Diabetes—2010. Diabetes Care 2010;33(Supplement_1):S11–61.
33. Oshima M, Shimizu M, Yamanouchi M, et al. Trajectories of kidney function in diabetes: a clinicopathological update. Nat Rev Nephrol 2021;17:740–50.
34. Feldman EL, Callaghan BC, Pop-Busui R, et al. Diabetic neuropathy. Nat Rev Dis Primers 2019;5:41.
35. Boulton AJM, Vinik AI, Arezzo JC, et al. Diabetic Neuropathies: A statement by the American Diabetes Association. Diabetes Care 2005;28(4):956–62.
36. Pop-Busui R, Boulton AJ, Feldman EL, et al. Diabetic Neuropathy: A Position Statement by the American Diabetes Association. Diabetes Care 2017;40(1):136–54.
37. Sharma H, Lencioni M, Narendran P. Cardiovascular disease in type 1 diabetes. Cardiovascular Endocrinology & Metabolism 2019;8(1):28–34.
38. Vergès B. Cardiovascular disease in type 1 diabetes: A review of epidemiological data and underlying mechanisms. Diabetes Metab 2020;46(6):442–9.
39. Nathan DM, Zinman B, Cleary PA, et al. Modern-Day Clinical Course of Type 1 Diabetes Mellitus after 30 Years' Duration: The Diabetes Control and Complications Trial/Epidemiology of Diabetes Interventions and Complications and Pittsburgh Epidemiology of Diabetes Complications Experience (1983–2005). Arch Intern Med 2009;169:1307–16.
40. Lind M, Svensson A-M, Kosiborod M, et al. Glycemic Control and Excess Mortality in Type 1 Diabetes. N Engl J Med 2014;371:1972–82.
41. Urbina EM, Dabelea D, D'Agostino RB Jr, et al. Effect of type 1 diabetes on carotid structure and function in adolescents and young adults: the SEARCH CVD study. Diabetes Care 2013;36(9):2597–9.
42. Christoforidis A, Georeli I, Dimitriadou M, et al. Arterial stiffness indices in children and adolescents with type 1 diabetes mellitus: A meta-analysis. Diabetes Metab Res Rev 2022;38(6):e3555.
43. Margeirsdottir HD, Larsen JR, Brunborg C, et al. High prevalence of cardiovascular risk factors in children and adolescents with type 1 diabetes: a population-based study. Diabetologia 2008;51(4):554–61.
44. Rodriguez BL, Fujimoto WY, Mayer-Davis EJ, et al. Prevalence of cardiovascular disease risk factors in U.S. children and adolescents with diabetes: the SEARCH for diabetes in youth study. Diabetes Care 2006;29(8):1891–6.
45. ElSayed Nuha A, Aleppo Grazia, Aroda Vanita R, et al. 10. Cardiovascular Disease and Risk Management: Standards of Care in Diabetes—2023. Diabetes Care 2023;46(Supplement_1):S158–90.
46. Schnell O, Cappuccio F, Genovese S, et al. Type 1 diabetes and cardiovascular disease. Cardiovasc Diabetol 2013;12:156.
47. Xu L, Wang W, Song W. A combination of metformin and insulin improve cardiovascular and cerebrovascular risk factors in individuals with type 1 diabetes mellitus. Diabetes Res Clin Pract 2022;191:110073.
48. Yapanis M, James S, Craig ME, et al. Complications of Diabetes and Metrics of Glycemic Management Derived From Continuous Glucose Monitoring. J Clin Endocrinol Metab 2022;107(6):e2221–36.
49. Yoo JH, Kim JH. Time in Range from Continuous Glucose Monitoring: A Novel Metric for Glycemic Control. Diabetes Metab J 2020;44(6):828–39.
50. ElSayed NA, Aleppo G, Aroda VR, et al. 7. Diabetes Technology: Standards of Care in Diabetes—2023. Diabetes Care 2023;46(Supplement_1):S111–27.

Type 1 and Covid-19: Diagnosis, Clinical Care, and Health Outcomes during the Pandemic

Emily Breidbart, MD*, Mary Pat Gallagher, MD

KEYWORDS

- COVID-19 telehealth • Type 1 diabetes disparities • Diabetes technology pandemic
- Remote monitoring health care delivery

KEY POINTS

- The coronavirus disease 2019 (COVID-19) pandemic permanently transformed clinical care models for people living with type 1 diabetes, primarily by accelerating the use of telemedicine.
- Remote patient monitoring and virtual health care allowed people with diabetes to maintain contact with health care providers without traveling to the office.
- Diabetes technology was associated with improved health outcomes in people with type 1 diabetes during the pandemic.
- Pre-existing health care disparities, including differences in diabetes technology use and access to telemedicine, persisted during the COVID-19 pandemic and were associated with worse health outcomes.
- Health care systems must work to create more flexible and equitable health care delivery models, to prepare for future pandemics and environmental disasters.
- While there is no strong evidence directly linking severe acute respiratory sndrome coronavirus-2 (SARS-CoV-2) infection with type 1 diabetes pathogenesis, pandemic-associated behaviors may have contributed to changes in the patterns of type 1 diabetes diagnosis.

BACKGROUND

When the World Health Organization declared coronavirus disease 2019 (COVID-19) a pandemic on March 11, 2020, the Centers for Disease Control identified people with diabetes as "high risk" for severe illness. Morbidity and mortality were

Department of Pediatrics, Division of Pediatric Endocrinology, NYU Grossman School of Medicine, Hassenfeld Children's Hospital at NYU Langone Health, 135 East 31st Street, Level 2, New York, NY 10016, USA
* Corresponding author.
E-mail address: emily.breidbart@nyulangone.org

Endocrinol Metab Clin N Am 53 (2024) 135–149
https://doi.org/10.1016/j.ecl.2023.11.001
0889-8529/24/© 2023 Elsevier Inc. All rights reserved.

higher for people with diabetes who identified as non-Hispanic Black (NHB) or Hispanic, highlighting existing health care disparities.[1] Health care services, including in-person appointments with diabetes providers and educators, as well as routine health screenings were put on hold. Access to essential medications and supplies was often interrupted. Limited access to health care facilities, reduced in-person appointments, and delays in necessary treatments often required people with diabetes to modify their diabetes care routines, sometimes rationing medication and supplies. In this review, we discuss the effects of the pandemic on people with type 1 diabetes, as well as the response of the health care system and how it transitioned rapidly to the use of telemedicine to provide virtual diabetes care during the pandemic.

DISCUSSION
Coronavirus Disease 2019

In early 2020, severe acute respiratory syndrome coronavirus-2(SARS-CoV-2) infection was associated with a high fatality rate. Initial publications reported increased hospitalization rates and mortality were associated with several factors, including advanced age, diabetes, hypertension, and renal failure.[2–4] These diagnoses are often comorbid and identifying the risk associated with each individual diagnosis is difficult. Subsequent studies evaluated outcomes in people with type 1 diabetes separately from people with type 2 diabetes, better characterizing the risk of COVID-related severe illness in each group.[5] This figure demonstrates the excess mortality that occurred in people with both type 1 and type 2 diabetes in England in early 2020 (**Fig. 1.**). Most excess deaths were related to documented SARS-CoV-2 infection. However, excess mortality in the absence of documented infection was also seen, possibly related to delays in seeking medical care for non-COVID illness during the pandemic.[5] Later studies further characterized risk factors for hospitalization and mortality in people with type 1 diabetes, including age, hemoglobin A1c level, and lack of diabetes technology use.[6–9]

The initial stay at home orders abruptly limited in-person health care in March 2020. This hastened the widespread adoption of telemedicine, with insurance companies paying for televisits, even across state lines in the United States, during the pandemic. One large pediatric diabetes center described that only 0.1% of diabetes visits were seen by telemedicine, versus 93.5% of visits during the pandemic[10]; this rapid shift was seen in other diabetes clinics,[11] with some proposing that the pediatric diabetes centers were advantaged because of more prevalent use of technology in the younger generation.[12,13]

Different measures of glycemia were often necessary during the pandemic. Due to decreased in-person visits, continuous glucose monitoring (CGM) measures and at-home hemoglobin A1c kits were frequently used in place of lab or point-of-care A1c levels. Some researchers predicted there would be more dysglycemia due to sedentary behavior, changes in dietary choices, and higher levels of stress.[14]

A meta-analysis of observational studies during stay at home showed that stable or even improved time in range (TIR) during stay at home occurred in more than two-thirds of their cohort (17 studies for a total of 3,441 individuals), inclusive of both individuals on multiple daily insulin (MDI) or continuous subcutaneous insulin infusion (CSII),[14] which was echoed by another large metanalysis.[15]

Diabetes care is particularly well suited for remote patient monitoring, with goals of care including a review of glucose levels and patterns, adjustment of medication doses, discussion of physical activity and food choices, and mental health.

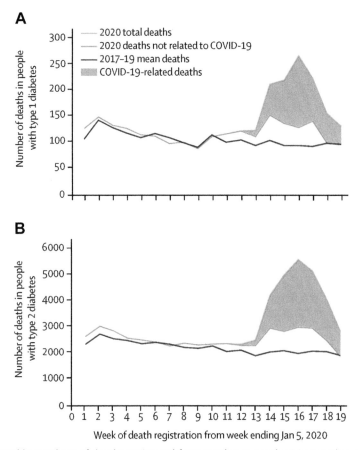

Fig. 1. Weekly numbers of deaths registered from week 1 to week 19 in people with type 1 (*A*) and type 2 (*B*) diabetes in England, 2017–19 and 2020. (Reprinted with permission from Elsevier. The Lancet Diabetes & Endocrinology. 2020; 8(10): 823-833.)[5]

Diabetes technology with cloud-based data sharing allows for the review of glucose levels and insulin delivery. Telehealth allowed people with diabetes to discuss dose adjustments, lifestyle, and mental health concerns with their diabetes team members, often after reviewing the data from their diabetes devices without any in-person visits (**Fig. 2**).

During the COVID-19 pandemic, diabetes technology was critical in improving diabetes outcomes for people unable to access traditional health care services. The use of CGM systems specifically was associated with improved outcomes during the pandemic.[9] Telemedicine also played a vital role in maintaining continuity of care, allowing individuals to consult with health care providers remotely, receive advice on diabetes management, and receive prescriptions without physical visits.[16] Diabetes technology has also facilitated remote education and support programs, empowering individuals to improve their self-care skills and enhance their diabetes management. By leveraging these innovative solutions, individuals with diabetes were able to proactively manage their condition, leading to glucose levels closer to target, reduced risk of complications, and improved overall diabetes outcomes during the COVID-19 pandemic.[17]

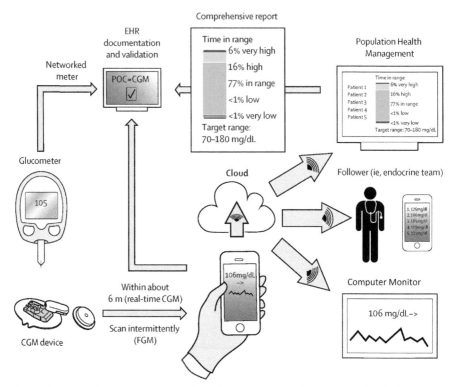

Fig. 2. Remote glucose management during the coronavirus disease 2019 (COVID-19) pandemic. (Reprinted with permission from Elsevier.The Lancet Diabetes & Endocrinology. 2020; 8(10): 823-833.)[70]

The pandemic was associated with increased symptoms of stress, anxiety, and other mental health concerns, which can adversely affect diabetes management. Health care providers and organizations attempted to adapt and offer support by providing online resources, virtual education programs, and remote monitoring technologies. Going forward, prioritizing diabetes care and addressing the pandemic's long-term effects will be crucial to supporting people living with diabetes.

Several studies examined the relationship between COVID-19-related stress and blood glucose levels. Two studies showed that stress and loss or furlough from work were predictors of lower TIR, with Bonora and colleagues reporting that improvements in TIR and time above range (TAR) were restricted to people who stayed at home during the stay-at-home orders, while those still experiencing stress of on-site working (essential workers) saw no change.[18,19] Though there was an overall improvement in CGM metrics in a large study of adults with type 1 diabetes in Scotland, socioeconomic deprivation (a measure of multiple domains such as employment, access to services, and housing) was associated with a lower TIR.[20]

Diabetes Technology and Telehealth

CGMs have enabled people with diabetes to remotely share blood glucose data with their diabetes teams. A 2017 review and meta-analysis of 38 randomized controlled trials found a mean A1C reduction of 0.18% with telemedicine and no effect on lipids, quality of life, or adverse diabetes events (demonstrating non-inferiority).[21] This small change in A1C was reported in several other studies before the pandemic.[22,23]

Before 2020, telemedicine was utilized in diabetes care but was mostly limited to rural areas, where people had to travel several hours to reach a specialist. Though a small number of studies pointed to positive results from telemedicine for type 1 diabetes,[24–26] its more widespread adoption was limited due to provider attitudes toward telemedicine, lack of access to technology for people with diabetes, inadequate health care infrastructure to support telemedicine, and lack of insurance reimbursement for televisits.

It is interesting to examine the small amount of data on telemedicine and diabetes available pre-pandemic, mainly in rural areas, where virtual visits were undertaken not due to a pandemic but to decrease the burden of travel. Wood and colleagues's group[24] published results of a telemedicine pilot at the Barbara Davis Center in Colorado from 2012 to 2014, designed to provide care to youth with type 1 diabetes in Wyoming, after identifying that even with access to outreach clinics closer to the families, youth often failed to attend the quarterly visits. It was one of the first published studies to examine the use of telemedicine in type 1 diabetes in youth. It found high satisfaction levels, increased number of visits per year, but no significant change between A1C levels at baseline and 1-year. Absenteeism has been estimated to cost over 3 billion dollars per/year for adults with diabetes, including missed work days for appointments.[27] Another study looking at veterans with type 1 diabetes conducted between 2014 and 2106 found that telemedicine visits were associated with time and cost savings, higher adherence rates to appointments, and a trend to lower A1C (0.6% decrease).[25] Perhaps the most novel design for an endocrine telemedicine program started in 2013 at the University of Nebraska, which serves 9 rural community hospitals.[26] Synchronous office visits occurred via secure video conferencing with the diabetes provider located at the academic medical center and the person with diabetes located in a clinical examination room at a rural community hospital. A certified diabetes care and education specialist (CDCES) employed by the local hospital was usually also present, and this practice continued during the pandemic with precautions in place.

Diabetes Technology and Telehealth During Coronavirus Disease 2019

The switch to telemedicine during the pandemic offered a way to monitor glucose data and assist people remotely. A worldwide study done by The International Society of Pediatric and Adolescent Diabetes (ISPAD)[28] that surveyed 215 diabetes centers in 75 countries (with the majority of providers from the United Kingdom, United States, and India) found that in-person visits continued in only 16.5% of the centers from April to May 2020, with the majority switching to telephone consults initially. The ISPAD ran another cross-sectional study analyzing surveys on telemedicine from 33 countries later in the pandemic (October 2020 to April 2021) and found that the proportion of people with diabetes receiving telemedicine visits increased from less than 10% to over 50% worldwide, triggered by changes in local regulations of data protection and privacy for telemedicine as well as insurance reimbursement.[29] At that point, most telemedicine visits used video call software instead of phone calls. The most utilized data-sharing platforms were Medtronic CareLink, Abbott Libreview, and Dexcom Clarity. Finally, a study by the Type 1 Diabetes Exchange Quality Improvement Collaborative (T1DX-QI)[30] surveyed 21 clinics in the United States about their telemedicine practices and found that the proportion of telemedicine visits before the pandemic was less than 1%, rising to an average of 95.2% in April 2020 and that by August 2020, after stay-at-home orders were relaxed, the proportion of telemedicine visits decreased to an average of 45% across T1DX-1 sites. Zoom was the most popular platform used for visits.

The most frequently used measures of glycemia in pandemic studies were CGM metrics. In Italian adults with type 1 diabetes, increased TIR, reduced glucose variability, reduced hyperglycemia, and reduced severe hypoglycemia were found during the stay-at-home order. The authors hypothesized that this was the result of a more regular lifestyle, more reproducible mealtimes, and more time for self-care and sleep.[31] A similar study, looking at children, found a similar increase in TIR and a reduction in mean glucose and TAR in the first 3 months of stay at home.[32] Interestingly, a small Italian study of pre-school and school-aged children with type 1 diabetes using CGM and semi-automated insulin delivery systems with Tandem Basal IQ directly after stay at home found that boluses were increased. They noted a statistically significant higher median value of TIR and decreased TAR.[33] Other studies found maintenance of glycemic measures comparing before and after the stay-at-home orders with more dysglycemia in young children.[34]

In a study of Italian children and adolescents receiving telemedicine visits during the stay-at-home order, median TIR increased, TAR decreased, and Time Below Range (TBR) decreased, with a trend toward decreased median glucose management indicator (GMI), which estimates HgA1C, without any changes in the total daily dose of insulin. There was a more significant effect in pre-pubertal youth compared to those who had started puberty.[35] Telemedicine had no effect on hemoglobin A1c in another small Italian study, though there was a statistically significant decrease in hemoglobin A1c during the stay-at-home period, virtual visits had no modulating effect.[36] Of note, CGM data waere not assessed in this study so changes in TIR, TAR, and TBR could not be assessed. Finally, a study in Finland found that measures of glycemia in children with type 1 diabetes did not deteriorate during the stay-at-home period. They also found that children using non-hybrid-closed-loop pumps spent more TIR, but interestingly no change was observed in children using hybrid closed loop (HCL) pumps.[37] Another study comparing conventional and new technology[38] found that TIR significantly increased from the first to the second virtual visit and that this increase was more marked among people with a baseline GMI of $\geq 7.5\%$.

The longest pediatric study of glucose metrics during the pandemic observed youth for 1 year and found that average glucose, glucose variability, and GMI were all significantly lower during the pandemic, with nearly 1 in 5 youth achieving the equivalent A1C goal of less than 7% versus 1 in 10 youth pre-pandemic.[10] Moreover, there were more frequent telemedicine visits than in-person visits before the pandemic, likely because of the easier access. The authors did note that the Tandem hybrid closed-loop system became available 1 month before the stay-at-home period and could have contributed to these improvements. In fact, another study demonstrated improved glycemic metrics during this period without telemedicine intervention.[33]

During the pandemic, a 6-week stay-at-home order in Saudi Arabia did not change glycemic measures among people with type 1 diabetes without telemedicine intervention. However, those with 1 televisit had an increase in TIR of 9% and a reduction in (time above range) TAR by 13%.[39] Another study of adults in Italy found that in the month following a structured telephone visit, mean glucose, TIR, and TAR also improved, regardless of MDI or CSII use.[40]

Even virtual pump starts were effective, with a similar increase in TIR and improvement in GMI, with some people reporting superior outcomes with virtual pump training compared to in-person training, in addition to high satisfaction in pump users.[41,42] Tele-ophthalmology, which had already demonstrated efficacy, increased during the pandemic allowing people to have virtual visits to monitor for progression of retinal disease.[43]

Health care Disparities and Coronavirus Disease 2019

The COVID-19 pandemic highlighted pre-existing inequalities in health care outcomes. People belonging to racial and ethnic minority groups, people with limited health care resources, and people who were socioeconomically disadvantaged were disproportionately impacted by the pandemic. They faced systemic barriers that interfered with their access to quality health care, including diabetes care. The pandemic intensified disparities by exacerbating challenges in social determinants of health, such as poverty, food insecurity, inadequate housing, and limited access to health care facilities.

People from disadvantaged backgrounds may have faced more challenges obtaining COVID-19 testing, timely medical advice, and diabetes management resources.[44] Although telemedicine allowed remote consultations and monitoring, not everyone had access to the necessary technology. Inequities in diabetes device use and internet and computer access determined whether telemedicine was accessible.

The pandemic has emphasized the urgent need for targeted interventions and equitable health care policies to address these disparities, improve access to diabetes care, and ensure that marginalized communities receive the necessary support and resources to manage their health effectively.

Youth and Adult User Perceptions of Telehealth

An international survey of 90 countries during the pandemic reported that 86% of people with diabetes found remote appointments helpful, and 75% wished to have remote appointments in the future.[45] Interestingly, age and level of education did not appear to influence the perception of telemedicine, but higher hemoglobin A1c affected perception negatively, especially in boys and men. While the perception of telemedicine was likely influenced by the pandemic itself (ie, worry about risk of in-person encounters), people who utilized telemedicine before the pandemic reported high satisfaction during the pandemic period as well, with 1 study noting that 42% of respondents reported that if their local telemedicine clinic were not an option, they would not have traveled hours to seek specialty care.[26]

Provider Perceptions of Telehealth

Most practitioners felt confident using digital tools, and general satisfaction was high. Only 17.3% of responders considered technology for telemedicine visits too complex to manage in clinical practice. They rated their skills "adequate" or "expert" in downloading data from glucose meters (93%), pumps (86%), and sensors (86%); analysis of glucose meter data (97%), pump data (92%), sensor data (95%), and platforms for data analysis (84%).[29] Through its survey, the ISPAD identified and categorized ways to improve the use of telemedicine (**Box 1**).

Incidence of Type 1 Diabetes and Coronavirus Disease 2019

Many practitioners anecdotally noted an increase in new diabetes diagnoses following the height of the pandemic. Based on pre-pandemic temporal trends in Europe, an annual increase of 3% to 4% in the incidence rate of type 1 diabetes was typical.[46] While several European studies—Scottish, Romanian, Danish, and German—as well as US studies[47–50] identified an increased incidence of T1D during the COVID-19 pandemic compared to pre-pandemic years, a larger, international, multicenter diabetes registry, SWEET (Pediatric and Adolescent diabeteS: Working to crEate CEnTers of Reference)[51] found that the increased number of T1D cases in 2020 and 2021 was similar to the trend observed in 2018 and 2019 without significant upward

Box 1
Highlights from International Society of Pediatric and Adolescent Diabetes survey of health care providers on ways to improve the use of telemedicine.

Improve technical aspects
  A single integrated platform to download all devices
  A platform that includes the possibility for video-consultations
  A platform with the possibility to share screen to analyze downloads together with the patient
  An integrated platform for the visit itself, for pumps, glucometers and sensors uploads and review, for screening questionnaires, for sharing of anthropometrics and blood test results
  Automatic download of the data without the need for patient to do it
  Interoperability among devices
  Availability of a single video-platform recognized and protected by privacy policies
  Possibility of using Wapp for video-calls

Improve training and education for caregivers
  Quick tutorials for platforms use available for all diabetes caregivers (doctors, nurses, dieticians, psychologists)
  Support available from industries for caregivers to use platforms
  Easier connection tools to download, send information, and keep in contact
  Better equipment available for caregivers to use telemedicine
  Training for data interpretation
  Increase experience within the team
  Possibility to share experiences with other teams
  More time available for analyzing patients' data
  Better and quicker internet connection in the hospital/office
  Multiple computer screens to allow for charting concurrently with the video portion of the tele-consultation
  Better electronic health records platforms available in the hospital and integrated with patients' data download platforms
  IT available in the team
  Time reserved to telemedicine
  More administrative staff dedicated to managing data downloads prior to tele-consultations, to ensure the connection to the platforms prior to Consultations, to integrate video-calls, phone-visits, mails and in person visits, to schedule the tele-consultations
  More nurses on the team
  Improve training and education for patients and families
  Multi-language resources available for patients
  Pre-existing standard forms for patients to be completed before the tele-consultation including all health records (eg, weight and blood pressure)
  Pre-existing tests to check the patient's knowledge on several diabetes aspects made available in the platforms
  Specific and easy to understand instructions about data download systems and platforms use
  Better trainings from companies for families to understand how to download data
  Short videos of diabetes self-care prior to consultation and discussing them with families during consultation
  Short therapeutic education sessions focused on the current main problem of the patient made available in the platform
  Improve regulatory, policy, and reimbursement
  Adequate reimbursement
  Adequate privacy rules to connect all the data of a patient in a single server
  Improve specific government policies
  Reduction of costs
  High-speed internet made available for all patients with diabetes from the health care system

(*Adapted from* [Giani, E, Dovc, K, Dos Santos, TJ, et al. Telemedicine and COVID-19 pandemic: The perfect storm to mark a change in diabetes care. Results from a world-wide cross-sectional web-based survey. Pediatr Diabetes. 2021; 22(8):1115- 1119.]; with permission)

or downward deviation, indicating no short-term influence of the COVID-19 pandemic or SARS-CoV-2. Similarly, reports from Saudia Arabia and Italy found no increase in the incidence of type 1 diabetes.[52,53] The typical seasonality of type 1 diabetes (more frequent during the winter season) was delayed, with the peak occurring in the summer and autumn months. While the seasonal incidence in Europe returned to pre-pandemic patterns in 2021, North America continued to report more summer cases in 2021.[51]

While there is controversy about the relationship of SARS-CoV-2 infection with the incidence of type 1 diabetes following the pandemic, studies have failed to find a direct association with SARS-CoV-2 infection based on antibody and/or polymerase chain reaction testing.[47,54–57] A large study from Colorado and Bavaria found the prevalence of high-affinity islet autoantibodies was similar in youth with and without a history of SARS-CoV-2 infection,[58] and another found no evidence of an increase in new cases of autoantibody-negative T1D in children, adolescents, and young adults.[59] In vitro studies have also showed that the infection is largely non-cytopathic and not found to favor pancreatic beta cells, challenging the idea that SARS-CoV-2 infection precipitates new-onset diabetes by directly affecting beta cells.[60]

While a direct effect of SARS-CoV-2 infection on the pathogenesis of type 1 diabetes has not been demonstrated, there may be pandemic-associated changes that may have had an impact. It is well known that autoimmunity and progressive B-cell function typically begin long before clinical diagnosis of T1D; the lockdown is likely to have substantially reduced the microbial exposure in children with typical respiratory and gastrointestinal illnesses.[57,59] The temporal association of lockdown with type 1 diagnosis lends credibility to the biodiversity hypothesis. While the hygiene hypothesis cites an inverse trend between the occurrence of infectious disease in early life and the occurrence of autoimmune disease, the biodiversity hypothesis extends this further, stating that decreased biodiversity of exposure increases the risk of immune-mediated disease.[59] Though common infections in early childhood have been shown to be risk factors for development of T1DM in children,[61,62] perhaps the abrupt change in socialization, contacts, and sanitization resulted in a dramatic decrease in biodiversity in children.[59] It is also possible that the social isolation and psychological stress from the pandemic and school closures could explain this uptick, as psychological stress has been linked to pathogenesis and onset of disease.[63,64] Finally, delay in diagnosis, as opposed to a real delay in disease onset may have contributed to this shift, as families may have hesitated to seek medical care, as reflected in the higher incidence of diabetic ketoacidosis (DKA) in diagnosis directly following the peak of the pandemic.[51]

SUMMARY

In summary, although a global worsening in metabolic parameters secondary to a dramatic reduction in access to medical services and laboratory testing was expected during COVID-19, surprisingly, most studies published throughout the pandemic demonstrated significant improvements in glucose metrics in adults and children.[65] Despite fewer organized sports and the more sedentary lifestyle that most individuals had during the pandemic's peak, it is possible that increased parental oversight, flexibility in schedules, and reductions in competing activities may have enhanced diabetes self-care.[10]

During the COVID-19 pandemic, diabetes technology was critical in improving diabetes outcomes for people unable to access traditional health care services. The use of CGM systems was associated with improved outcomes during the pandemic.[9]

Telemedicine also played a vital role in maintaining continuity of care, allowing individuals to consult with health care providers remotely, receive advice on diabetes management, and receive prescriptions without physical visits. Diabetes technology also facilitated remote education and support programs, supporting self-care skills during a challenging period during the COVID-19 pandemic.

In addition to increased age and increased hemoglobin A1c level, disparities in diabetes technology access and use, along with other social determinants of health, were risk factors for severe illness during the COVID-19 pandemic.

Those who had to go to work during the height of the pandemic or who had an unstable socioeconomic situation did not see this benefit.[18–20] Many studies, however, included only CGM users to assess glycemia in the absence of laboratory measurements, and this likely represents a more advantaged group of individuals. Excluding non-CGM users limits the generalizability of the findings, given recognized disparities in diabetes technology use.[10] Several researchers also pointed out that data have predominantly come from larger, well-resourced diabetes programs with populations that have good access to health care and technology, and the data cannot be extrapolated to under-resourced centers or developing countries.[15]

Thus, though telemedicine is an attractive option for diabetes care, the potential limitations of telemedicine use must be acknowledged. Telemedicine is not always feasible, especially in under-resourced countries where consistent internet connections, necessary equipment, and technical knowledge may not be available. While the adoption of telemedicine for type 1 diabetes care was rapid across the United States and most of Europe, lack of access to technology and the unequal payer coverage of video and telephone visits exacerbated disparities in diabetes care even in well-resourced countries.[66,67] The health outcomes reported for people with type 1 diabetes during the COVID-19 pandemic highlight the need for health care systems to develop flexible and more equitable methods of health care delivery.[68,69]

There appeared to be at least a transient increase in the incidence of type 1 diabetes in many countries following the peak of the COVID-19 pandemic. While there is no strong evidence directly linking SARS-CoV-2 infection with type 1 diabetes pathogenesis, pandemic-associated behaviors may have contributed to changes in the patterns of type 1 diabetes diagnosis.

CLINICS CARE POINTS

- Risk factors for serious illness during the COVID-19 pandemic (either diabetes related or COVID-related illnesses) for people with type 1 diabetes were increased age, increased hemoglobin A1c level, and decreased use of CGMs.

- People with type 1 diabetes who had access to, and utilized, diabetes technology and telemedicine during the COVID-19 pandemic had better health outcomes.

- People with type 1 diabetes who identified as non-Hispanic Black or Black had higher hemoglobin A1c levels, less CGM use, and worse health outcomes during the COVID-19 pandemic than their non-Hispanic White peers.

- Disparities in health outcomes included increased risk for hospitalization and DKA in children and increased risk of hospitalization and mortality in adults.

- While there is no strong evidence directly linking SARS-CoV-2 infection with type 1 diabetes pathogenesis, pandemic-associated behaviors may have contributed to changes in the patterns of type 1 diabetes diagnosis.

DISCLOSURE

The authors have no commercial or financial conflicts of interest.

REFERENCES

1. Ebekozien O, Agarwal S, Noor N, et al. Inequities in diabetic ketoacidosis among patients with type 1 diabetes and COVID-19: data from 52 us clinical centers. J Clin Endocrinol Metab 2021;106(4):e1755–62.
2. Richardson S, Hirsch JS, Narasimhan M, et al. Presenting characteristics, comorbidities, and outcomes among 5700 patients hospitalized with COVID-19 in the New York City Area. JAMA 2020;323(20):2052–9.
3. Grasselli G, Zangrillo A, Zanella A, et al. Baseline characteristics and outcomes of 1591 patients infected with SARS-CoV-2 admitted to ICUs of the Lombardy Region, Italy. JAMA 2020;323(16):1574–81.
4. Xiong S, Liu L, Lin F, et al. Clinical characteristics of 116 hospitalized patients with COVID-19 in Wuhan, China: a single-centered, retrospective, observational study. BMC Infect Dis 2020;20(1):787.
5. Holman N, Knighton P, Kar P, et al. Risk factors for COVID-19-related mortality in people with type 1 and type 2 diabetes in England: a population-based cohort study. Lancet Diabetes Endocrinol 2020;8(10):823–33.
6. O'Malley G, Ebekozien O, Desimone M, et al. COVID-19 hospitalization in adults with type 1 diabetes: results from the T1D exchange multicenter surveillance study. J Clin Endocrinol Metab 2021;106(2):e936–42.
7. Demeterco-Berggren C, Ebekozien O, Rompicherla S, et al. Age and hospitalization risk in people with type 1 diabetes and COVID-19: data from the T1D exchange surveillance study. J Clin Endocrinol Metab 2022;107(2):410–8.
8. Noor N, Ebekozien O, Levin L, et al. Diabetes technology use for management of type 1 diabetes is associated with fewer adverse COVID-19 outcomes: findings from the T1D exchange COVID-19 surveillance registry. Diabetes Care 2021; 44(8):e160–2.
9. Alonso GT, Ebekozien O, Gallagher MP, et al. Diabetic ketoacidosis drives COVID-19 related hospitalizations in children with type 1 diabetes. J Diabetes 2021;13(8):681–7.
10. Kaushal T, Tinsley L, Volkening LK, et al. Improvement in mean CGM glucose in young people with type 1 diabetes during 1 year of the COVID-19 pandemic. Diabetes Technol Ther 2022;24(2):136–9.
11. March CA, Flint A, DeArment D, et al. Paediatric diabetes care during the COVID-19 pandemic: Lessons learned in scaling up telemedicine services. Endocrinol Diabetes Metab 2021;4(1):e00202.
12. Danne T, Limbert C, Puig Domingo M, et al. Telemonitoring, telemedicine and time in range during the pandemic: paradigm change for diabetes risk management in the post-COVID future. Diabetes Ther 2021;12(9):2289–310.
13. DeSalvo DJ, Miller KM, Hermann JM, et al. Continuous glucose monitoring and glycemic control among youth with type 1 diabetes: international comparison from the T1D Exchange and DPV Initiative. Pediatr Diabetes 2018;19(7):1271–5.
14. Garofolo M, Aragona M, Rodia C, et al. Glycaemic control during the lockdown for COVID-19 in adults with type 1 diabetes: A meta-analysis of observational studies. Diabetes Res Clin Pract 2021;180:109066.
15. O'Mahoney LL, Highton PJ, Kudlek L, et al. The impact of the COVID-19 pandemic on glycaemic control in people with diabetes: a systematic review and meta-analysis. Diabetes Obes Metab 2022;24(9):1850–60.

16. Kaushal T, Ambler-Osborn L, Turcotte C, et al. Rapid adoption of telemedicine along with emergent use of continuous glucose monitors in the ambulatory care of young persons with new-onset type 1 diabetes in the time of covid-19: a case series. Telemed J e Health 2022;28(1):107–14.

17. Kaushal T, Tinsley LJ, Volkening LK, et al. Improved CGM glucometrics and more visits for pediatric type 1 diabetes using telemedicine during 1 year of COVID-19. J Clin Endocrinol Metab 2022;107(10):e4197–202.

18. Bonora BM, Boscari F, Avogaro A, et al. Glycaemic control among people with type 1 diabetes during lockdown for the SARS-CoV-2 Outbreak in Italy. Diabetes Therapy 2020;11(6):1369–79.

19. Barchetta I, Cimini FA, Bertoccini L, et al. Effects of work status changes and perceived stress onglycaemiccontrol in individuals with type 1 diabetes during COVID-19 lockdown in Italy. Diabetes Res Clin Pract 2020;170:108513.

20. Dover AR, Ritchie SA, McKnight JA, et al. Assessment of the effect of the COVID-19 lockdown on glycaemic control in people with type 1 diabetes using flash glucose monitoring. Diabet Med 2021;38(1):e14374.

21. Lee SWH, Ooi L, Lai YK. Telemedicine for the management of glycemic control and clinical outcomes of type 1 diabetes mellitus: a systematic review and meta-analysis of randomized controlled studies. Front Pharmacol 2017;8:330.

22. Faruque LI, Wiebe N, Ehteshami-Afshar A, et al. Effect of telemedicine on glycated hemoglobin in diabetes: a systematic review and meta-analysis of randomized trials. CMAJ (Can Med Assoc J) 2017;189(9):E341–64.

23. Tchero H, Kangambega P, Briatte C, et al. Clinical effectiveness of telemedicine in diabetes mellitus: a meta-analysis of 42 randomized controlled trials. Telemed J e Health 2019;25(7):569–83.

24. Wood CL, Clements SA, McFann K, et al. Use of telemedicine to improve adherence to american diabetes association standards in pediatric type 1 diabetes. Diabetes Technol Ther 2016;18(1):7–14.

25. Xu T, Pujara S, Sutton S, et al. Telemedicine in the management of type 1 diabetes. Prev Chronic Dis 2018;15:E13.

26. Eiland LA, Drincic A. Rural telehealth visits in the management of type 1 diabetes. J Diabetes Sci Technol 2022;16(4):852–7.

27. American Diabetes A. Economic costs of diabetes in the U.S. in 2017. Diabetes Care 2018;41(5):917–28.

28. Elbarbary NS, Dos Santos TJ, de Beaufort C, et al. COVID-19 outbreak and pediatric diabetes: Perceptions of health care professionals worldwide. Pediatr Diabetes 2020;21(7):1083–92.

29. Giani E, Dovc K, Dos Santos TJ, et al. Telemedicine and COVID-19 pandemic: The perfect storm to mark a change in diabetes care. results from a worldwide cross-sectional web-based survey. Pediatr Diabetes 2021;22(8):1115–9.

30. Lee JM, Carlson E, Albanese-O'Neill A, et al. Adoption of telemedicine for type 1 diabetes care during the COVID-19 pandemic. Diabetes Technol Ther 2021; 23(9):642–51.

31. Capaldo B, Annuzzi G, Creanza A, et al. Blood glucose control during lockdown for COVID-19: CGM Metrics in italian adults with type 1 diabetes. Diabetes Care 2020;43(8):e88–9.

32. Marigliano M, Maffeis C. Glycemic control of children and adolescents with type 1 diabetes improved after COVID-19 lockdown in Italy. Acta Diabetol 2021;58(5): 661–4.

33. Schiaffini R, Barbetti F, Rapini N, et al. School and pre-school children with type 1 diabetes during Covid-19 quarantine: the synergic effect of parental care and technology. Diabetes Res Clin Pract 2020;166:108302.

34. Brener A, Mazor-Aronovitch K, Rachmiel M, et al. Lessons learned from the continuous glucose monitoring metrics in pediatric patients with type 1 diabetes under COVID-19 lockdown. Acta Diabetol 2020;57(12):1511–7.

35. Predieri B, Leo F, Candia F, et al. Glycemic control improvement in italian children and adolescents with type 1 diabetes followed through telemedicine during lockdown due to the COVID-19 pandemic. Front Endocrinol 2020;11:595735.

36. Cognigni M, D'Agostin M, Schiulaz I, et al. HbA1c and BMI after lockdown for COVID-19 in children and adolescents with type 1 diabetes mellitus. Acta Paediatr 2021;110(7):2206–7.

37. Hakonen E, Varimo T, Tuomaala AK, et al. The effect of COVID-19 lockdown on the glycemic control of children with type 1 diabetes. BMC Pediatr 19 2022; 22(1):48.

38. Parise M, Tartaglione L, Cutruzzola A, et al. Teleassistance for patients with type 1 diabetes during the covid-19 pandemic: results of a pilot study. J Med Internet Res 2021;23(4):e24552.

39. Alharthi SK, Alyusuf EY, Alguwaihes AM, et al. The impact of a prolonged lockdown and use of telemedicine on glycemic control in people with type 1 diabetes during the COVID-19 outbreak in Saudi Arabia. Diabetes Res Clin Pract 2021; 173:108682.

40. Boscari F, Ferretto S, Uliana A, et al. Efficacy of telemedicine for persons with type 1 diabetes during Covid19 lockdown. Nutr Diabetes 2021;11(1):1.

41. Vigersky RA, Velado K, Zhong A, et al. The effectiveness of virtual training on the minimed 670g system in people with type 1 diabetes during the COVID-19 pandemic. Diabetes Technol Ther 2021;23(2):104–9.

42. Bozzetto L, De Angelis R, Calabrese I, et al. Clinical outcomes of remote training for advanced diabetes technologies during the COVID-19 pandemic. J Diabetes Sci Technol 2022;16(1):264–5.

43. Galiero R, Pafundi PC, Nevola R, et al. The importance of telemedicine during covid-19 pandemic: a focus on diabetic retinopathy. J Diabetes Res 2020; 2020:9036847.

44. Haynes SC, Kompala T, Neinstein A, et al. Disparities in telemedicine use for subspecialty diabetes care during COVID-19 shelter-in-place orders. J Diabetes Sci Technol 2021;15(5):986–92.

45. Scott SN, Fontana FY, Zuger T, et al. Use and perception of telemedicine in people with type 1 diabetes during the COVID-19 pandemic-Results of a global survey. Endocrinol Diabetes Metab 2021;4(1):e00180.

46. Patterson CC, Harjutsalo V, Rosenbauer J, et al. Trends and cyclical variation in the incidence of childhood type 1 diabetes in 26 European centres in the 25 year period 1989-2013: a multicentre prospective registration study. Diabetologia 2019;62(3):408–17.

47. McKeigue PM, McGurnaghan S, Blackbourn L, et al. Relation of Incident Type 1 Diabetes to Recent COVID-19 Infection: Cohort Study Using e-Health Record Linkage in Scotland. Diabetes Care 2023;46(5):921–8.

48. Vlad A, Serban V, Timar R, et al. Increased Incidence of Type 1 Diabetes during the COVID-19 Pandemic in Romanian Children. Medicina (Kaunas) 2021;57(9). https://doi.org/10.3390/medicina57090973.

49. Zareini B, Sorensen KK, Eiken PA, et al. Association of COVID-19 and development of type 1 diabetes: a danish nationwide register study. Diabetes Care 2023;46(8):1477–82.
50. Wolf RM, Noor N, Izquierdo R, et al. Increase in newly diagnosed type 1 diabetes in youth during the COVID-19 pandemic in the United States: A multi-center analysis. Pediatr Diabetes 2022;23(4):433–8.
51. Reschke F, Lanzinger S, Herczeg V, et al. The COVID-19 Pandemic Affects Seasonality, With Increasing Cases of New-Onset Type 1 Diabetes in Children, From the Worldwide SWEET Registry. Diabetes Care 2022;45(11):2594–601.
52. Alaqeel A, Aljuraibah F, Alsuhaibani M, et al. The Impact of COVID-19 Pandemic Lockdown on the Incidence of New-Onset Type 1 Diabetes and Ketoacidosis Among Saudi Children. Front Endocrinol 2021;12:669302.
53. Mameli C, Scaramuzza A, Macedoni M, et al. Type 1 diabetes onset in Lombardy region, Italy, during the COVID-19 pandemic: The double-wave occurrence. EClinicalMedicine 2021;39:101067.
54. Ata A, Jalilova A, Kirkgoz T, et al. Does COVID-19 predispose patients to type 1 diabetes mellitus? Clin Pediatr Endocrinol 2022;31(1):33–7.
55. Kamrath C, Rosenbauer J, Eckert AJ, et al. Incidence of type 1 diabetes in children and adolescents during the COVID-19 pandemic in Germany: results from the DPV registry. Diabetes Care 2022;45(8):1762–71.
56. Novoa-Medina Y, Pavlovic-Nesic S, Gonzalez-Martin JM, et al. Role of the SARS-CoV-2 virus in the appearance of new onset type 1 diabetes mellitus in children in Gran Canaria, Spain. J Pediatr Endocrinol Metab 2022;35(3):393–7.
57. Knip M, Parviainen A, Turtinen M, et al. SARS-CoV-2 and type 1 diabetes in children in Finland: an observational study. Lancet Diabetes Endocrinol 2023;11(4):251–60.
58. Rewers M, Bonifacio E, Ewald D, et al. SARS-CoV-2 infections and presymptomatic type 1 diabetes autoimmunity in children and adolescents from Colorado, USA, and Bavaria, Germany. JAMA 2022;328(12):1252–5.
59. Kamrath C, Rosenbauer J, Tittel SR, et al. Frequency of autoantibody-negative type 1 diabetes in children, adolescents, and young adults during the first wave of the COVID-19 pandemic in Germany. Diabetes Care 2021;44(7):1540–6.
60. van der Heide V, Jangra S, Cohen P, et al. Limited extent and consequences of pancreatic SARS-CoV-2 infection. Cell Rep 2022;38(11):110508.
61. Hyoty H. Viruses in type 1 diabetes. Pediatr Diabetes 2016;17(Suppl 22):56–64.
62. Stene LC, Oikarinen S, Hyoty H, et al. Enterovirus infection and progression from islet autoimmunity to type 1 diabetes: the diabetes and autoimmunity study in the young (DAISY). Diabetes 2010;59(12):3174–80.
63. Sipetic S, Vlajinac H, Marinkovi J, et al. Stressful life events and psychological dysfunctions before the onset of type 1 diabetes mellitus. J Pediatr Endocrinol Metab 2007;20(4):527–34.
64. Nygren M, Carstensen J, Koch F, et al. Experience of a serious life event increases the risk for childhood type 1 diabetes: the ABIS population-based prospective cohort study. Diabetologia 2015;58(6):1188–97.
65. de Kreutzenberg SV. Telemedicine for the clinical management of diabetes; implications and considerations after COVID-19 experience. High Blood Press Cardiovasc Prev 2022;29(4):319–26.
66. Alvarez-Risco A, Del-Aguila-Arcentales S, Yanez JA. Telemedicine in peru as a result of the covid-19 pandemic: perspective from a country with limited internet access. Am J Trop Med Hyg 2021;105(1):6–11.

67. Garcia-Villasante E, Baca-Carrasco V, Gutierrez-Ortiz C, et al. Diabetes care during COVID 19: Experience in telemedicine from a developing country. Diabetes Metab Syndr 2020;14(5):1519.
68. Phillip M, Bergenstal RM, Close KL, et al. The digital/virtual diabetes clinic: the future is now-recommendations from an international panel on diabetes digital technologies introduction. Diabetes Technol Ther 2021;23(2):146–54.
69. Cobry EC, Wadwa RP. The future of telehealth in type 1 diabetes. Curr Opin Endocrinol Diabetes Obes 2022;29(4):397–402.
70. Pasquel FJ, Lansang MC, Dhatariya K, et al. Management of diabetes and hyperglycaemia in the hospital. Lancet Diabetes Endocrinol 2021;9(3):174–88.

Type 1 Diabetes and Cardiovascular Health

Maria Pesantez, MD[a], Osagie Ebekozien, MD[b],
Francesco Vendrame, MD, PhD[c],*

KEYWORDS

- Type 1 diabetes • Cardiovascular health • Cardiovascular disease risk • Prevention

KEY POINTS

- Type 1 diabetes (T1D) is associated with an increased risk of cardiovascular disease (CVD), which is higher in those diagnosed at early age and with longer disease duration.
- Glycemia is the strongest modifiable risk factor for CVD, although traditional CVD risk factors are involved as well.
- There is an undertreatment of CVD risk factors in T1D, particularly in young adults.
- To promote cardiovascular health (CVH) in T1D, the eight CVH metrics proposed for the general population should adopt targets specific for the T1D population.

INTRODUCTION

In 2010, the American Health Association introduced the concept of cardiovascular health (CVH).[1] The definition was updated in 2022 and now includes four health behaviors and four health factors which, when optimal, are associated with increased longevity and better quality of life.[2] Ideal CVH is defined by the presence of health behaviors such as DASH- and Mediterranean-style eating patterns, physical activity ≥150 min/week of moderate-(or greater) intensity activity, never smoking, sleeping 7 -< 9 hours per night, and health factors such as a body mass index (BMI) less than 25 kg/m^2, non-high-density lipoprotein (HDL) cholesterol less than 130 mg/dL, fasting blood glucose less than 100 mg/dL or glycated hemoglobin test (HbA1c) less than 5.7%, and blood pressure less than 120/80 mm Hg[2]. Currently, there are no specific recommendations about the use of these metrics in type 1 diabetes (T1D) management. To address this, a comprehensive approach to CVH in T1D is needed, which requires understanding the impact of the disease on the occurrence

^{a} Jackson Memorial Hospital, 1450 Northwest 10 Avenue, Miami, FL 33136, USA; ^{b} T1D Exchange, 101 Federal Street Suite 440, Boston, MA 02110, USA; ^{c} Department of Medicine, Division of Endocrinology, Diabetes and Metabolism, University of Miami Miller School of Medicine, 1450 Northwest 10 Avenue, Room 1086, Miami, FL 33136, USA
* Corresponding author.
E-mail address: fvendrame@med.miami.edu

Endocrinol Metab Clin N Am 53 (2024) 151–163
https://doi.org/10.1016/j.ecl.2023.07.003
0889-8529/24/© 2023 Elsevier Inc. All rights reserved.

of CVD, identifying cardiovascular disease (CVD) risk factors and T1D individuals who are at increased risk, and identifying CVH treatment targets and approaches/implementation strategies to reach these goals.

EPIDEMIOLOGY OF CARDIOVASCULAR DISEASE IN TYPE 1 DIABETES

Mortality rates for people with T1D vary by geographic location but are 3 to 18 times higher than what would be expected in their respective countries.[3] CVD is the leading cause of death, although renal disease is another contributor factor.[3] Although few studies have directly compared CVD mortality in people with T1D and people with type 2 diabetes (T2D), T1D seems to have an impact on mortality which is at least comparable if not higher than T2D.[4,5]

A meta-analysis which included 10 observational studies involving 166,027 patients with T1D and controls from the general population has shown that for people with T1D, the relative risk of coronary artery disease (CAD) is 9.38 (95% CI, 5.56–15.82), and of myocardial infarction is 6.37 (95% CI, 3.81–10.66).[6] In the European Diabetes Prospective Complication Study which analyzed a cohort of 3250 individuals with T1D, the incidence of a cerebrovascular accident was 0.74% per year, almost double of what is reported in the general population which is reported at 0.2% to 0.3% per year.[7] This finding was also supported by Nurses' Health Study.[8] Data about peripheral artery disease (PAD) are mostly derived from studies which focused on amputation. People with T1D have a rate of nontraumatic amputation of 0.4% to 7.2% per year.[9] In a meta-analysis of five studies of people with T1D, each 1% increase in mean HbA1c was associated with an 18% increased risk of PAD.[10]

RISK FACTORS FOR CARDIOVASCULAR DISEASE IN TYPE 1 DIABETES

Several factors increase the risk of CVD in T1D. They are listed in **Box 1** and the most relevant discussed below.

Glycemic Control

Hyperglycemia is a recognized risk factor for the development of both microvascular and macrovascular complications.[11] Hyperglycemia is associated with preclinical atherosclerosis as shown in the Oslo study where a 1% increase in mean HbA1c was associated with a 6.4% increase in coronary vessel stenosis.[12] In the Pittsburgh

---

Box 1
Factors associated with increased risk of cardiovascular disease in type 1 diabetes

Traditional risk factors
  Poor glycemic control
  Dyslipidemia
  High blood pressure
  Diabetic kidney disease
  Obesity
  Smoking

Additional risk factors
  Genetics
  Age of T1D onset
  Female sex
  Cardiac autonomic neuropathy
  Cardiac autoimmunity

Epidemiology of Diabetes Complications (EDC) study for every 1% increase in mean HbA1c, the risk of CVD over 25 years after adjusting for risk factors was increased between 1.13- and 1.26-fold.[13] In the EDC study and Diabetes Control and Complications Trial and follow-up Epidemiology of Diabetes Interventions and Complications study (DCCT/EDIC), HbA1c was the strongest risk factor for the first and subsequent CVD event.[11] Hyperglycemia however is not the only determinant of CVD risk in T1D because additional analyses have revealed that other risk factors such as systolic blood pressure and lipids attenuated up to ~50% the effect of glycemia on the risk of CVD in the DCCT/EDIC study.[14,15] Besides hyperglycemia, there is also some evidence that glycemic variability including hypoglycemia can contribute to future CVD events.[16–18]

Dyslipidemia

Poor glycemic control is associated with hypertriglyceridemia, elevated low-density lipoprotein cholesterol (LDL-C), and lower HDL cholesterol (HDL-C).[19] Data from the Swedish National Registry suggest that LDL-C is a significant predictor of CVD and mortality in T1D, with each 1 mmol/L (38.7 mg/dL) increase in LDL-C associated with 35% to 50% greater risk.[20] An association between LDL-C and CVD in people with T1D has been also reported in studies such as the DCCT/EDIC study and the EDC study.[21,22] In addition, in people with T1D, small dense LDL-C particle size is associated with CVD risk and dysfunctional HDL particles which may become proatherogenic have been reported.[23,24]

High Blood Pressure

Hypertension is a risk factor for CVD in the general population and people with T1D in the DCCT/EDIC study and EDC study.[21,22,25] Hypertension can be a consequence of diabetic kidney disease, but T1D is associated with higher prevalence of hypertension, also in the absence of diabetic kidney disease being three times more common in people with T1D compared with the nondiabetic population.[26]

Diabetic Kidney Disease

Several studies indicate that the diabetic kidney defined as the presence of albuminuria and/or reduced glomerular filtration rate is associated with an increased CVD risk in people with T1D.[22,27,28] The risk of all-cause mortality also increases with the severity of chronic kidney disease.[29] In addition, the Coronary Artery Calcification in Type 1 Diabetes (CACTI) study showed that an increasing albumin excretion and declining glomerular filtration rate predicted the progression of coronary artery calcification in 1066 participants with T1D compared with nondiabetic adults.[30]

Obesity

There is an increasing prevalence of overweight and obesity in people with T1D as shown by the DCCT/EDIC study where the prevalence of obesity increased from 1% of subjects at baseline to 31% after 12 years of follow-up in 2005.[31] This finding is comparable to the one of the EDC study and more recently the T1D Exchange Clinic Network.[32,33] The association of T1D with obesity and comorbidities such as hypertension and dyslipidemia has led to the definition of "double diabetes" to indicate people with T1D and with features of T2D, a condition which increases the CVD risk.[34]

Genetics

A major candidate gene for CVD risk in T1D is the haptoglobin (Hp), an acute phase protein with anti-oxidative properties. Hp is polymorphic with two major alleles and three genotypes.[35] The Hp 2-2 genotype has been associated with the occurrence of CAD in the DCCT/EDIC study.[36,37] However, the Hp 2-2 genotype has not been identified by genome-wide association studies which instead found associations between increased CVD risk in T1D and single nucleotide polymorphisms, which, however, were weak or not replicated.[38,39]

Age of Type 1 Diabetes Onset

CVD occurs much earlier in people with T1D than in the general population, and premature atherosclerosis may be present in 50% to 70% of individuals by age 45 years.[40–42] In the Swedish National Diabetes registry which included 27,195 people with T1D, those with the disease onset before 10 years of age experienced a 30-fold increased risk of CAD and acute myocardial infarction compared with general population and had increased CVD mortality compared with those who were diagnosed between 26 and 30 years of age after adjusting for diabetes duration.[40]

Female Sex

Women with T1D have a higher risk for CVD than men.[40,41] In the general population, the rates of CAD in premenopausal women are lower than men, but in women with T1D age less than 40 years, the CVD rates are equal in both sex.[43–45] The reasons for these differences are unclear but may be secondary to the undertreatment of risk factors, different fat distribution, and different lipoprotein profiles. Nondiabetic women have a more favorable lipid profile than nondiabetic men, but women with T1D have concentration of LDL-C particles similar to men with T1D.[46–49]

PREDICTION OF CARDIOVASCULAR DISEASE IN TYPE 1 DIABETES

Different approaches have been used to identify people who are at an increased risk of CVD disease and to detect early signs of CVD.

Risk Predication Models

CVD risk calculators are available for the general population and people with T2D, but both the Framingham Risk Score and UK Prospective Diabetes Study (UKPDS) Risk Engine underestimate the CVD risk in T1D.[50] Models which have been developed to address the CVD risk in T1D include the Swedish National Diabetes Register (NDR), the Pittsburgh CHD in Type 1 Diabetes Risk Model, the Steno Type 1 Risk Engine, and the QRISK model.[51–54] Among these models, the Danish Steno Type 1 Risk Engine was externally validated and was superior to the NDR and UKPDS models in predicting the 5-year risk of first fatal or non-fatal CVD event in people with T1D.[53] The British QRISK latest version QRISK3, which accounts for the T1D or T2D status, predicts the 10-year CVD risk with a performance which is higher for people with T1D than T2D.[55] However, CVD risk prediction models for T1D are not widely adopted or recommended by guideline because of lack of international validation.[56]

Imaging to Detect Cardiovascular Disease

Imaging-based tests have been used to detect early signs of CVD.

- Diastolic dysfunction has been reported in adolescents, younger, and older adults with T1D.[57,58] Subclinical systolic dysfunction, which manifests subsequently, can occur in people with T1D but may not be detected by assessing the ejection fraction, which can be normal in the early stages of the disease.[59] Tissue Doppler imaging, speckle tracking echocardiography, and cardiac MRI can be used as screening methods but their use to predict CVD events has not been validated yet.[59–61]

- Arterial stiffness has been described in people with T1D. In particular, aortic stiffness has been identified as an independent maker of all-cause mortality in this population and can be assessed by carotid-femoral pulse wave velocity.[62,63]
- Carotid intima-media thickness (CIMT) is a surrogate marker of CVD disease. However, the DCCT/EDIC study failed to find a significant association between CIMT and subsequent coronary events after adjusting for traditional CVD risk factors.[64]
- Coronary Artery Calcium (CAC) test. Computed tomography is used to measure CAC in the four major coronary arteries. The Multi-Ethnic Study of Atherosclerosis cohort study has demonstrated that the CAC score has a prognostic value in determining the CVD risk in people with T2D.[65] In people with T1D in the EDC study, a score greater than 400 Agatston was the most efficient coronary calcium correlate of CAD.[66] More recent data from the DCCT/EDIC study found that a CAC score greater than 100 Agatston units was significantly associated with an increased risk of the subsequent occurrence of CVD and major cardiovascular events.[67] CAC score could detect asymptomatic atherosclerotic disease in T1D and in the clinical practice favor an aggressive therapy to reduce LDL-C to change the natural course of CVD.[68]

CARDIOVASCULAR DISEASE PREVENTION IN TYPE 1 DIABETES

No randomized trials have been specifically designed to assess the impact of CVD risk reduction strategies in T1D. Recommendations for the reduction of CVD risk in T1D are then mostly derived from data obtained from studies conducted in patients with T2D.

- The DCCT/EDIC study showed that hyperglycemia is modifiable risk factor for CVD in T1D.[69,70] The intensive glycemic control over a mean 6.5 years resulting in a mean HbA1c of 7.2% compared with 9.1% in the conventional therapy group determined a reduction of CVD which persisted beyond the completion of the intervention trial and despite the initial difference in glycemic control was not maintained on follow-up. During the 30 years of follow-up, the incidence of CVD in the former intensive treatment group decreased by 30% and the incidence of major cardiovascular events such as nonfatal myocardial infarction, stroke, or cardiovascular dearth by 32% compared with the former conventional therapy group.[70] Additional analyses have revealed that other risk factors such as systolic blood pressure and lipids attenuated up to ~50% of the effect of glycemia on the risk of CVD, but the association between HbA1c and the risk of CVD remained highly significant even after adjustment for these risk factors.[14,15] Maintaining an optimal glycemic control is then necessary to reduce the risk of CVD. Targeting HbA1c less than 7% or lower if this is not associated with hypoglycemia or adverse effects, or a time in range of 70 to 180 mg/dL greater than 70% is therefore recommended for most people with T1D.[71]
- Some trials investigating the effect of statin therapy in people with T2D have also included people with T1D. A meta-analysis, which included 18,686 people with diabetes from 14 randomized trials of statin therapy, inclusive of 17,220 participants with T2D and 1466 with T1D, has shown a 9% proportional reduction in all-cause mortality and 21% reduction in major vascular events, defined as the composite outcome of myocardial infarction or coronary death, stroke, or coronary revascularization, for each 1 mmol/L (39 mg/dL) reduction in LDL-C.[72] The evidence of benefit in adults with T1D was limited but not different from what

observed in patients with T2D. Recommendations for starting statin treatment for primary prevention in people with T1D are present in different guidelines.[73–75]

- In the EDC study, 605 participants with T1D without known CVD at baseline and followed for 25 years, the optimal blood pressure threshold associated with minimal CVD risk was 120/80 mm Hg.[73,76,77] People with T1D and hypertension should be treated with antihypertensive medications if the blood pressure is persistently above 130/80. The initial treatment can include any of the drug classes demonstrated to reduce CVD in people with diabetes: angiotensin-converting enzyme inhibitors, angiotensin receptor blockers, thiazide-like diuretics, or dihydropyridine calcium channel blockers.
- Strategies for weight reduction can include medical nutrition therapy, physical activity, behavioral counseling, pharmacologic therapy, and bariatric surgery. People with T1D may benefit from eating plans that result in an energy deficit and that are lower in carbohydrate and glycemic index and higher in fiber and lean protein.[78] Mediterranean, DASH, vegetarian, or plant-based eating patterns have been shown to be beneficial in T2D, but there is limited evidence to support one specific eating pattern in T1D.[79] Physical activity is associated with weight loss, improved metabolic profile, and reduced CVD mortality in people with T1D.[80,81] The use of adjunct therapies, including glucagon-like peptide-1 analogs in particular, has been associated with weight loss and improved glycemic control but more studies are needed.[82] It is unclear at this time if bariatric surgery and weight loss medications in people with T1D are associated with improved glycemic control or reduced CVD risk.[83]
- Individuals with T1D should engage in 150 minute or more or moderate to vigorous intensity aerobic activity per week and in two to three sessions per week of resistance exercise on nonconsecutive days noting that blood glucose responses to physical activity in T1D are highly variable.[84,85]
- People with T1D should not use cigarettes, other tobacco products and e-cigarettes.[79]

CARDIOVASCULAR HEALTH IN TYPE 1 DIABETES

Better CVH scores are associated with lower risks of CVD disease.[86] CVH metrics can then be applied to people with T1D, but current CVH targets which are recommended for the general population should be modified to reflect the characteristics of T1D and goals associated with lower CVD risk in this population. For example, the measure for blood glucose should the HbA1c less than 7% or lower if this is not associated with hypoglycemia or adverse effect. Ideal blood lipids should be based on LDL-C and reflect the duration of disease and presence of additional risk factors. **Table 1** lists the ideal health behaviors and factors for CVH in adults with T1D.

CONSIDERATIONS

As the incidence of T1D in increasing worldwide and with the constant improvement in medical care and diabetes technology, the expectation is an increased number of older adults living with T1D who were diagnosed when they were children. Data from international registries such as the Type 1 Diabetes Exchange registry in United States and the German/Austrian diabetes-patienten-verlaufsdokumentation (DPV) Registry revealed that less than 40% of people with T1D reached HbA1c, blood pressure, and lipid goals.[87] In addition, more than 80% of young adults aged less than 26 years were not receiving antihypertensive or lipid-lowering medications despite

Table 1
Cardiovascular health goals for adults with type 1 diabetes

Domain	CVH Metric	Quantification
Health behaviors	Diet	Mediterranean-, DASH-style
	Physical activity	$\geq$ 150 min/wk
	Nicotine exposure	Never/quit
	Sleep health	7-<9 h per night
Health factors	BMI	<25 Kg/m^2
	Blood lipids (76)	• LDL-C <100 mg/dL, if age <35 years or T1D duration <10 years
		• LDL-C <70 mg/dL and LDL-C reduction $\geq$50%, if T1D duration $\geq$10 years or another additional risk factor
		• LDL-C< 55 mg/dL and LDL-C reduction $\geq$50%, if T1D duration >20 years or target organ damage or $\geq$3 risk factors
	Blood glucose	HbA1c <7%, time in range 70–180 mg/dL >70%; target can be individualized
	Blood pressure	<120/80 mg/dL; if treated <130/80 mg/dL

Adapted from Lloyd-Jones DM, Allen NB, Anderson CAM, et al. Life's Essential 8: Updating and Enhancing the American Heart Association's Construct of Cardiovascular Health: A Presidential Advisory From the American Heart Association. Circulation 2022;146(5):e18-e43.

meeting criteria.[87] The presence of guidelines with different recommendations particularly in younger age groups is another factor which can contribute to different management and clinical inertia for younger people with T1D.[87,88] Strategies to improve CVH should then involve more education for both health care providers and people with diabetes. The development and distribution of educational tools could improve patients' health literacy. An alignment of the different guidelines can also help providers to better navigate the complex process of treatment decision-making. Finally, there is a need to reduce health inequities because with the recent advancements in diabetes technology, health care disparities in T1D treatment have also become more evident.[89]

SUMMARY

As the incidence of T1D in increasing worldwide and with improvements in medical care and diabetes technology, there is an increasing number of people with T1D at risk of CVD. Several CVD risk factors have been identified and therapeutic targets established to promote CVH in T1D. Tools such as risk prediction models and imaging-based tests have not been well validated in T1D, but the CAC test could detect asymptomatic atherosclerotic disease. CVD risk factors are also undertreated. Increased awareness about CVD risk in T1D for both health care providers and individuals with T1D and harmonization of different guidelines are recommended.

CLINICS CARE POINTS

- Discuss with people with type 1 diabetes (T1D) the increased risk of cardiovascular disease (CVD).

- Routinely address CVD risk factors such as elevated blood pressure and lipids in addition to glycemic control.

- Consider the Coronary Artery Calcium (CAC) screening test for better CVD risk stratification.
- Consider early treatment of CVD risk factors, in particular in young adults and women age less than 40 years.

DISCLOSURE

No competing financial interests exist.

REFERENCES

1. Lloyd-Jones DM, Hong Y, Labarthe D, et al. Defining and Setting National Goals for Cardiovascular Health Promotion and Disease Reduction. Circulation 2010; 121(4):586–613.
2. Lloyd-Jones DM, Allen NB, Anderson CAM, et al. Life's Essential 8: Updating and Enhancing the American Heart Association's Construct of Cardiovascular Health: A Presidential Advisory From the American Heart Association. Circulation 2022; 146(5):e18–43.
3. Secrest AM, Washington RE, Orchard TJ. Mortality in Type 1 Diabetes. In: Cowie CC, Casagrande SS, Menke A, et al, editors. Diabetes in America. Bethesda (MD): National Institute of Diabetes and Digestive and Kidney Diseases (US); 2018.
4. Juutilainen A, Lehto S, Rönnemaa T, et al. Similarity of the impact of type 1 and type 2 diabetes on cardiovascular mortality in middle-aged subjects. Diabetes Care 2008;31(4):714–9.
5. Kristófi R, Bodegard J, Norhammar A, et al. Cardiovascular and Renal Disease Burden in Type 1 Compared With Type 2 Diabetes: A Two-Country Nationwide Observational Study. Diabetes Care 2021;44(5):1211–8.
6. Cai X, Li J, Cai W, et al. Meta-analysis of type 1 diabetes mellitus and risk of cardiovascular disease. J Diabetes Complicat 2021;35(4):107833.
7. Schram MT, Chaturvedi N, Fuller JH, et al. Pulse pressure is associated with age and cardiovascular disease in type 1 diabetes: the Eurodiab Prospective Complications Study. J Hypertens 2003;21(11):2035–44.
8. Janghorbani M, Hu FB, Willett WC, et al. Prospective study of type 1 and type 2 diabetes and risk of stroke subtypes: the Nurses' Health Study. Diabetes Care 2007;30(7):1730–5.
9. Moss SE, Klein R, Klein BE. The 14-year incidence of lower-extremity amputations in a diabetic population. The Wisconsin Epidemiologic Study of Diabetic Retinopathy. Diabetes Care 1999;22(6):951–9.
10. Adler AI, Erqou S, Lima TA, et al. Association between glycated haemoglobin and the risk of lower extremity amputation in patients with diabetes mellitus-review and meta-analysis. Diabetologia 2010;53(5):840–9.
11. Bebu I, Schade D, Braffett B, et al. Risk Factors for First and Subsequent CVD Events in Type 1 Diabetes: The DCCT/EDIC Study. Diabetes Care 2020;43(4): 867–74.
12. Larsen J, Brekke M, Sandvik L, et al. Silent coronary atheromatosis in type 1 diabetic patients and its relation to long-term glycemic control. Diabetes 2002;51(8): 2637–41.
13. Miller RG, Anderson SJ, Costacou T, et al. Hemoglobin A1c Level and Cardiovascular Disease Incidence in Persons With Type 1 Diabetes: An Application of Joint

Modeling of Longitudinal and Time-to-Event Data in the Pittsburgh Epidemiology of Diabetes Complications Study. Am J Epidemiol 2018;187(7):1520–9.

14. Bebu I, Braffett BH, Pop-Busui R, et al. The relationship of blood glucose with cardiovascular disease is mediated over time by traditional risk factors in type 1 diabetes: the DCCT/EDIC study. Diabetologia 2017;60(10):2084–91.

15. Bebu I, Braffett BH, Orchard TJ, et al. Mediation of the Effect of Glycemia on the Risk of CVD Outcomes in Type 1 Diabetes: The DCCT/EDIC Study. Diabetes Care 2019;42(7):1284–9.

16. Snell-Bergeon JK, Roman R, Rodbard D, et al. Glycaemic variability is associated with coronary artery calcium in men with Type 1 diabetes: the Coronary Artery Calcification in Type 1 Diabetes study. Diabet Med 2010;27(12):1436–42.

17. Fährmann ER, Adkins L, Loader CJ, et al. Severe hypoglycemia and coronary artery calcification during the diabetes control and complications trial/epidemiology of diabetes interventions and complications (DCCT/EDIC) study. Diabetes Res Clin Pract 2015;107(2):280–9.

18. Khunti K, Davies M, Majeed A, et al. Hypoglycemia and risk of cardiovascular disease and all-cause mortality in insulin-treated people with type 1 and type 2 diabetes: a cohort study. Diabetes Care 2015;38(2):316–22.

19. Vergès B. Dyslipidemia in Type 1 Diabetes: AMaskedDanger. Trends Endocrinol Metab 2020;31(6):422–34.

20. Rawshani A, Rawshani A, Sattar N, et al. Relative Prognostic Importance and Optimal Levels of Risk Factors for Mortality and Cardiovascular Outcomes in Type 1 Diabetes Mellitus. Circulation 2019;139(16):1900–12.

21. Risk Factors for Cardiovascular Disease in Type 1 Diabetes. Diabetes 2016;65(5): 1370–9.

22. Miller RG, Costacou T, Orchard TJ. Risk Factor Modeling for Cardiovascular Disease in Type 1 Diabetes in the Pittsburgh Epidemiology of Diabetes Complications (EDC) Study: A Comparison With the Diabetes Control and Complications Trial/Epidemiology of Diabetes Interventions and Complications Study (DCCT/EDIC). Diabetes 2019;68(2):409–19.

23. Erbey JR, Robbins D, Forrest KY, et al. Low-density lipoprotein particle size and coronary artery disease in a childhood-onset type 1 diabetes population. Metabolism 1999;48(4):531–4.

24. Chapman MJ. HDL functionality in type 1 and type 2 diabetes: new insights. Curr Opin Endocrinol Diabetes Obes 2022;29(2):112–23.

25. Miller RG, Orchard TJ, Costacou T. Risk factors differ by first manifestation of cardiovascular disease in type 1 diabetes. Diabetes Res Clin Pract 2020;163: 108141.

26. Rönnback M, Fagerudd J, Forsblom C, et al. Altered age-related blood pressure pattern in type 1 diabetes. Circulation 2004;110(9):1076–82.

27. Soedamah-Muthu SS, Chaturvedi N, Toeller M, et al. Risk factors for coronary heart disease in type 1 diabetic patients in Europe: the EURODIAB Prospective Complications Study. Diabetes Care 2004;27(2):530–7.

28. de Boer IH, Gao X, Cleary PA, et al. Albuminuria Changes and Cardiovascular and Renal Outcomes in Type 1 Diabetes: The DCCT/EDIC Study. Clin J Am Soc Nephrol 2016;11(11):1969–77.

29. Groop PH, Thomas MC, Moran JL, et al. The presence and severity of chronic kidney disease predicts all-cause mortality in type 1 diabetes. Diabetes 2009; 58(7):1651–8.

30. Maahs DM, Jalal D, Chonchol M, et al. Impaired renal function further increases odds of 6-year coronary artery calcification progression in adults with type 1 diabetes: the CACTI study. Diabetes Care 2013;36(9):2607–14.
31. Diabetes C, Nathan DM, Zinman B, et al. Complications Trial/Epidemiology of Diabetes I, Complications Research G, et al. Modern-day clinical course of type 1 diabetes mellitus after 30 years' duration: the diabetes control and complications trial/epidemiology of diabetes interventions and complications and Pittsburgh epidemiology of diabetes complications experience (1983-2005). Arch Intern Med 2009;169(14):1307–16.
32. Shah VN, Wu M, Polsky S, et al. Gender differences in diabetes self-care in adults with type 1 diabetes: Findings from the T1D Exchange clinic registry. J Diabetes Complicat 2018;32(10):961–5.
33. Conway B, Miller RG, Costacou T, et al. Temporal patterns in overweight and obesity in Type 1 diabetes. Diabet Med 2010;27(4):398–404.
34. Kietsiriroje N, Pearson S, Campbell M, et al. Double diabetes: A distinct high-risk group? Diabetes Obes Metab 2019;21(12):2609–18.
35. Asleh R, Levy AP. In vivo and in vitro studies establishing haptoglobin as a major susceptibility gene for diabetic vascular disease. Vasc Health Risk Manag 2005; 1(1):19–28.
36. Costacou T, Ferrell RE, Orchard TJ. Haptoglobin genotype: a determinant of cardiovascular complication risk in type 1 diabetes. Diabetes 2008;57(6):1702–6.
37. Orchard TJ, Backlund JC, Costacou T, et al. Haptoglobin 2-2 genotype and the risk of coronary artery disease in the Diabetes Control and Complications Trial/ Epidemiology of Diabetes Interventions and Complications study (DCCT/EDIC). J Diabetes Complicat 2016;30(8):1577–84.
38. Charmet R, Duffy S, Keshavarzi S, et al. Novel risk genes identified in a genome-wide association study for coronary artery disease in patients with type 1 diabetes. Cardiovasc Diabetol 2018;17(1):61.
39. Antikainen AAV, Sandholm N, Trégouët DA, et al. Genome-wide association study on coronary artery disease in type 1 diabetes suggests beta-defensin 127 as a risk locus. Cardiovasc Res 2021;117(2):600–12.
40. Rawshani A, Sattar N, Franzén S, et al. Excess mortality and cardiovascular disease in young adults with type 1 diabetes in relation to age at onset: a nationwide, register-based cohort study. Lancet 2018;392(10146):477–86.
41. Livingstone SJ, Levin D, Looker HC, et al. Estimated life expectancy in a Scottish cohort with type 1 diabetes, 2008-2010. JAMA 2015;313(1):37–44.
42. Chiesa ST, Marcovecchio ML. Preventing Cardiovascular Complications in Type 1 Diabetes: The Need for a Lifetime Approach. Front Pediatr 2021;9:696499.
43. Laing SP, Swerdlow AJ, Slater SD, et al. Mortality from heart disease in a cohort of 23,000 patients with insulin-treated diabetes. Diabetologia 2003;46(6):760–5.
44. Laing SP, Swerdlow AJ, Slater SD, et al. The British Diabetic Association Cohort Study, II: cause-specific mortality in patients with insulin-treated diabetes mellitus. Diabet Med 1999;16(6):466–71.
45. Skrivarhaug T, Bangstad HJ, Stene LC, et al. Long-term mortality in a nationwide cohort of childhood-onset type 1 diabetic patients in Norway. Diabetologia 2006; 49(2):298–305.
46. Miller RG, Costacou T. Glucose Management and the Sex Difference in Excess Cardiovascular Disease Risk in Long-Duration Type 1 Diabetes. Curr Diabetes Rep 2019;19(12):139.

47. Larkin ME, Backlund JY, Cleary P, et al. Disparity in management of diabetes and coronary heart disease risk factors by sex in DCCT/EDIC. Diabetic Med 2010; 27(4):451–8.
48. Krishnan S, Fields DA, Copeland KC, et al. Sex differences in cardiovascular disease risk in adolescents with type 1 diabetes. Gend Med 2012;9(4):251–8.
49. Amor AJ, Castelblanco E, Hernández M, et al. Advanced lipoprotein profile disturbances in type 1 diabetes mellitus: a focus on LDL particles. Cardiovasc Diabetol 2020;19(1):126.
50. Zgibor JC, Piatt GA, Ruppert K, et al. Deficiencies of cardiovascular risk prediction models for type 1 diabetes. Diabetes Care 2006;29(8):1860–5.
51. Cederholm J, Eeg-Olofsson K, Eliasson B, et al. A new model for 5-year risk of cardiovascular disease in Type 1 diabetes; from the Swedish National Diabetes Register (NDR). Diabet Med 2011;28(10):1213–20.
52. Zgibor JC, Ruppert K, Orchard TJ, et al. Development of a coronary heart disease risk prediction model for type 1 diabetes: the Pittsburgh CHD in Type 1 Diabetes Risk Model. Diabetes Res Clin Pract 2010;88(3):314–21.
53. Vistisen D, Andersen GS, Hansen CS, et al. Prediction of First Cardiovascular Disease Event in Type 1 Diabetes Mellitus: The Steno Type 1 Risk Engine. Circulation 2016;133(11):1058–66.
54. Hippisley-Cox J, Coupland C, Vinogradova Y, et al. Derivation and validation of QRISK, a new cardiovascular disease risk score for the United Kingdom: prospective open cohort study. BMJ 2007;335(7611):136.
55. Hippisley-Cox J, Coupland C, Brindle P. Development and validation of QRISK3 risk prediction algorithms to estimate future risk of cardiovascular disease: prospective cohort study. BMJ 2017;357:j2099.
56. McGurnaghan SJ, McKeigue PM, Read SH, et al. Development and validation of a cardiovascular risk prediction model in type 1 diabetes. Diabetologia 2021; 64(9):2001–11.
57. Ifuku M, Takahashi K, Hosono Y, et al. Left atrial dysfunction and stiffness in pediatric and adult patients with Type 1 diabetes mellitus assessed with speckle tracking echocardiography. Pediatr Diabetes 2021;22(2):303–19.
58. Hajdu M, Knutsen MO, Vértes V, et al. Quality of glycemic control has significant impact on myocardial mechanics in type 1 diabetes mellitus. Sci Rep 2022;12(1):20180.
59. Schäfer M, Nadeau KJ, Reusch JEB. Cardiovascular disease in young People with Type 1 Diabetes: Search for Cardiovascular Biomarkers. J Diabetes Complicat 2020;34(10):107651.
60. Palmieri V, Capaldo B, Russo C, et al. Uncomplicated type 1 diabetes and preclinical left ventricular myocardial dysfunction: insights from echocardiography and exercise cardiac performance evaluation. Diabetes Res Clin Pract 2008; 79(2):262–8.
61. von Bibra H, John Sutton M. Diastolic dysfunction in diabetes and the metabolic syndrome: promising potential for diagnosis and prognosis. Diabetologia 2010; 53(6):1033–45.
62. Llauradó G, Ceperuelo-Mallafré V, Vilardell C, et al. Arterial stiffness is increased in patients with type 1 diabetes without cardiovascular disease: a potential role of low-grade inflammation. Diabetes Care 2012;35(5):1083–9.
63. Helleputte S, Van Bortel L, Verbeke F, et al. Arterial stiffness in patients with type 1 diabetes and its comparison to cardiovascular risk evaluation tools. Cardiovasc Diabetol 2022;21(1):97.

64. Polak JF, Backlund JC, Budoff M, et al. Coronary Artery Disease Events and Carotid Intima-Media Thickness in Type 1 Diabetes in the DCCT/EDIC Cohort. J Am Heart Assoc 2021;10(24):e022922.

65. Malik S, Zhao Y, Budoff M, et al. Coronary Artery Calcium Score for Long-term Risk Classification in Individuals With Type 2 Diabetes and Metabolic Syndrome From the Multi-Ethnic Study of Atherosclerosis. JAMA Cardiol 2017;2(12): 1332–40.

66. Olson JC, Edmundowicz D, Becker DJ, et al. Coronary calcium in adults with type 1 diabetes: a stronger correlate of clinical coronary artery disease in men than in women. Diabetes 2000;49(9):1571–8.

67. Budoff M, Backlund JC, Bluemke DA, et al. The Association of Coronary Artery Calcification With Subsequent Incidence of Cardiovascular Disease in Type 1 Diabetes: The DCCT/EDIC Trials. JACC Cardiovasc Imaging 2019;12(7 Pt 2): 1341–9.

68. Burge MR, Eaton RP, Schade DS. The Role of a Coronary Artery Calcium Scan in Type 1 Diabetes. Diabetes Technol Therapeut 2016;18(9):594–603.

69. Nathan DM, Cleary PA, Backlund JY, et al. Intensive diabetes treatment and cardiovascular disease in patients with type 1 diabetes. N Engl J Med 2005;353(25): 2643–53.

70. Intensive Diabetes Treatment and Cardiovascular Outcomes in Type 1 Diabetes: The DCCT/EDIC Study 30-Year Follow-up. Diabetes Care 2016;39(5):686–93.

71. ElSayed NA, Aleppo G, Aroda VR, et al. 6. Glycemic Targets: Standards of Care in Diabetes-2023. Diabetes Care 2023;46(Suppl 1):S97–110.

72. Kearney PM, Blackwell L, Collins R, et al. Efficacy of cholesterol-lowering therapy in 18,686 people with diabetes in 14 randomised trials of statins: a meta-analysis. Lancet 2008;371(9607):117–25.

73. ElSayed NA, Aleppo G, Aroda VR, et al. Cardiovascular Disease and Risk Management: Standards of Care in Diabetes-2023. Diabetes Care 2023;46(Suppl 1): S158–90, 10.

74. de Ferranti SD, de Boer IH, Fonseca V, et al. Type 1 diabetes mellitus and cardiovascular disease: a scientific statement from the American Heart Association and American Diabetes Association. Circulation 2014;130(13):1110–30.

75. Authors/Task Force Members, ESC Committee for Practice Guidelines CPG, ESC National Cardiac Societies. 2019 ESC/EAS guidelines for the management of dyslipidaemias: Lipid modification to reduce cardiovascular risk. Atherosclerosis 2019;290:140–205. https://doi.org/10.1016/j.atherosclerosis.2019.08.014.

76. Cosentino F, Grant PJ, Aboyans V, et al. 2019 ESC Guidelines on diabetes, pre-diabetes, and cardiovascular diseases developed in collaboration with the EASD. Eur Heart J 2020;41(2):255–323.

77. Guo J, Brooks MM, Muldoon MF, et al. Optimal Blood Pressure Thresholds for Minimal Coronary Artery Disease Risk in Type 1 Diabetes. Diabetes Care 2019; 42(9):1692–9.

78. Evert AB, Dennison M, Gardner CD, et al. Nutrition Therapy for Adults With Diabetes or Prediabetes: A Consensus Report. Diabetes Care 2019;42(5):731–54.

79. ElSayed NA, Aleppo G, Aroda VR, et al. 5. Facilitating Positive Health Behaviors and Well-being to Improve Health Outcomes: Standards of Care in Diabetes-2023. Diabetes Care 2023;46(Supple 1):S68–96.

80. Tikkanen-Dolenc H, Wadén J, Forsblom C, et al. Physical Activity Reduces Risk of Premature Mortality in Patients With Type 1 Diabetes With and Without Kidney Disease. Diabetes Care 2017;40(12):1727–32.

81. Ostman C, Jewiss D, King N, et al. Clinical outcomes to exercise training in type 1 diabetes: A systematic review and meta-analysis. Diabetes Res Clin Pract 2018; 139:380–91.
82. Mathieu C, Zinman B, Hemmingsson JU, et al. Efficacy and Safety of Liraglutide Added to Insulin Treatment in Type 1 Diabetes: The ADJUNCT ONE Treat-To-Target Randomized Trial. Diabetes Care 2016;39(10):1702–10.
83. Vendrame F, Calhoun P, Bocchino LE, et al. Impact of bariatric surgery and weight loss medications in adults with type 1 diabetes in the T1D Exchange Clinic Registry. J Diabetes Complicat 2021;35(6):107884.
84. Colberg SR, Sigal RJ, Yardley JE, et al. Physical Activity/Exercise and Diabetes: A Position Statement of the American Diabetes Association. Diabetes Care 2016; 39(11):2065–79.
85. Biankin SA, Jenkins AB, Campbell LV, et al. Target-seeking behavior of plasma glucose with exercise in type 1 diabetes. Diabetes Care 2003;26(2):297–301.
86. Bundy JD, Zhu Z, Ning H, et al. Estimated Impact of Achieving Optimal Cardiovascular Health Among US Adults on Cardiovascular Disease Events. J Am Heart Assoc 2021;10(7):e019681.
87. Shah VN, Grimsmann JM, Foster NC, et al. Undertreatment of cardiovascular risk factors in the type 1 diabetes exchange clinic network (United States) and the prospective diabetes follow-up (Germany/Austria) registries. Diabetes Obes Metab 2020;22(9):1577–85.
88. Varkevisser RDM, Birnie E, Vollenbrock CE, et al. Cardiovascular risk management in people with type 1 diabetes: performance using three guidelines. BMJ Open Diabetes Res Care 2022;10(4). https://doi.org/10.1136/bmjdrc-2022-002765.
89. Majidi S, Ebekozien O, Noor N, et al. Inequities in Health Outcomes in Children and Adults With Type 1 Diabetes: Data From the T1D Exchange Quality Improvement Collaborative. Clin Diabetes 2021;39(3):278–83.

Stakeholder Engagement in Type 1 Diabetes Research, Quality Improvement, and Clinical Care

Nicole Rioles, MA[a], Christine March, MD, MS[b],
Cynthia E. Muñoz, PhD, MPH[c], Jeniece Ilkowitz, RN, MA[d],
Amy Ohmer[e], Risa M. Wolf, MD[f],*

KEYWORDS

- Stakeholder engagement • Type 1 diabetes • Quality improvement
- Partnership approaches • Public and patient involvement

KEY POINTS

- The integration of stakeholder engagement in diabetes research, quality improvement (QI), and clinical care is growing.
- Many funding organizations promote partnerships with key stakeholders in the planning and conduct of research to ensure that research outcomes match the values of the patient and provider communities.
- The creation of family and youth stakeholder committees has furthered the integration of the patient and caregiver voice in implementation and dissemination of research findings in the clinical setting. The T1D Exchange QI Consortium is an example of a national QI organization that has fostered a strong Patient/Parent Advisory Committee that contributes to research design, implementation, and dissemination of research findings.

INTRODUCTION

The management of type 1 diabetes (T1D) is complex and requires the collaboration of patients, parents/caregivers, multidisciplinary care teams, and other community

Funding statement: No funding was secured for this study.
[a] T1D Exchange, Boston, MA, USA; [b] Division of Pediatric Endocrinology and Diabetes, University of Pittsburgh, UPMC Children's Hospital of Pittsburgh, Pittsburgh, PA, USA; [c] Department of Pediatrics, Keck School of Medicine, University of Southern California, Los Angeles, CA, USA; [d] Pediatric Diabetes Center, NYU Langone Health, New York, NY, USA; [e] International Children's Advisory Network, Atlanta, GA, USA; [f] Department of Pediatrics, Division of Endocrinology, Johns Hopkins University School of Medicine, Baltimore, MD, USA
* Corresponding author. Department of Pediatrics, Division of Endocrinology, 200 North Wolfe Street, Baltimore, MD 21287.
E-mail address: RWolf@jhu.edu

supports.[1] As an integral part of clinical care, quality improvement (QI) and research, stakeholder perspectives, and stakeholder engagement (SE) require effective approaches and strategies to ensure all voices are integrated. The concept of SE, defined as the engagement of patients, caregivers, and other health care stakeholders as partners in planning, conducting, and disseminating clinical interventions, QI, and research, was first initiated by the Patient-Centered Outcomes Research Institute (PCORI) in 2010.[2–4] The increasing amount of literature and funding opportunities involving SE clearly demonstrates an increased acceptance of SE in all aspects of patient care and health outcomes, including a more patient-focused research agenda.[5] Over the last decade, the integration of SE has gained significant traction, yet there is a limited body of literature on SE in T1D scholarship, specifically.

In this article, the authors describe the current framework for SE and its application to T1D research, QI, and clinical care across the lifespan, highlighting efforts by the T1D Exchange (T1DX).

FUNDAMENTALS AND FRAMEWORK OF STAKEHOLDER ENGAGEMENT

Since the inception of the PCORI initiative, the mission of PCORI has been to shift the paradigm of clinical research such that patients are not just participants, but active collaborators in the design, implementation, and formulation of outcomes, so that the research better matches values meaningful to the patient community. The PCORI mission statement suggests active and sustained engagement of patients and other key stakeholders in determining research priorities as well as recommendations for research funding.[3,6] To do this, PCORI developed a rubric to provide a framework for engaging patients and other stakeholders in all phases of research.[3] It includes definitions of stakeholder types, examples of stakeholder roles, and considerations in the planning, conducting, and dissemination of stakeholder-engaged research.[3,5]

Stakeholders include patients, providers, and both community and commercial partners.[3] Patient stakeholders include individuals with the lived experience of the condition of interest, in addition to their caregivers and family members, as well as advocacy or community organizations that represent patients and caregivers.[7,8] Provider stakeholders include clinical health care professionals and their institutions (hospitals and health care systems), researchers of the condition of interest, health care industry players (purchasers and payers), and policymakers. Adequate diversity in stakeholder representation is important to ensure that the research endeavors and outcomes reflect the values of the patient community.

STAKEHOLDER ENGAGEMENT IN RESEARCH

It is recommended to include stakeholders in all stages of the research process, from conception to dissemination. Researchers should partner with stakeholders, allowing for open dialogue, bidirectional sharing, and meaningful contributions from stakeholders, as well as establishing expectation of roles at the outset to ensure a productive and meaningful working relationship.[9–11] PCORI researchers have recommended that stakeholders have a collaborative role and partnership rather than a consulting or advisory role.[12–15] A review by Harrison and colleagues[15] summarized foundational principles of SE, including respect, equitable power between all team members, open discussion forums, and creating trust between stakeholders and researchers. Experienced programs in engaging stakeholders have also suggested providing compensation and/or reimbursements to patients and other stakeholders contributing time and expertise.[16,17] Stakeholders should be engaged early in the process to help with the conceptualization and prioritization of the research questions and to codesign the research protocol and can also contribute to developing optimal strategies for recruitment and retention of study participants, as well as engaging representative and hard-to-reach populations for greater external validity.[18,19]

When involving SE in research design, it may be helpful to the patient or family member to better understand research methodology, recruitment, and participant characteristics. Some institutions have created training programs for stakeholders to introduce them to the purpose of research, research ethics, and human subject protections.[20] Such training helps to prepare stakeholders and may also help to sustain ongoing engagement.[21] Regardless of how SE is being used to contribute to the overall applicability and success of a project, efforts to include stakeholders that have been well planned and continually monitored are necessary for optimal SE and adequate representation among patient communities.[22] Outreaching to stakeholders from diverse backgrounds that include representation across age groups, income and education levels, and races and ethnicities can help to ensure that traditionally underrepresented stakeholders have a voice at the table. Bringing patient stakeholders to research and opening dialogue to allow bidirectional teaching can help to create an environment of true collaboration, where patient knowledge and experience are valued as a subject matter expertise, fostering an environment of co-design and collaboration.

Dissemination of research findings supported by community engagement can lead to expanded applicability of the findings particularly in hard-to-reach populations, and accelerated uptake in communities through community ambassadors. Furthermore, some argue that SE in research design and execution results in better quality research and engages and empowers patients to play a more active role in their care and that of their community. Furthermore, the integration of SE ensures that research and clinical initiatives are, by design, more appropriate for the community.[19,22]

As SE in research becomes increasingly prioritized, investigators and funding bodies need to consider its quality and effectiveness. Although there are many published best practices for SE, methods to evaluate the processes and outcomes of stakeholder inclusion in research are varied in scope and content.[3,23–26] SE evaluations have spanned which stakeholders were represented, characteristics of engagement, stakeholders' experiences with the collaboration and perceptions of their contributions, and descriptions of how stakeholders affected the research plans.[26] The inconsistency across studies highlights the lack of a common framework by which to appraise the impact of SE. The need remains for consensus on how to partner with all stakeholders equitably, selection of valid measures for SE assessment, and the identification of reportable outcomes for stakeholder-engaged research.[27,28] Regardless, there is widespread initiative from funding organizations to enhance meaningful SE with patient and community-based organizations in order to meet the needs and priorities of stakeholders and to promote health equity among all stakeholders in the long term.

In addition to PCORI, other funding bodies have promoted SE in their funding announcements and research partnerships, including the Institute for Patient and Family Centered Care, the Agency for Health Care Research and Quality, the National Institute of Diabetes and Digestive and Kidney Disease (NIDDK), and the American Diabetes Association (ADA).[29–32]

STAKEHOLDER ENGAGEMENT IN DIABETES RESEARCH

In chronic disease conditions like diabetes, the use of SE to guide and inform research at the design stage, through the implementation, recruitment, and retention as well as the dissemination of results can lead to more relevant and meaningful outcomes for both the patient and the provider.[7,33] Schmittdiel and colleagues[33] describe their experience in engaging stakeholders in comparative effectiveness research in the field of diabetes, and their five-step process for assessing data gaps and translating gaps into critical concepts to be addressed in pilot studies of patient-centered research outcomes. This process entails a survey to elicit ideas for a research agenda, followed by a representative stakeholder in-person meeting to discuss which topics can translate into potential studies. Step 3 involves the refinement of ideas into a smaller number of pilot projects that are innovative, feasible, sustainable, and patient-centered while advancing diabetes knowledge and care. These ideas are further narrowed in step 4, with the final projects selected by the stakeholders in step 5. Other studies have used engagement logs, interviews, focus groups, and surveys in diabetes research studies at singular or repeated intervals and to different ends as a means to evaluate outcomes related to SE.[26,34–36]

Patient-reported outcomes (PROs) and advisory committees can also inform the development, implementation, and interpretation of pediatric research, as previously mentioned, and can promote positive health outcomes.[37–41] The use of parent or proxy reports is commonly used to gain insight of the child, youth, and family experience. Researchers have identified possible limitations in this use of data and have suggested that self-report by children with T1D may provide important subjective data from the child's perspective.[42] In a study involving children aged 10 to 15 years, Wiebe and colleagues[43] evaluated the impact of maternal involvement on coping with T1D from the child's perspective. In a study of the T1D pediatric experience with the use of PROs, Lassen and colleagues[39] similarly concluded that the inclusion of self-report measures is valuable and also recommended consideration of the child's age as well as their reading and writing skills.

In a more formalized process, the Development and Evaluation of a Psycho-social Intervention in Children and Teenagers Experiencing Diabetes (DEPICTED) study created a stakeholder action group (SAG) to inform their research intervention.[8] The planned research intervention was to be deployed in the context of routine diabetes care, so they needed to ensure acceptability by all stakeholders involved, including children and teenagers with diabetes. The DEPICTED SAG participated in meetings, as experts by experience, to actively collaborate on the design of a research and clinical care intervention for patients with diabetes. The funding body for this study required SE, and the investigators cited benefits of stakeholder involvement in contributions to the research intervention design as well as the promise of acceptability of the intervention. In a similar project aimed at personalizing evidence-based interventions to meet individual families' needs, the Achieving control, Connecting resources, and Empowering families (ACE) study also engaged stakeholders in the research process.[44] This study randomized children and their parents to a family-centered approach for diabetes care and measured outcomes of HbA_{1c} and Quality of Life (QoL). Recognizing the importance of SE and collaboration in the generalizability to real-world implementation, the investigators used SE to optimize trial recruitment, retention, and integration into routine clinical diabetes care.[44]

Across every disease state there are patients and families with varying demographics, including culture, gender, language, ethnicity, race, age, education level, socioeconomic status, and setting (urban vs rural).[45] Therefore, when engaging with stakeholders, a diverse group should be included. Engagement logs, interviews, focus groups, and surveys have been used in diabetes research studies at singular or repeated intervals and to different ends.[26,34–36,46] In addition, diverse representation among those who provide feedback is important (eg, patient vs the parent or legal guardian, a single parent, sibling). When using SE in a research project, special attention must also be given to ensure that SE groups involve members beyond the "usual contributors."[47] If this occurs, the risk for marginalization may be minimized when the effort is to tailor the interventions to the entire patient population and not just one subset.[47] As an example, there are inequities in diabetes care and management with regard to diabetes technology prescription and utilization. To this end, Agarwal and colleagues[48] address the needs of the diverse population of people with diabetes (PWD) and further diabetes disparities research by using intervention ideas recommended by multidisciplinary stakeholders to reduce inequities in diabetes technology use among people with T1D.

STAKEHOLDER ENGAGEMENT IN DIABETES AND DIVERSITY

SE may help mitigate underrepresentation of individuals from diverse racial/ethnic backgrounds and disparities in T1D research.[48-53] In general, individuals from diverse racial/ethnic and/or low-income backgrounds are underrepresented in clinical trials, and reporting of study results by racial/ethnic subgroup populations is also inconsistent.[54] For example, there is a wide body of literature describing underrepresentation of racial/ethnic populations in diabetic eye disease intervention trials. A review of clinical intervention trials for diabetic retinopathy and diabetic macular edema (DME) from 2001 to 2020 demonstrated that black patients with DME were 3 times less likely to be represented in National Institutes of Health (NIH) trials and 4.5 times less likely to be represented in industry trials, despite this population bearing a significant burden of diabetic eye disease in the United States.[51] Furthermore, clinical trial participants are often supported by the study team and by financial compensation in maintaining adherence to trial therapies, which may overrepresent the efficacy of treatments, thereby limiting the generalizability, especially in communities with fewer clinical and social supports.[52] Clinical trials of diabetes technology are also overrepresented by white participants with few individuals from diverse racial/ethnic backgrounds represented.[55,56] Given the known disparities in glycemic control, where non-white individuals have up to 2% higher HbA_{1c} levels than their white peers, the larger improvements in HbA_{1c} seen in these automated insulin delivery trials may have greater applicability to black and Hispanic individuals.[57,58] Especially in diseases with known disparities, such as diabetes, it is even more important to include PWD from diverse racial/ethnic backgrounds so that results are generalizable and applicable to all populations.

Increasing representative SE, particularly in underrepresented communities, can help guide advancement in diabetes care and research.[48] Given the stark disparities in advanced diabetes technology use with white individuals more likely to use continuous glucose monitors (CGM) and insulin pumps than black and Hispanic individuals with T1D, Agarwal and colleagues[48,58-60] convened a multidisciplinary stakeholder group of patients and providers to develop solutions to increase technology uptake in diverse and underresourced communities. They determined that providing standard and equitable diabetes technology recommendations, offering hands-on and visual demonstrations of technology, providing peer and social supports, and assisting in navigating insurance and financial coverage would be helpful in increasing technology use among racially and ethnically underrepresented populations with T1D. Similarly, the NIDDK has prioritized SE in informing trial interventions and enhancing participation in communities generally underrepresented in NIH-funded research.

STAKEHOLDER ENGAGEMENT IN QUALITY IMPROVEMENT OF DIABETES CARE

In addition to research, there is also QI work in the health care setting that seeks to systematically plan and implement actions that lead to measurable improvement in the quality and safety of health care services. There are several examples of SE in the QI process in general pediatrics and T1D care. The Roadmap Project was initiated in 2017 by the American Board of Pediatrics after 3 parents of children with chronic conditions requested the creation of a roadmap to improve the emotional health of their children and their families. Through this effort, clinicians, psychologists, and subject matter experts, including patients and families living with a chronic condition, developed a roadmap to identify tools and strategies that could help improve emotional health among children with chronic disease.[61] Family and youth advisory committees have been increasingly created and relied on in research and initiatives associated with diabetes care and QI. In an example in medical education to engage stakeholders with chronic disease, and specifically, T1D, a curriculum was established to engage PWD to learn about research and clinical care at their institution to engage them as meaningful stakeholders.[62]

One of the largest efforts to incorporate SE into QI for diabetes is through the T1D Exchange Quality Improvement Collaborative (T1DX-QI). This is a national consortium of 55 health care institutions working together in QI initiatives to improve care and outcomes for PWD.[63] SE, including patients with diabetes, parents/guardians, clinical collaborators, and industry partners, governs the framework of the T1DX-QI in research design, and qualitative and quantitative surveys. The T1DX-QI also has a Patient/Parent Advisory Committee (PPAC) that includes representation from patients with diabetes and their families to support patient engagement and shared decision making for the Collaborative. The PPAC offers personal expertise on diabetes management and insights on person-centered approach to care in all QI initiatives. Health equity work is governed by members of the Health Equity Advancement Lab Committee, which is composed of clinicians, researchers, industry partners, and PWD working together to design the strategy for the Collaborative' s equity work.

Clinical centers that join the T1DX-QI are encouraged to engage PWD and their family members in QI work and interventions. PWD and parent team representatives complete online training in QI fundamentals. They are also invited to attend in-person semiannual learning sessions to supplement the fundamentals training, as well as provide advice and input on the design and development of QI goals and objectives. They provide feedback for educational materials designed for clinician training and PWD/family education sessions. The partnership seeks to better understand the patient and family perspective and experience to prioritize and improve comprehensive and compassionate person-centered and family-centered health care.

The T1D Exchange Registry is an online, longitudinal research study designed to capture the experiences and challenges of individuals living with T1D. It tracks disease progress over time and includes more than 18,000 people living with T1D in the United States. The T1D Exchange Registry gathers information directly from PWD, including data on disease management, CGM data, and self-reported outcomes. Participants of the registry can also complete an annual questionnaire and subsequently have the option to participate in additional research studies that are shared on behalf of industry and academic health care partners throughout the year.

The T1D Exchange Registry provides participants with an online dashboard of curated T1D research opportunities, which can facilitate research participation among people with T1D, and has contributed to thousands of people engaging in research studies through the T1D Exchange Registry. The T1DX also manages an

Online Community with more than 50,000 participants that represent an anonymous, uncharacterized population who can participate in research surveys. In addition, the T1DX's Web site hosts The Question of the Day, a survey that is answered by an average of 500 people daily from the Online Community. These surveys consist of daily queries, and responses are received from a diverse stakeholder group, composed of PWD, parents and caregivers of PWD, and health care professionals who care for PWD.

STAKEHOLDER ENGAGEMENT IN DIABETES CLINICAL CARE

SE and the involvement of patients as partners extend to the implementation and dissemination of clinical care initiatives. Considering diverse patient perspectives and experiences of communities with varied backgrounds in the delivery of health care can ensure that patients and their supports (caregiver/family) receive optimal clinical care.[64] Various questionnaires have measured patients' experiences with both outpatient and inpatient health care and have highlighted several components that are meaningful to patients, including physical comfort, quality of care, emotional support, communication and education, involvement of supports such as family and friends, scheduling and timeliness of appointments, organization and coordination of care, and the physical environment.[65–67] In clinical care, SE has been used with patients and families to co-design, involving patients in the operational and process improvement goals of the practice with the long-term goals of improving patient experiences and health outcomes. In diabetes care, considering the patient experience at diagnosis and throughout ongoing treatment across the lifespan is critical to ensure that the needs and priorities at each stage and transition are addressed.

Essential forms of SE have included the use of PROs, Parent Advisory Committees, and Patient and Family Advisory Councils. These types of SE promote the consideration of pediatric and adolescent patient and parent perspectives and engagement in shared decision making throughout the course of pediatric patients' health care. Hospitals, for example, are more commonly using family/parent or patient advisory committees to comment on or suggest adjustments to all areas of hospital care and research by creating child- and family-centered programs and services.[68] These committees provide a space to identify a wide range of personal biases and obstacles that should be discussed to better support self-management behaviors and therefore have a positive impact on clinical outcomes.[69] In the next section, the importance of SE throughout childhood and adolescence and the unique aspects of adulthood and elder care in diabetes care are expanded upon.

Pediatric and Adolescent Care

Caregiver and parent support as well as team decision making are critical for children with T1D and require communication between many stakeholders, including endocrinologists, pediatricians, and daycare or school team members. For children with additional special health care needs, communication with special education and mental health care team members is also important to promote both informed and shared decision making.

The development of optimal pediatric and adolescent treatment models and research programs is complex, as physiologic and psychosocial issues shift over time. Better understanding the experience of children and adolescents with diabetes is critical to achieve optimal diabetes management during these stages of development, which has remained a challenge despite improvements in diabetes treatment options.[70,71] Developmentally appropriate diabetes care is complex and, according to the ADA Position Statement on Type 1 Diabetes in Children and Adolescents, "Diabetes management for children must not be extrapolated from adult diabetes care."[72]

Stakeholder engagement in pediatric clinical care

In another example of patient-centered care, Davis and MacKay[73] qualitatively interviewed a group of young adults and adolescents with T1D to understand their use of the electronic medical record (EMR) to design it with their input.

In a study focused on the health care transition for young adults with T1D to adult care, Pierce and colleagues included the perspectives of young adults with T1D, parents, providers, and other health care transition experts to develop a measure for evaluating outcomes. Before this study, the focus of health care transition outcomes was often on glycemic control, hospitalization rates, and loss to follow-up.[74] However, by involving all key stakeholders in qualitative interviews, Pierce and colleagues[75] determined that in addition to markers of glycemic control, other important aspects of transition to adult care included navigating a new health care system, confidence in self-management skills, integration of care in the adult role, and autonomy and ownership in T1D management.

Stakeholder engagement in pediatric research

PROs and advisory committees can also inform the development, implementation, and interpretation of pediatric research, as previously mentioned, and can promote positive health outcomes.[37–41] The use of parent or proxy reports is commonly used to gain insight of the child, youth, and family experience. Researchers have identified possible limitations in this use of data and have suggested that self-report by children with T1D may provide important subjective data from the child's perspective.[42] In a study involving children aged 10 to 15 years, Wiebe and colleagues[43] evaluated the impact of maternal involvement on coping with T1D from the child's perspective. In a study of the T1D pediatric experience with the use of PROs, Lassen and colleagues[39] similarly concluded that the inclusion of self-report measures is valuable and also recommended consideration of the child's age as well as their reading and writing skills.

In a more formalized process, the DEPICTED study created a SAG to inform their research intervention.[8] The planned research intervention was to be deployed in the context of routine diabetes care, so they needed to ensure acceptability by all stakeholders involved, including children and teenagers with diabetes. The DEPICTED SAG participated in meetings, as experts by experience, to actively collaborate on the design of a research and clinical care intervention for patients with diabetes. The funding body for this study required SE, and the investigators cited benefits of stakeholder involvement in contributions to the research intervention design as well as the promise of acceptability of the intervention. In a similar project aimed at personalizing evidence-based interventions to meet individual families' needs, the ACE study also engaged stakeholders in the research process.[44] This study randomized children and their parents to a family-centered approach for diabetes care and measured outcomes of HbA_{1c} and QoL. Recognizing the importance of SE and collaboration in the generalizability to real-world implementation, the investigators used SE to optimize trial recruitment, retention, and integration into routine clinical diabetes care.[44]

Stakeholder engagement in the pediatric school setting

The close collaboration and coordination of care between the student with T1D and their family, diabetes care team, and school team members responsible for supporting a student's diabetes care during school activities are necessary, as children often spend significant amounts of time at school. School team members involved with a student's diabetes care may include a school nurse, health aide, teacher, administrator, 504 Plan or IEP team members, school psychologist, coach, school bus driver, and/or other designated trained adults.[76,77]

As SE in research naturally leads to team science, another useful application is in studies involving community-based services or programs, such as in schools, childcare programs, camps, or other settings. Indeed, several studies on diabetes care in the school setting have integrated the perspectives of parent, school staff, and diabetes provider stakeholders to varying degrees. In a qualitative study by March and colleagues[78] on school nurse experiences with modern diabetes technologies, vested stakeholders participated in the design of study materials (eg, interview guide), subject recruitment, and the analysis of emerging themes.[35] A similar approach has been applied to subsequent studies examining other aspects of school-based diabetes care delivery, including surveys targeting both school health staff and diabetes care providers.[79-81] In these studies, partnering with community members purportedly strengthened the study's validity, as the stakeholders provided input on whether the findings resonated with their real-world experiences.

Women's Health in Diabetes Care

Women with T1D who are planning for pregnancy or who become pregnant face morbidity and mortality risks that are 2 to 3 times higher than women without diabetes.[82] The health risks and complications associated with T1D include preeclampsia, hyperglycemia, hypoglycemia, macrosomia, preterm labor, miscarriage, birth injury, macrosomia, C-section, retinopathy, postpartum hemorrhaging, and perinatal mortality.[83,84] These pregnancies require frequent follow-up and close monitoring by specialty care; fetal movement counting, ultrasounds, and nonstress testing are managed solely or co-managed by endocrinology, primary care, maternal-fetal medicine (MFM), and obstetrics. Adults with T1D who are not pregnant are recommended to have 2 diabetes care visits annually, whereas prenatal women with T1D require monthly to multiple visits per week, depending on the gestational age and the risk of complications.[31,85]

The chronic disease nature of diabetes means that people will often receive care from the same clinic or practice for long periods of time, sometimes decades, whereas the pregnancy remains a relatively short, critical period of approximately 40 weeks, plus postpartum care. There is a quintuple impact on women experiencing one of the most challenging times for diabetes management: (1) her diabetes care team often changes completely, with care transitioning from diabetes and endocrinology to obstetrics and/or MFM; (2) she experiences rapid changes in insulin resistance and insulin requirements; (3) blood glucose goals change drastically from 70 to 180 mg/dL time in range (TIR) to less than 95 mg/dL fasting and 120 mg/dL 2 hours postprandial; (4) many diabetes devices are not US Food and Drug Administration approved for use during pregnancy; and finally, (5) she manages the stress of knowing that the daily decision making of diabetes impacts her health and the health of her fetus, and this may influence treatment decisions that result in hypoglycemia, which may lead to further challenges.[86,87]

It is critical that, throughout the pregnancy period, women should not be sequestered to a single specialty area for their care needs. Instead, they should have access to the expertise of all their subspecialists and specialists, including their endocrinologists and diabetologists. SE communication can be used to empower teams and support women during pregnancy planning, the pregnancy term, and perinatal care. Building communication paths that flow between endocrine, primary, MFM, obstetrics, and PWD will lessen opportunities for errors or gaps in care. Instead, collaborating care teams that build a true multidisciplinary network that extends beyond the walls of a practice and specialty can understand and communicate changes, needs, and patient preferences that evolve over pregnancies.

Patient and provider collaboration in perinatal care

One of the greatest challenges at this time is the confluence of change and uncertainty.[88] During pregnancy, PWD will often defer to medical decision making because of their concern for the health and safety of the fetus, especially women experiencing pregnancy for the first time.[89,90] Endocrine and diabetes providers are often out of the loop for the pregnancy term and may believe that the PWD's health is best managed by the obstetrics teams during pregnancy. Obstetrics and MFM teams often struggle with diabetes management owing, in part, to limited knowledge about the PWD's diabetes management style and diabetes-related experiences. This time of transition and lack of care continuity can lead to many challenges that impact patient-provider trust.[91]

There are opportunities to build relationships, SE, and continuity during the prenatal, perinatal, and postnatal periods.[85] Understanding that, sometimes, new and additional specialty care teams are necessary to support PWD during their pregnancies, the authors suggest these 5 following steps be taken to improve PWD experience and support their engagement[92]:

1. Optimize communication between care provider teams: Facilitate teamwork by hosting a (virtual or in-person) hand-off meeting between the diabetes care team and MFM/obstetrics specialist; PWD should be central in the decision making and communications of preferences, priorities, and concerns, whereas the logistics of communicating and follow-up between care teams should remain the responsibility of the care team, not the PWD.
2. Facilitate ongoing communication: If the department managing the pregnancy term uses an EMR system that is separate from the diabetes care EMR system, make the follow-up appointment notes accessible for all.
3. Coordination of care: Make staff introductions between members of the MFM, diabetes, endocrinology, obstetrics, and primary care teams to improve communication, coordination, and continuity.
4. Postpartum hand-off: Host a second hand-off meeting postpartum to communicate priorities with the endocrinology and primary care team members so that they can continue the PWD's care management informed by the pregnancy period and support the PWD's postpartum health.
5. Include PWD in all decision making and communications.

Postpartum diabetes care also brings many transition periods with PWD experiencing a change in insulin sensitivity and additional risks for hypoglycemia during breastfeeding.[85] This may also be a time that PWD transition their care back to their primary care or Endocrinology teams while they are still experiencing postpartum symptoms and concerns. It is important to maintain open communication between MFM, obstetrics, primary, and endocrine care providers to best support the PWD.

Diabetes and Elder Care

T1D management becomes more complex for people over the age of 65 years and for people with long diabetes duration. High HbA_{1c} and high glucose variability are associated with a decline in cognitive function.[93] ADA Standards of Care recommend using assessments to identify appropriate targets and therapeutic approaches for older adults (OA). It is appropriate to screen for risks that are prevalent for OA with diabetes, including cognitive impairment, vision and hearing loss, falls, depression, and cardiovascular diseases.[31,94]

Hypoglycemia unawareness is more common for people over the age of 65 years, and glucose targets should be personalized appropriately for QoL and safety.[95] HbA_{1c} targets of 7.5% to 8% may be more appropriate for adults over the age of 80 years and adults aged 65 to 80 years who are managing comorbidities and/or hypoglycemia unawareness. CGM use is recommended for OA, considering the dangers of severe hypoglycemia events that are exacerbated by hypoglycemia unawareness.[96] Minimizing hypoglycemia, maximizing QoL, and reducing burden of disease management should all be considered with age-related changes.[97] OA with T1D also experience changes in dexterity, vision, hearing, and strength and are diagnosed with Alzheimer disease and dementia at higher rates than peers without diabetes.[98]

Engaging OA in their health care and involving family members and caregivers, and empowering them to support the well-being of the OA with diabetes are important ways to build SE in this population.[99] Patients and caregivers should be the decision makers in how and at what level they engage with their health care teams.[99] Assessment and reassessment of OA diabetes management needs should be considered often because of the potential for acute changes in health. Care teams should consider the goals and wishes of OA with diabetes by involving them directly in considering the advantages and disadvantages of care management and QoL decisions. Teams should be intentional to avoid bias and age discrimination and to avoid making assumptions about OA capacity.

Active listening and asking open-ended questions help care teams understand where they can match support and resources to PWD and family preferences.[100] Devices should accommodate OA needs and preferences; care teams should help to make them accessible, knowing that OA with arthritis or OA who have experienced a stroke may have more challenges with devices that require fine dexterity and fine motor skills. Small print and small screens may be additional barriers where OA may need more accommodations. Events like falls have significant health impacts for OA. Addressing individual needs to accommodate health changes with age and involving family members and caregivers in education and training sessions can support SE and increase participation in diabetes management through the lifespan.[101]

Because OA can transition to a more fragile state that requires additional support, it is critical to periodically reassess to understand what the new needs, goals, and preferences are, as they may change over time and after acute health events. These events may also change the OA outlook such that they may benefit from mental health counseling. Offering psychosocial support and communicating referrals to psychosocial professionals may benefit OA mental health, supporting overall diabetes management and whole person health.[102]

OA have complex needs in managing their diabetes and their overall health. Collaborating with them and their caregivers to know their preferences and priorities is paramount. Care teams can help support their needs by communicating across primary, specialty, and tertiary care providers to improve care coordination, safety, and satisfaction. Clinicians and other stakeholders in OA diabetes care should advocate for OA needs with public and private insurers to ensure that care is comprehensive, supporting medication and device access so that costs are not overwhelming barriers.[103] This is especially critical for a population with a fixed income and limited financial resources. Comprehensive care should also include free/affordable occupational therapy/physical therapy, behavioral and mental health, as well as prevention services.[104] Diabetes care teams should communicate OA needs with device manufacturers to ensure that devices and products are designed to meet the needs of the population. The health of OA and their self-management capacity can change rapidly.[105] Staying up-to-date with their needs by assessing changes in the domains of their health is essential; communicating across stakeholder groups to have agreement and understanding of health priorities and approaches is also important. For successful engagement, barriers should be removed by making the clinic and hospital spaces accessible and comfortable for older people, ensuring that lighting, text/print size, floor spaces, seating, and tables do not limit OA. Spaces and materials should be designed to match the requirements and preferences of the people receiving care.[94,106]

SUMMARY

The engagement of stakeholders in T1D research has increased over the last 10 years and has led to patient-centered research and interventions, as well as wider representation among diverse populations in research. Dissemination of clinical interventions has further expanded the role of stakeholders in QI initiatives and the clinical care setting. The management of diabetes across the lifespan is dynamic and changes with each life stage, which further highlights the importance of engaging stakeholders in the design and implementation of multidisciplinary clinical care from childhood, through adolescence, adulthood, pregnancy care, and elder care. The addition of patient and family advisory panels has facilitated a focus on patient-centered care and PROs that ensure research, QI, and clinical interventions match the values and goals of the patient populations. Although funding agencies are increasingly requiring SE in diabetes research, the integration of stakeholders in QI and clinical care is still in the early stages. The T1DX has facilitated a robust engagement of patient and provider stakeholders in their QI efforts that can provide a framework for other programs and initiatives, as well as in the clinical realm. Although currently there is a limited body of literature on SE in T1D, the authors anticipate that future collaboration among funding agencies, QI consortiums, health care systems and providers, community organizations, and PWD will facilitate growth of SE initiatives that will have a significant impact on outcomes for PWD. By providing a voice to all those involved in the care of PWD, the care and outcomes for PWD can be advanced.

ACKNOWLEDGMENTS

The authors acknowledge Neha Parimi for her assistance with formatting and references.

AUTHORS' DISCLOSURES

R.M. Wolf receives research support from Novo Nordisk as the site PI of a clinical trial.

REFERENCES

1. ElSayed NA, Aleppo G, Aroda VR, et al. Classification and diagnosis of diabetes: standards of care in diabetes-2023. Diabetes Care 2023;46(Suppl 1): S19–40.
2. Institute, P.C.O.R. PCORI engagement rubric for applicants. 2014 06/06/2016 (cited 2023, 10 July 2023); Available at: https://www.pcori.org/sites/default/files/Engagement-Rubric.pdf. .
3. Sheridan S, Schrandt S, Forsythe L, et al. The PCORI engagement rubric: promising practices for partnering in research. Ann Fam Med 2017;15(2):165–70.
4. STROKOFF SL. Compilation of patient protection and affordable care act. In: Subtitle D of Title VI. U.S.H.O. Representatives; 2010.

5. PCORI. patient centered outcome institute (cited 2023 06/16/2023); Available at: https://www.pcori.org/.

6. PCORI Methodology Committee. The PCORI Methodology Report. Patient-Centered Outcomes Research Institute (PCORI). Washington, DC; 2013.

7. Hoddinott P, Pollock A, O'Cathain A, et al. How to incorporate patient and public perspectives into the design and conduct of research. F1000Res 2018;7:752.

8. Lowes L, Robling MR, Bennert K, et al. Involving lay and professional stakeholders in the development of a research intervention for the DEPICTED study. Health Expect 2011;14(3):250–60.

9. Forsythe L, Heckert A, Margolis MK, et al. Methods and impact of engagement in research, from theory to practice and back again: early findings from the patient-centered outcomes Research Institute. Qual Life Res 2018;27(1):17–31.

10. Forsythe LP, Ellis LE, Edmundson L, et al. Patient and stakeholder engagement in the PCORI pilot projects: description and lessons learned. J Gen Intern Med 2016;31(1):13–21.

11. Manafo E, Petermann L, Vandall-Walker V, et al. Patient and public engagement in priority setting: A systematic rapid review of the literature. PLoS One 2018; 13(3):e0193579.

12. Bennett LM, Gadlin H. Collaboration and team science: from theory to practice. J Investig Med 2012;60(5):768–75.

13. Motu'apuaka M, Whitlock E, Kato E, et al. Defining the benefits and challenges of stakeholder engagement in systematic reviews. Comp Eff Res 2015;5:13.

14. Hahn DL, Hoffmann AE, Felzien M, et al. Tokenism in patient engagement. Fam Pract 2017;34(3):290–5.

15. Harrison JD, Anderson WG, Fagan M, et al. Patient and family advisory councils (PFACs): identifying challenges and solutions to support engagement in research. Patient 2018;11(4):413–23.

16. Arkind J, Likumahuwa-Ackman S, Warren N, et al. Lessons learned from developing a patient engagement panel: an OCHIN Report. J Am Board Fam Med 2015;28(5):632–8.

17. Sheridan S, S.S. A framework for financial compensation for patient partners in research. 2018, (cited 2023, July 11, 2023); Available from: https://www.pcori.org/blog/framework-financial-compensation-patient-partners-research.

18. CD M, Integrating patients' voices in study design elements with a focus on hard-to-reach populations, 2012, Patient-Centered Outcomes Research Institute, (PCORI). Accessed July 10, 2023.

19. Viswanathan M, Ammerman A, Eng E, et al. Community-based participatory research: assessing the evidence. Evid Rep Technol Assess 2004;(99):1–8.

20. Yonas MA, Jaime MC, Barone J, et al. Community partnered research ethics training in practice: a collaborative approach to certification. J Empir Res Hum Res Ethics 2016;11(2):97–105.

21. Petkovic J, Riddle A, Lytvyn L, et al. PROTOCOL: Guidance for stakeholder engagement in guideline development: A systematic review. Campbell Syst Rev 2022;18(2):e1242.

22. O'Haire C., McPheeters M., Nakamoto E., et al., Engaging Stakeholders To Identify and Prioritize Future Research Needs [Internet]. Rockville (MD): Agency for Healthcare Research and Quality (US); 2011. (Methods Future Research Needs Reports, No. 4.) Executive Summary. Available at: https://www.ncbi.nlm.nih.gov/books/NBK62559/.

23. Concannon TW, Fuster M, Saunders T, et al. A systematic review of stakeholder engagement in comparative effectiveness and patient-centered outcomes research. J Gen Intern Med 2014;29(12):1692–701.

24. Concannon TW, Grant S, Welch V, et al. Practical guidance for involving stakeholders in health research. J Gen Intern Med 2019;34(3):458–63.

25. Esmail L, Moore E, Rein A. Evaluating patient and stakeholder engagement in research: moving from theory to practice. J Comp Eff Res 2015;4(2):133–45.

26. Martinez J, Wong C, Piersol CV, et al. Stakeholder engagement in research: a scoping review of current evaluation methods. J Comp Eff Res 2019;8(15):1327–41.

27. Bowen DJ, Hyams T, Goodman M, et al. Systematic review of quantitative measures of stakeholder engagement. Clin Transl Sci 2017;10(5):314–36.

28. Ray KN, Miller E. Strengthening stakeholder-engaged research and research on stakeholder engagement. J Comp Eff Res 2017;6(4):375–89.

29. (IPFCC), I.o.p.a.f.c.c. Effective patient and family advisory councils. Available from: https://www.ipfcc.org/bestpractices/sustainable-partnerships/engaging/effective-pfacs.html. Accessed July 10, 2023.

30. AHRQ. Agency for Healthcare Research and Quality (AHRQ). (cited 2023 7/11/2023); Available at: https://www.ahrq.gov/.

31. ElSayed NA, Aleppo G, Aroda VR, et al. Summary of revisions: standards of care in diabetes-2023. Diabetes Care 2023;46(Suppl 1):S5–9.

32. NIDDK. National Institute of Diabetes and Digestive and Kidney Diseases (cited 2023 7/11/23); Available from: https://www.niddk.nih.gov/.

33. Schmittdiel JA, Desai J, Schroeder EB, et al. Methods for engaging stakeholders in comparative effectiveness research: a patient-centered approach to improving diabetes care. Healthc (Amst) 2015;3(2):80–8.

34. Greenwood DA, Litchman ML, Ng AH, et al. Development of the intercultural diabetes online community research council: codesign and social media processes. J Diabetes Sci Technol 2019;13(2):176–86.

35. March CA, Kazmerski TM, Moon C, et al. Evaluating the impact of stakeholder engagement in a school-based type 1 diabetes study. Diabetes Spectr 2021;34(4):419–24.

36. McElfish PA, Ayers BL, Felix HC, et al. How stakeholder engagement influenced a randomized comparative effectiveness trial testing two Diabetes Prevention Program interventions in a Marshallese Pacific Islander Community. J Transl Med 2019;17(1):42.

37. Gianini A, Suklan J, Skela-Savič B, et al. Patient reported outcome measures in children and adolescents with type 1 diabetes using advanced hybrid closed loop insulin delivery. Front Endocrinol 2022;13:967725.

38. Hannon TS, Moore CM, Cheng ER, et al. Codesigned shared decision-making diabetes management plan tool for adolescents with type 1 diabetes mellitus and their parents: prototype development and pilot test. J Particip Med 2018;10(2):e8.

39. Lassen RB, Abild CB, Kristensen K, et al. Involving children and adolescents with type 1 diabetes in health care: a qualitative study of the use of patient-reported outcomes. Journal of Patient-Reported Outcomes 2023;7(1):20.

40. Lassen RB, Abild CB, Kristensen K, et al. Patient-reported outcome instruments for assessing the involvement of children and adolescents with type 1 diabetes in their treatment: a scoping review protocol. JBI Evid Synth 2023;21(3):609–16.

41. Yu CH, Ivers NM, Stacey D, et al. Impact of an interprofessional shared decision-making and goal-setting decision aid for patients with diabetes on

decisional conflict–study protocol for a randomized controlled trial. Trials 2015; 16:286.

42. Nieuwesteeg AM, Pouwer F, van Bakel HJ, et al. Quality of the parent-child interaction in young children with type 1 diabetes mellitus: study protocol. BMC Pediatr 2011;11:28.

43. Wiebe DJ, Berg CA, Korbel C, et al. Children's appraisals of maternal involvement in coping with diabetes: enhancing our understanding of adherence, metabolic control, and quality of life across adolescence. J Pediatr Psychol 2005;30(2):167–78.

44. Fiallo-Scharer R, Palta M, Chewning BA, et al. Design and baseline data from a PCORI-funded randomized controlled trial of family-centered tailoring of diabetes self-management resources. Contemp Clin Trials 2017;58:58–65.

45. Rolfe DE, Ramsden VR, Banner D, et al. Using qualitative Health Research methods to improve patient and public involvement and engagement in research. Res Involv Engagem 2018;4:49.

46. Poger JM, Yeh HC, Bryce CL, et al. PaTH to partnership in stakeholder-engaged research: A framework for stakeholder engagement in the PaTH to Health Diabetes study. Healthc (Amst) 2020;8(1):100361.

47. Bonet Olivencia S, Rao AH, Smith A, et al. Eliciting requirements for a diabetes self-management application for underserved populations: a multi-stakeholder analysis. Int J Environ Res Public Health 2021;19(1).

48. Agarwal S, Crespo-Ramos G, Leung SL, et al. Solutions to address inequity in diabetes technology use in type 1 diabetes: results from multidisciplinary stakeholder co-creation workshops. Diabetes Technol Ther 2022;24(6):381–9.

49. Berkowitz ST, Groth SL, Gangaputra S, et al. Racial/ethnic disparities in ophthalmology clinical trials resulting in US Food and Drug Administration Drug Approvals From 2000 to 2020. JAMA Ophthalmol 2021;139(6):629–37.

50. Bowe T, Salabati M, Soares RR, et al. Racial, ethnic, and gender disparities in diabetic macular edema clinical trials. Ophthalmol Retina 2022;6(6):531–3.

51. Sanjiv N, Osathanugrah P, Harrell M, et al. Race and ethnic representation among clinical trials for diabetic retinopathy and diabetic macular edema within the United States: A review. J Natl Med Assoc 2022;114(2):123–40.

52. Sherman RE, Anderson SA, Dal Pan GJ, et al. Real-world evidence - what is it and what can it tell us? N Engl J Med 2016;375(23):2293–7.

53. Soares RR, Parikh D, Shields CN, et al. Geographic access disparities to clinical trials in diabetic eye disease in the United States. Ophthalmol Retina 2021;5(9): 879–87.

54. Corbie-Smith G, St George DMM, Moody-Ayers S, et al. Adequacy of reporting race/ethnicity in clinical trials in areas of health disparities. J Clin Epidemiol 2003;56(5):416–20.

55. Beck RW, Kanapka LG, Breton MD, et al. A meta-analysis of randomized trial outcomes for the t:slim X2 insulin pump with control-IQ technology in youth and adults from age 2 to 72. Diabetes Technol Ther 2023;25(5):329–42.

56. Ruedy KJ, Parkin CG, Riddlesworth TD, et al. Continuous glucose monitoring in older adults with type 1 and type 2 diabetes using multiple daily injections of insulin: results from the DIAMOND Trial. J Diabetes Sci Technol 2017;11(6): 1138–46.

57. Agarwal S, Kanapka LG, Raymond JK, et al. Racial-ethnic inequity in young adults with type 1 diabetes. J Clin Endocrinol Metab 2020;105(8):e2960–9.

58. Willi SM, Miller KM, DiMeglio LA, et al. Racial-ethnic disparities in management and outcomes among children with type 1 diabetes. Pediatrics 2015;135(3): 424–34.

59. Agarwal S, Schechter C, Gonzalez J, et al. Racial-ethnic disparities in diabetes technology use among young adults with type 1 diabetes. Diabetes Technol Therapeut 2021;23(4):306–13.

60. Foster NC, Beck RW, Miller KM, et al. State of type 1 diabetes management and outcomes from the T1D exchange in 2016-2018. Diabetes Technol Ther 2019; 21(2):66–72.

61. PEDIATRICS, A.B.o. Roadmap to Resilience, Emotional, and Mental Health. (Website) 05/22/2023 (cited 2023 06/16/2023); Available from: https://www.abp.org/foundation/roadmap.

62. Walker AF, Atkinson MA, Lee AM, et al. Teaching type 1 diabetes: creating stakeholder engagement in biomedical careers through undergraduate research curriculum. Med Sci Educ 2020;30(1):69–73.

63. Exchange, T.D. T1D Exchange Available at: https://t1dexchange.org/. Accessed July 24, 2023.

64. Schroeder K, Bertelsen N, Scott J, et al. Building from patient experiences to deliver patient-focused healthcare systems in collaboration with patients: a call to action. Ther Innov Regul Sci 2022;56(5):848–58.

65. Benson T, Potts HW. A short generic patient experience questionnaire: howRwe development and validation. BMC Health Serv Res 2014;14:499.

66. Jenkinson C, Coulter A, Bruster S. The picker patient experience questionnaire: development and validation using data from in-patient surveys in five countries. Int J Qual Health Care 2002;14(5):353–8.

67. Kemp K, McCormack B, Chan N, et al. Correlation of inpatient experience survey items and domains with overall hospital rating. J Patient Exp 2015;2(2): 29–36.

68. Hospital, H.C.s. Family partnership programs. Available at: https://nyulangone.org/locations/hassenfeld-childrens-hospital/sala-child-family-support/family-partnership-programs. Accessed July 10, 2023.

69. Hamilton K, Stanton-Fay SH, Chadwick PM, et al. Sustained type 1 diabetes self-management: Specifying the behaviours involved and their influences. Diabet Med 2021;38(5):e14430.

70. Demeterco-Berggren C, Ebekozien O, Noor N, et al. Factors associated with achieving target A1C in children and adolescents with type 1 diabetes: findings from the T1D exchange quality improvement collaborative. Clin Diabetes 2022; 41(1):68–75.

71. Miller KM, Beck RW, Foster NC, et al. HbA1c levels in type 1 diabetes from early childhood to older adults: a deeper dive into the influence of technology and socioeconomic status on HbA1c in the T1D exchange clinic registry findings. Diabetes Technol Ther 2020;22(9):645–50.

72. Chiang JL, Maahs DM, Garvey KC, et al. Type 1 diabetes in children and adolescents: a position statement by the American Diabetes Association. Diabetes Care 2018;41(9):2026–44.

73. Davis S, MacKay L. Moving beyond the rhetoric of shared decision-making: designing personal health record technology with young adults with type 1 diabetes. Can J Diabetes 2020;44(5):434–41.

74. Lyons SK, Becker DJ, Helgeson VS. Transfer from pediatric to adult health care: effects on diabetes outcomes. Pediatr Diabetes 2014;15(1):10–7.

75. Pierce JS, Aroian K, Schifano E, et al. Health care transition for young adults with type 1 diabetes: stakeholder engagement for defining optimal outcomes. J Pediatr Psychol 2017;42(9):970–82.
76. ADA. Training Resources for School Staff. 06/21/2023; Available at: https://diabetes.org/tools-support/know-your-rights/safe-at-school-state-laws/training-resources-school-staff. Accessed July 11, 2023.
77. Jackson CC, Albanese-O'Neill A, Butler KL, et al. Diabetes care in the school setting: a position statement of the American Diabetes Association. Diabetes Care 2015;38(10):1958–63.
78. March CA, Nanni M, Kazmerski TM, et al. Modern diabetes devices in the school setting: Perspectives from school nurses. Pediatr Diabetes 2020;21(5):832–40.
79. March C, Siminerio LM, Kazmerski TM, et al. School-based diabetes care: a national survey of U.S. pediatric diabetes providers. Pediatr Diabetes 2023; 2023:1–10.
80. March CA, Hill A, Kazmerski TM, et al. Development and psychometric analysis of the Diabetes Device Confidence Scale for school nurses. Pediatr Diabetes 2022;23(6):820–30.
81. March CA, Hill A, Kazmerski TM, et al. School nurse confidence with diabetes devices in relation to diabetes knowledge and prior training: a study of convergent validity. Pediatr Diabetes 2023;2023:2162900.
82. Knorr S, Juul S, Bytoft B, et al. Impact of type 1 diabetes on maternal long-term risk of hospitalisation and mortality: a nationwide combined clinical and register-based cohort study (The EPICOM study). Diabetologia 2018;61(5):1071–80.
83. Alexopoulos AS, Blair R, Peters AL. Management of preexisting diabetes in pregnancy: a review. JAMA 2019;321(18):1811–9.
84. Jaffar F, Laycock K, Huda MSB. Type 1 diabetes in pregnancy: a review of complications and management. Curr Diabetes Rev 2022;18(7). e051121197761.
85. Feldman AZ, Brown FM. Management of type 1 diabetes in pregnancy. Curr Diab Rep 2016;16(8):76.
86. Crimmins SD, Ginn-Meadow A, Jessel RH, et al. Leveraging technology to improve diabetes care in pregnancy. Clin Diabetes 2020;38(5):486–94.
87. Kitzmiller JL, Block JM, Brown FM, et al. Managing preexisting diabetes for pregnancy: summary of evidence and consensus recommendations for care. Diabetes Care 2008;31(5):1060–79.
88. Watkins V, Nagle C, Kent B, et al. Labouring Together: Women's experiences of "Getting the care that I want and need" in maternity care. Midwifery 2022;113: 103420.
89. McCance DR. Pregnancy and diabetes. Best Pract Res Clin Endocrinol Metab 2011;25(6):945–58.
90. Murugesu L, Damman OC, Derksen ME, et al. Women's participation in decision-making in maternity care: a qualitative exploration of clients' health literacy skills and needs for support. Int J Environ Res Public Health 2021;18(3).
91. Nicoloro-SantaBarbara J, Rosenthal L, Auerbach MV, et al. Patient-provider communication, maternal anxiety, and self-care in pregnancy. Soc Sci Med 2017;190:133–40.
92. Goldberg H. Informed decision making in maternity care. J Perinat Educ 2009; 18(1):32–40.
93. Yaffe K, Falvey C, Hamilton N, et al. Diabetes, glucose control, and 9-year cognitive decline among older adults without dementia. Arch Neurol 2012;69(9): 1170–5.

94. McNeil H, Elliott J, Huson K, et al. Engaging older adults in healthcare research and planning: a realist synthesis. Res Involv Engagem 2016;2:10.
95. Carlson AL, Kanapka LG, Miller KM, et al. Hypoglycemia and glycemic control in older adults with type 1 diabetes: baseline results from the WISDM study. J Diabetes Sci Technol 2021;15(3):582–92.
96. Pratley RE, Kanapka LG, Rickels MR, et al. Effect of continuous glucose monitoring on hypoglycemia in older adults with type 1 diabetes: a randomized clinical trial. JAMA 2020;323(23):2397–406.
97. Dhaliwal R, Weinstock RS. Management of type 1 diabetes in older adults. Diabetes Spectr 2014;27(1):9–20.
98. Jacobson AM, Ryan CM, Braffett BH, et al. Cognitive performance declines in older adults with type 1 diabetes: results from 32 years of follow-up in the DCCT and EDIC Study. Lancet Diabetes Endocrinol 2021;9(7):436–45.
99. Elliott J, McNeil H, Ashbourne J, et al. Engaging older adults in health care decision-making: a realist synthesis. Patient 2016;9(5):383–93.
100. Frost H, Campbell P, Maxwell M, et al. Effectiveness of motivational interviewing on adult behaviour change in health and social care settings: a systematic review of reviews. PLoS One 2018;13(10):e0204890.
101. Bennett WL, et al. Strategies for Patient, Family, and Caregiver Engagement. Rockville (MD). Agency for Healthcare Research and Quality (US); AHRQ Comparative Effectiveness Technical Briefs; 2020. https://pubmed.ncbi.nlm.nih.gov/32924385/.
102. Pennbrant S, Berg A, Fohlin Johansson L. Self-care experiences of older patients with diabetes mellitus: A qualitative systematic literature review. Nord J Nurs Res 2020;40(2):64–72.
103. Fitzpatrick AL, Powe NR, Cooper LS, et al. Barriers to health care access among the elderly and who perceives them. Am J Public Health 2004;94(10):1788–94.
104. Nicholas JA, Hall WJ. Screening and preventive services for older adults. Mt Sinai J Med 2011;78(4):498–508.
105. Taboada Gjorup AL, Snoek FJ, van Duinkerken E. Diabetes self-care in older adults with type 1 diabetes mellitus: how does cognition influence self-management. Front Clin Diabetes Healthc 2021;2:727029.
106. Sharma AE, Willard-Grace R, Willis A, et al. How can we talk about patient-centered care without patients at the table?" lessons learned from patient advisory councils. J Am Board Fam Med 2016;29(6):775–84.

Moving?

Make sure your subscription moves with you!

To notify us of your new address, find your **Clinics Account Number** (located on your mailing label above your name), and contact customer service at:

Email: journalscustomerservice-usa@elsevier.com

800-654-2452 (subscribers in the U.S. & Canada)
314-447-8871 (subscribers outside of the U.S. & Canada)

Fax number: 314-447-8029

Elsevier Health Sciences Division
Subscription Customer Service
3251 Riverport Lane
Maryland Heights, MO 63043

*To ensure uninterrupted delivery of your subscription, please notify us at least 4 weeks in advance of move.

Printed and bound by CPI Group (UK) Ltd, Croydon, CR0 4YY

08/05/2025

01864724-0013